Clinical Trial
Data Analysis
Using R and SAS
Second Edition

Chapman & Hall/CRC Biostatistics Series

Published Titles

Published Titles

Bayesian Modeling in Bioinformatics
Dipak K. Dey, Samiran Ghosh,
and Bani K. Mallick

Benefit-Risk Assessment in Pharmaceutical Research and Development
Andreas Sashegyi, James Felli,
and Rebecca Noel

Benefit-Risk Assessment Methods in Medical Product Development: Bridging Qualitative and Quantitative Assessments
Qi Jiang and Weili He

Bioequivalence and Statistics in Clinical Pharmacology, Second Edition
Scott Patterson and Byron Jones

Biosimilar Clinical Development: Scientific Considerations and New Methodologies
Kerry B. Barker, Sandeep M. Menon,
Ralph B. D'Agostino, Sr., Siyan Xu, and Bo Jin

Biosimilars: Design and Analysis of Follow-on Biologics
Shein-Chung Chow

Biostatistics: A Computing Approach
Stewart J. Anderson

Cancer Clinical Trials: Current and Controversial Issues in Design and Analysis
Stephen L. George, Xiaofei Wang,
and Herbert Pang

Causal Analysis in Biomedicine and Epidemiology: Based on Minimal Sufficient Causation
Mikel Aickin

Clinical and Statistical Considerations in Personalized Medicine
Claudio Carini, Sandeep Menon, and Mark Chang

Clinical Trial Data Analysis Using R
Ding-Geng (Din) Chen and Karl E. Peace

Clinical Trial Data Analysis Using R and SAS, Second Edition
Ding-Geng (Din) Chen, Karl E. Peace,
and Pinggao Zhang

Clinical Trial Methodology
Karl E. Peace and Ding-Geng (Din) Chen

Computational Methods in Biomedical Research
Ravindra Khattree and Dayanand N. Naik

Computational Pharmacokinetics
Anders Källén

Confidence intervals for Proportions and Related Measures of Effect Size
Robert G. Newcombe

Controversial Statistical Issues in Clinical Trials
Shein-Chung Chow

Data Analysis with Competing Risks and Intermediate States
Ronald B. Geskus

Data and Safety Monitoring Committees in Clinical Trials, Second Edition
Jay Herson

Design and Analysis of Animal Studies in Pharmaceutical Development
Shein-Chung Chow and Jen-pei Liu

Design and Analysis of Bioavailability and Bioequivalence Studies, Third Edition
Shein-Chung Chow and Jen-pei Liu

Design and Analysis of Bridging Studies
Jen-pei Liu, Shein-Chung Chow,
and Chin-Fu Hsiao

Design & Analysis of Clinical Trials for Economic Evaluation & Reimbursement: An Applied Approach Using SAS & STATA
Iftekhar Khan

Design and Analysis of Clinical Trials for Predictive Medicine
Shigeyuki Matsui, Marc Buyse,
and Richard Simon

Design and Analysis of Clinical Trials with Time-to-Event Endpoints
Karl E. Peace

Design and Analysis of Non-Inferiority Trials
Mark D. Rothmann, Brian L. Wiens,
and Ivan S. F. Chan

Difference Equations with Public Health Applications
Lemuel A. Moyé and Asha Seth Kapadia

Published Titles

Published Titles

Noninferiority Testing in Clinical Trials: Issues and Challenges
Tie-Hua Ng

Optimal Design for Nonlinear Response Models
Valerii V. Fedorov and Sergei L. Leonov

Patient-Reported Outcomes: Measurement, Implementation and Interpretation
Joseph C. Cappelleri, Kelly H. Zou, Andrew G. Bushmakin, Jose Ma. J. Alvir, Demissie Alemayehu, and Tara Symonds

Quantitative Evaluation of Safety in Drug Development: Design, Analysis and Reporting
Qi Jiang and H. Amy Xia

Quantitative Methods for Traditional Chinese Medicine Development
Shein-Chung Chow

Randomized Clinical Trials of Nonpharmacological Treatments
Isabelle Boutron, Philippe Ravaud, and David Moher

Randomized Phase II Cancer Clinical Trials
Sin-Ho Jung

Repeated Measures Design with Generalized Linear Mixed Models for Randomized Controlled Trials
Toshiro Tango

Sample Size Calculations for Clustered and Longitudinal Outcomes in Clinical Research
Chul Ahn, Moonseong Heo, and Song Zhang

Sample Size Calculations in Clinical Research, Second Edition
Shein-Chung Chow, Jun Shao, and Hansheng Wang

Statistical Analysis of Human Growth and Development
Yin Bun Cheung

Statistical Design and Analysis of Clinical Trials: Principles and Methods
Weichung Joe Shih and Joseph Aisner

Statistical Design and Analysis of Stability Studies
Shein-Chung Chow

Statistical Evaluation of Diagnostic Performance: Topics in ROC Analysis
Kelly H. Zou, Aiyi Liu, Andriy Bandos, Lucila Ohno-Machado, and Howard Rockette

Statistical Methods for Clinical Trials
Mark X. Norleans

Statistical Methods for Drug Safety
Robert D. Gibbons and Anup K. Amatya

Statistical Methods for Healthcare Performance Monitoring
Alex Bottle and Paul Aylin

Statistical Methods for Immunogenicity Assessment
Harry Yang, Jianchun Zhang, Binbing Yu, and Wei Zhao

Statistical Methods in Drug Combination Studies
Wei Zhao and Harry Yang

Statistical Testing Strategies in the Health Sciences
Albert Vexler, Alan D. Hutson, and Xiwei Chen

Statistics in Drug Research: Methodologies and Recent Developments
Shein-Chung Chow and Jun Shao

Statistics in the Pharmaceutical Industry, Third Edition
Ralph Buncher and Jia-Yeong Tsay

Survival Analysis in Medicine and Genetics
Jialiang Li and Shuangge Ma

Theory of Drug Development
Eric B. Holmgren

Translational Medicine: Strategies and Statistical Methods
Dennis Cosmatos and Shein-Chung Chow

Chapman & Hall/CRC Biostatistics Series

Clinical Trial Data Analysis Using R and SAS

Second Edition

Ding-Geng (Din) Chen

Karl E. Peace

Pinggao Zhang

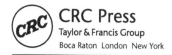

CRC Press
Taylor & Francis Group
Boca Raton London New York

CRC Press is an imprint of the
Taylor & Francis Group, an **informa** business
A CHAPMAN & HALL BOOK

CRC Press
Taylor & Francis Group
6000 Broken Sound Parkway NW, Suite 300
Boca Raton, FL 33487-2742

First issued in paperback 2020

© 2017 by Taylor & Francis Group, LLC
CRC Press is an imprint of Taylor & Francis Group, an Informa business

No claim to original U.S. Government works

ISBN-13: 978-1-4987-7952-4 (hbk)
ISBN-13: 978-0-367-73621-7 (pbk)

Library of Congress Cataloging-in-Publication Data

Names: Chen, Ding-Geng. | Peace, Karl E., 1941- | Zhang, Pinggao. | Chen,
Ding-Geng. Clinical trial data analysis using R.
Title: Clinical trial data analysis using R and SAS.
Other titles: Clinical trial data analysis using R
Description: Second edition / Ding-Geng Chen, Karl E. Peace, Pinggao Zhang. |
Boca Raton : CRC Press, 2017. | "Major updates to include SAS
programs"--Preface. | Previous edition: Clinical trial data analysis using
R / Ding-Geng Chen, Karl E. Peace (Boca Raton, Florida : CRC Press, 2011).
Identifiers: LCCN 2016057399 | ISBN 9781498779524 (hardback)
Subjects: LCSH: Clinical trials--Statistical methods. | R (Computer program
language) | SAS (Computer program language)
Classification: LCC R853.C55 C43 2017 | DDC 610.72/7--dc23
LC record available at https://lccn.loc.gov/2016057399

Visit the Taylor & Francis Web site at
http://www.taylorandfrancis.com

and the CRC Press Web site at
http://www.crcpress.com

Dedication

To my parents and parents-in-law who value high education and hard work, and to my wife, Ke, my son, John D. Chen, and my daughter, Jenny K. Chen, for their love and support.

Ding-Geng(Din) Chen

To the memory of my late mother, Elsie Mae Cloud Peace, my late wife, Jiann-Ping Hsu (JP), and to my son, Christopher K. Peace, daughter-in-law, Ashley Hopkins Peace, granddaughter, Camden, and grandson, Henry. Memories of my mom and wife JP continue to sustain me. My son, Chris, and his family provide much joy and esteem.

Karl E. Peace

To my wife, Jenny Z. Yang, and my sons, Andrew Y. Zhang and Anthony Y. Zhang, for their love and support. I am particularly thankful to my wife for her patience and understanding while I worked on the book.

Pinggao Zhang

Contents

List of Figures

List of Tables

Preface for the Second Edition

Since the publication of the first edition of this book in 2011, we have received extensive compliments on how well it was structured for use by clinical trial statisticians and analysts in analyzing their own clinical trial data following the detailed step-by-step illustrations using R. We have also received suggestions and comments for further improvement among which is to add SAS to the new edition. A feature of this second edition is to also illustrate data analyses using the SAS system. Therefore, in this second edition, we have incorporated all suggestions and comments from enthusiastic readers and corrected all errors and typos in addition to including SAS programs for data analysis. The SAS programs appear in the appendix of each chapter corresponding to the sections where analyses using R were performed.

Another major update is to change the way data are loaded into R. In the first edition, we used RODBC to read the dataset from an Excel book (named as `datR4CTDA.xlsx`) where all data are stored. Many readers communicated to us that they had difficulties in using RODBC. Therefore, in this edition, we saved all the datasets into `.csv` (comma separated values) files and use the R command `read.csv` to read the data into R. Readers can also use `read.table` to read the data into R for analysis.

We have updated the chapters. In Chapter 3, we included the clinical trial data analysis for correlated data using multivariate analysis of variance (MANOVA) in Section 3.2.1.4 with R implementation of this MANOVA approach in Section 3.3.1.6. The associated SAS programs are included in an appendix at the end of the chapter. In Chapter 4, we also included the clinical trial data analysis for correlated data using multivariate analysis of covariance (MANCOVA) in Section 4.3.1.3. The associated SAS programs are included in an appendix at the end of the chapter.

In Chapter 5, the `IntCox` package is no longer supported, but can be obtained from `https://cran.r-project.org/web/packages/intcox/index.html`. So we kept Section 5.4.3 for the description of this method as well as the R implementation in Section 5.5.2.4. However, we updated the analysis using another R package of `ictest` to test treatment effect using semiparametric estimation in Section 5.5.2.5. In addition, we updated the analysis using yet another R package for interval-censored data (i.e., `interval`) to fit Turnbull's nonparametric estimator in Section 5.5.2.2. The SAS programs for all the analyses are included in an appendix at the end of this chapter.

In Chapter 6, we updated the analysis using *lmerTest*. In analysis of longitudinal data using mixed-effects modeling, typically two R packages of *nlme* and *lme4* are used with more updates from *lme4*. However, this package does not list the p-values for their fixed-effects estimates as discussed by the creator, Professor Bates in `https://stat.ethz.ch/pipermail/r-help/2006-May/094765.html`. Dr. Alexandra Kuznetsova (`alku@dtu.dk`) expanded *lme4* to *lmerTest* with F-tests of types I-III hypotheses for the fixed-effects, likelihood-ratio tests for the random-effects, least squares means (population means), and differences of least squares means for the fixed effects factors with corresponding plots. In this edition, we updated the analyses with this package to illustrate longitudinal data analysis where all parameter estimates are the same for both editions and p-values are given in this second edition.

We updated Chapter 7 to include power analysis using SAS. The SAS procedure `proc power` is a very powerful and commonly used procedure for statistical power analysis and sample size determination. In this chapter, we updated all the power calculations from R in the first edition this book to include SAS programs in this second edition. In Chapter 8 for meta-analysis, we programmed the meta-analysis using SAS `proc iml` following the theory of meta-analysis since there is no existing SAS procedure for this purpose. We used the example in Section 8.3.3 for illustration purposes. Based on our experience, we recommend interested readers use R for their meta-analysis due to its extensive functionalities and ease of use of all the R packages designed for meta-analysis. We also recommend our book (Chen and Peace (2013)) for this purpose.

In Chapter 9 for Bayesian analysis, we make use of the SAS procedure `proc MCMC` which is commonly used in SAS for Bayesian modeling. We also illustrated the `proc genmod` with the option `bayes` to implement Bayes modeling corresponding to the data analysis in R in this chapter. Bioequivalence clinical trials have been commonly analyzed in SAS and there are many SAS programs online to be used. Therefore, we do not duplicate this effort in Chapter 10. Instead, we refer the reader to the following online link: `http://onbiostatistics.blogspot.com/2012/04/cookbook-sas-codes-for-bioequivalence.html` from Dr. Deng in his "Cookbook SAS Codes for Bioequivalence Test in $2 \times 2 \times 2$ Crossover Design", which is for the bioequivalence trials used in this chapter.

For analysis of adverse events in clinical trials in Chapter 11, there is no SAS procedure specifically designed for this analysis. We thus made use of SAS procedures of `proc iml` and `proc model` and programmed step-by-step for the examples in the chapter for illustration. In Chapter 12 for analysis of DNA microarray, we still highly recommend using R Bioconductor from `http://www.bioconductor.org` described in this chapter to analyze DNA microarray data. For readers who really like to use SAS, there is an experimental procedure `HPMIXED` in SAS for this purpose as seen in `https://support.sas.com/documentation/cdl/en/statug/63033/HTML/default/viewer.htm#hpmixed_toc.htm`.

With these updates, the book is more suitable as a text for a course in clinical trial data analysis at the graduate level (Master's or Doctorate's) using R and SAS. In addition, the book should be a valuable reference for self-study and a learning tool for clinical trial practitioners and biostatisticians in public health, medical research universities, governmental agencies, and the pharmaceutical industry, particularly those with little or no experience in using R and SAS.

Readers may use the computer programs and datasets and modify the R and SAS programs for their own applications. To facilitate the understanding of implementation in R and SAS, we annotated all the R and SAS programs with comments and explanations so that readers can easily understand the meaning of the corresponding R and SAS programs.

We would like to express our gratitude to many individuals. First, thanks to David Grubbs from Taylor & Francis for his encouragement in producing this second edition. Thanks also go to our research assistant Lin Nie who helped greatly with the SAS programs. Special thanks are due to professors Robert Gentleman and Ross Ihaka who created the R language with visionary open source, as well as to the developers and contributing authors in the R community for their endless efforts and contributed packages.

As a special note to interested readers, all the datasets, R, and SAS programs in this book can be obtained from the first author (Professor Chen) by email at: `DrDG.Chen@gmail.com`.

Ding-Geng(Din) Chen, Ph.D.
University of North Carolina, Chapel Hill, NC, USA
University of Pretoria, Pretoria, South Africa

Karl E. Peace, Ph.D.
Jiann-Ping Hsu College of Public Health
Georgia Southern University, Statesboro, GA, USA

Pinggao Zhang, Ph.D.
Shire Pharmaceuticals, Boston, MA, USA

Preface for the First Edition

With the exception of two chapters, our first book: "Clinical Trial Methodology" (Peace and Chen (2010)) contained no statistical analysis software code for the analysis results presented therein. In this book we provide a thorough presentation of biostatistical analyses of clinical trial data with detailed step-by-step illustrations on their implementation using R. In each chapter, examples of clinical trials based on the authors' actual experience in many areas of clinical drug development are presented. After understanding the application, various biostatistical methods appropriate for analyzing data from the clinical trials are identified. Then analysis code is developed using appropriate R packages and functions to analyze the data. Analysis code development and results are presented in a stepwise fashion. This stepwise approach should enable readers to follow the logic and gain an understanding of the analysis methods and the R implementation so that they may use R to analyze their own clinical trial data.

Based on their experience in biostatistical research and working in clinical development, the authors understand that there are gaps between developed statistical methods and applications of statistical methods by students and practitioners. This book is intended to fill this gap by illustrating the implementation of statistical methods using R applied to real clinical trial data following a step-by-step presentation style.

With this style, the book is suitable as a text for a course in clinical trial data analysis at the graduate level (Master's or Doctorate's), particularly for students seeking degrees in statistics or biostatistics. In addition, the book should be a valuable reference for self-study and a learning tool for clinical trial practitioners and biostatisticians in public health, medical research universities, governmental agencies and the pharmaceutical industry, particularly those with little or no experience in using R.

R has become widely used in statistical modeling and computing since its creation in the mid 1990s and it is now an integrated and essential software for statistical analyses. Becoming familiar with R is then an imperative for the next generation of statistical data analysts. In Chapter 1, we present a basic introduction to the R system, where to get R, how to install R and how to upgrade R packages. Readers who are already familiar with R may skip this chapter and go directly to any of the remaining chapters.

In Chapter 2, we provide an overview of the phases and objectives of clinical trials as well as biostatistical aspects of clinical trials.

In Chapter 3, we consider basic treatment comparisons in clinical trials using the R system. Datasets from two clinical efficacy trials are introduced; "Diastolic Blood Pressure" data from a hypertension trial and "Duodenal Ulcer Healing" data from a large duodenal ulcer trial. Statistical methods, such as Student's t-test, analysis of variance (ANOVA), bootstrapping, Pearson's χ^2 and other contingency table methods, appropriate for the type of data are identified followed by step-by-step statistical analyses using R.

In Chapter 4, we present data analysis methods for treatment comparisons in clinical trials adjusting for covariates using R. In addition to the "Diastolic Blood Pressure" dataset in Chapter 3, datasets from two additional clinical trials are introduced; one from a large trial of "Beta-Blockers" and one from a trial of "Familial Andenomatous Polyposis". We present statistical methods such as analysis of covariance (ANCOVA), logistic regression for binomial data and Poisson regression for count data appropriate for analyzing these types of data using R. In the application of logistic regression, we emphasize diagnostics for detecting overdispersion for correct modeling and present several remedies whenever overdispersion is pinpointed.

Analysis methods using R for data from clinical trials with time-to-event endpoints are presented in Chapter 5. In this chapter, we use data from a Phase II trial of patients with Stage-2 breast carcinoma as an example of right-censored time-to-event data. In addition, data from a publically available breast cancer trial is used as an example of interval-censored time-to-event data. We then present the associated statistical models for analyzing these data with appropriate R packages. Methods for right-censored data are typically well-known; e.g. the nonparametric Kaplan-Meier estimator, semi-parametric Cox regression and full parametric models such as the exponential, Weibull or other distributions. However, methods for analyzing interval-censored data are less-known and sometimes not available in statistical software packages. In this chapter, we include some up-to-date statistical methods as well as the R packages for analyzing this type of data.

Analysis methods appropriate for data from longitudinal clinical trials are presented in Chapter 6. Two datasets are used as examples in this chapter. The first dataset is the "Diastolic Blood Pressure" used in Chapters 3 and 4 and reflects continuous data. The second dataset is from the clinical trial of Duodenal Ulcer Healing of which a subset was analyzed in Chapter 3, and reflects categorical data. These datasets are analyzed using longitudinal statistical methods, such as linear mixed models, generalized linear mixed models and generalized estimating equations and implemented in R packages.

Chapter 7 discusses sample size determination and power analysis in clinical trials. We present an extensive list of methods as well as the R packages to calculate sample size required under different data types and protocol design.

Meta-analysis of data from clinical trials is presented in Chapter 8. In this chapter, we present both fixed-effects and random-effects models used in meta-analysis with several R packages to implement these models.

Since Bayesian methods are being increasingly used in the design and analysis of clinical trials, Chapter 9 explores relevant Bayesian models with a Markov-chain Monte-Carlo approach and application of R packages. Chapter 10 introduces bioequivalence clinical trials. In this Chapter, we use a dataset from Chow and Liu (2009) to illustrate the step-by-step implementation in R and the reproducibility of their results using the R system. We then analyze a dataset from a bioequivalence trial comparing different tablet formulations of a commercially available drug.

The analysis of adverse events in clinical trials is outlined in Chapter 11. Similarly to other chapters, we introduce a clinical trial data and present statistical models using confidence interval and significance level methods to analyze this type of data as well as the step-by-step implementation using the R system.

In recent years, microarray technologies have been used extensively to study molecular differences among different types of diseases which lead to identification of new drugs in the biopharmaceutical industry. Along with the development of microarray technology, many new statistical methods and models have been developed in parallel and incorporated in software to analyze high-throughput data. We think it is important to introduce some of these methods and software as an introductory Chapter. Chapter 12 then serves this purpose to introduce the analysis of microarray data derived from samples collected in clinical trials using the `bioconductor` project.

All R programs and datasets used in this book are available in authors' webpages at `http://jphcoph.georgiasouthern.edu/Faculty.php`. Readers may download the programs and datasets and modify the R programs for their own applications. To facilitate the understanding of implementation in R, we annotated all the R programs with comments and explanations started with `#` (i.e. the R command for "comment") so that the readers can understand exactly the meaning of the corresponding R programs.

We would like to express our gratitude to many individuals. First, thanks to David Grubbs from Taylor & Francis for his interest in the book and to Shashi Kumar for assistance in LaTeX. Thanks also go to Professors Jianguo Sun and Lili Yu for their suggestions to Chapter 5 and to Professor Xijin Ge for his suggestions to Chapter 12 which significantly improved these chapters. Special thanks are due to Professors Robert Gentleman and Ross Ihaka who created the R language with visionary open source, as well as to the developers and contributing authors in the R community for their endless efforts and contributed packages. Finally, from the Jiann-Ping Hsu College of Public Health at Georgia Southern University, thanks go to Macaulay Okwakenye, our graduate assistant, for assistance in proofing some of the chapters, and to Dean Charlie Hardy for his support and encouragement to finish the book.

Statesboro, GA,

Ding-Geng (Din) Chen
Karl E. Peace
July 23, 2010

About the Authors

Ding-Geng (Din) Chen is a fellow of ASA and currently the Wallace H. Kuralt Distinguished Professor at the University of North Carolina-Chapel Hill and an extraordinary professor at the University of Pretoria, South Africa. Formerly, he was the Karl E. Peace Endowed Eminent Scholar Chair in Biostatistics and Professor of Biostatistics in the Jiann-Ping Hsu College of Public Health at Georgia Southern University (GSU), and Professor of Biostatistics at the University of Rochester. Dr. Chen's research interests 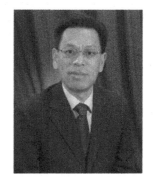 include clinical trial biostatistical methodological development in Bayesian models, survival analysis, and statistics in biological assays. He has published more than 150 refereed papers and co-authored/co-edited 12 book in statistics.

Karl E. Peace is the Georgia Cancer Coalition Distinguished Cancer Scholar, Founding Director of the Center for Biostatistics, Professor of Biostatistics, and Senior Research Scientist in the Jiann-Ping Hsu College of Public Health at GSU. Dr. Peace has made pivotal contributions in the development and approval of drugs to treat numerous diseases and disorders. A fellow of the ASA, he has been a recipient of many honors, including the Drug Information Association Outstanding Service Award, the American Public Health Association Statistics Section 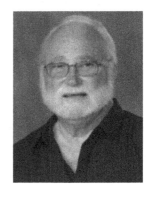 Award, the first recipient of the President's Medal for Outstanding Contributions to GSU, and recognition by the Georgia and US Houses of Representatives, and the Virginia House of Delegates.

Pinggao Zhang has 20 years of experience in the pharmaceutical/biotech industries. He joined Shire in 2004 and previously worked for Aventis, Scirex, and Purdue Pharma. He has led biostatistics activities in support of clinical development across all phases, regulatory submissions, and publications. He has worked in various therapeutic areas including vaccine, oncology, CNS, analgesics, and hematology, and has contributed to several successful drug approvals. As Director 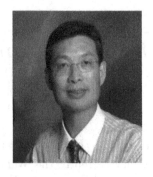 of Biostatistics, Pinggao is currently responsible for biostatistics activities in relation to medical affairs. Dr. Zhang received his MSc in Statistics and PhD in Epidemiology from the University of Guelph.

Drs. Chen and Peace previously collaborated on other books in the CRC Press Series in Biostatistics: *Clinical Trial Methodology*, *Clinical Trial Data Analysis Using R*, and *Applied Meta-Analysis with R*.

Chapter 1

Introduction to R

In this chapter, we provide a basic introduction to the R system (R Development Core Team (2005)): where to get R, how to install R and upgrade R packages. We also show how easy it is to use R to simulate and analyze data from a simple clinical trial. We conclude the chapter with a brief summary and some recommendations for further reading and references. Readers who already know and have familiarity with R can skip this chapter and go directly to any of the remaining chapters.

1.1 What is R?

To obtain an introduction to R, go to the official homepage of the R project at

`http://www.R-project.org`

and click "About R" under "R Project":

R is a language and environment for statistical computing and graphics. It is a GNU project which is similar to the S language and environment which was developed at Bell Laboratories (formerly AT&T, now Lucent Technologies) by John Chambers and colleagues. R can be considered as a different implementation of S. There are some important differences, but much code written for S runs unaltered under R.

According to a NY Times article, R first appeared in 1996, when statistics professors Ross Ihaka and Robert Gentleman of the University of Auckland in New Zealand released the code as a free software package (`http://www.nytimes.com/2009/01/07/technology/business-computing/07program.html?pagewanted=all&_r=`

1

0). Based on a recent IEEE spectrum publication, R currently occupies 5th place among top programming languages (`http://blog.revolutionanalytics.com/popularity/`).

R provides a wide variety of statistical (linear and nonlinear modelling, classical statistical tests, time-series analysis, classification, clustering, ...) and graphical techniques, and is highly extensible. The S language is often the vehicle of choice for research in statistical methodology, and R provides an Open Source route to participation in that activity.

One of R's strengths is the ease with which well-designed publication-quality plots can be produced, including mathematical symbols and formulae where needed. Great care has been taken over the defaults for the minor design choices in graphics, but the user retains full control.

R is available as Free Software under the terms of the Free Software Foundation's GNU General Public License in source code form. It compiles and runs on a wide variety of UNIX platforms and similar systems (including FreeBSD and Linux), Windows and MacOS.

To some users, "free" software may be a "negative" word for software that is difficult to use, has lower quality or utilizes procedures that have not been validated or verified, etc. However, to other users, "free" software means software from an open source that not only allows use of the software, but also permits modifications to handle a variety of applications. This latter description is the fundamental principle for R system.

We now proceed to the steps for installing and using R.

1.2   Steps on Installing **R** and Updating **R** Packages

In general, the R system consists of two parts. One is the so-called R *base system* for the core R language and associated fundamental libraries. The other consists of user contributed *packages* that are more specialized applications. Both the *base system* and the *packages* may be obtained from the Comprehensive R Archive Network (CRAN) from the weblink:

`http://CRAN.r-project.org`

Installation of R system is described in the following sections.

1.2.1   First Step: Install **R** *Base System*

The *base system* can be downloaded from

<code>http://CRAN.r-project.org</code>

for different platforms of "Linux", "MacOS X" and "Windows". In this book, we illustrate the use of R for "Windows". "Windows" users can download the latest verison of R using the link:

<code>http://CRAN.r-project.org/bin/windows/base/release.htm</code>

(At the writing of this book, version *R 3.3.1* is available.) To download and install R to your computer, simply follow the instructions from the installer to install R to the "Program Files" subdirectory in your C. You are ready to use R for statistical computing and data analysis.

Note to LaTeX and *R/Sweave* users: LaTeX will complain about the extra space in the path as in "Program Files". Therefore if you want to use R along with LaTeX, you need to make a subdirectory *without* space in the path to install R.

You should now have an icon with a shortcut to R. Simply click the icon to start R. You should see some introductory information about R and a command prompt '>':

```
>
```

To illustrate R computation, suppose we wish to calculate the sum of 1 and 2. The first line of R computation is:

```
> x = 1+2
```

The computed value may be printed using:

```
> print(x)
```

```
[1] 3
```

You should get "3".

1.2.2   Second Step: Installing and Updating **R** Packages

The R *base system* contains a variety of standard statistical functions, descriptive and inferential statistical analysis methods, and graphics which are appropriate for many statistical computing and data analysis requirements.

However, the *packages* are more specialized applications that are contributed by advanced R developers and users who are experts in their field. From our view, *packages* in R is the most important component in R development and upgrading. At the time of writing this second edition of our book, there are more than 9203 packages in the R system spanning almost all fields of statistical computing and methodology.

You may install any *packages* from the R prompt by clicking `install.packages` from the R menu *Packages* .

For example, for researchers and practitioners who are interested in designing group sequential clinical trials, the *gsDesign* contributed by *Keaven Anderson* from Merck and Company can be installed from this pull-down manual. All the functionality of this package is then available by loading it to R as:

```
> library(gsDesign)
```

For first-time users for this package, information about its use may be obtained by invoking:

```
> library(help=gsDesign)
```

A help page is then available which explains all the functionality of this package. For readers who desire a comprehensive list of available packages, go to

http://CRAN.R-project.org/src/contrib/PACKAGES.html

1.2.3   Steps to Get Help and Documentation

A striking feature of R is the easy access of its "Help and Documentation" which may distinguish it from other software systems. There are several ways to access "Help and Documentation".

The general reference may be obtained from *RGui* in R. When R is started, click "Help" to access R help items on "FAQ on R", "FAQ on R on Windows", "Manuals (in PDF)", etc. We recommend that readers print the online PDF manual "Introduction to R" for future reference.

Additional "Help and Documentation" may be obtained from the R homepage. Many documentations and online discussions on R are available from the R homepage http://www.r-project.org/. The online "Documentation" section consists of almost all the manuals, FAQs, R Journal, books and other related. We recommend readers spend some time in reviewing the online documents to gain familiarity with R.

The most convenient way to access is from the R command prompt. You can always obtain specific help information from the R command prompt by using "help()". For example, if you want help on "Conditional Power Computation" in the library *gsDesign*, type:

```
> help(gsCP)
```

This will load an information page on "Conditional Power Computation" containing relevant information. This includes the description of the function, detailed usage for the function and some examples on how to use this function.

1.3 R for Clinical Trials

Since its release, R has been used in academia, government agencies and the pharmaceutical industry in the design and analysis of clinical trials. There are numerous R packages that have been written for clinical trial applications. We use some of them in this book. For reference to the R system for clinical trials, readers are referred to the online documentation titled as

R: Regulatory Compliance and Validation Issues

A Guidance Document for the Use of R in Regulated Clinical Trial Environments is available from the R homepage (http://www.r-project.org/) by pointing the web browser to "Certification" under "Documentation" on the left side, or it may be directly downloaded from

http://www.r-project.org/doc/R-FDA.pdf

This online documentation was prepared by "The R Foundation for Statistical Computing" on August 17, 2008.

This guidance discusses aspects of the use of R for human clinical trials conducted by the pharmaceutical industry in compliance with regulations of the United States Food and Drug Administration (hereafter referred to as the FDA) and the International Conference on Harmonisation of Technical Requirements for Registration of Pharmaceuticals in Human Use (hereafter referred to as the ICH).

Ed Zhang maintains a R online **CRAN Task View** available via

http://cran.r-project.org/web/views/ClinicalTrials.html

containing specific packages for design, monitoring and analysis of data from clinical trials.

This **CRAN Task View** gathers "packages for clinical trial design and monitoring in general plus data analysis packages for specific types of design. Also, it gives a brief introduction to important packages for analyzing clinical trial data."

To illustrate use of **CRAN Task View**, we emphasize and copy several packages that we often use. Readers are encouraged to visit **CRAN Task View** to gain familiarity.

In **Design and Monitoring**

- *Blockrand* creates randomizations for clinical trials using blocked randomization. It can also produce a PDF file of randomization cards.

- *GroupSeq* performs computations related to group sequential designs via the alpha spending approach, i.e., interim analyses need not be equally spaced, and their number need not be specified in advance.

- *gsDesign* derives group sequential designs and describes their properties.

- *ldBand* from *Hmisc* computes and plots group sequential stopping boundaries from the Lan-DeMets method with a variety of α-spending functions using the ld98 program from the Department of Biostatistics, University of Wisconsin written by DM Reboussin, DL DeMets, KM Kim, and KKG Lan.

- *PwrGSD* is a set of tools to compute power in a group sequential design.

- *seqmon* computes the probability of crossing sequential efficacy and futility boundaries in a clinical trial. It implements the Armitage-McPherson and Rowe Algorithm using the method described in Schoenfeld (2001).

In **Analysis for Specific Design**

- *clinfun* has functions for both design and analysis of clinical trials. For phase II trials, it has functions to calculate sample size, effect size, and power based on Fisher's exact test, the operating characteristics of a two-stage boundary, Optimal and Minimax 2-stage Phase II designs given by Richard Simon (Simon (1989)), the exact 1-stage Phase II design and can compute a stopping rule and its operating characteristics for toxicity monitoring based on repeated significance testing. For Phase III trials, sample size for group sequential designs may also be computed.

- *bifactorial* makes global and multiple inferences for specified bi- and trifactorial clinical trial designs using bootstrap methods and a classical approach.

- *ClinicalRobustPriors* can be employed for computing distributions (prior, likelihood, and posterior) and moments of robust models: Cauchy/Binomial, Cauchy/Normal and Berger/Normal. Furthermore, the assessment of the hyperparameters and the posterior analysis can be processed.

- *MChtest* performs hypothesis tests using Monte Carlo methods. It allows a couple of different sequential stopping boundaries (a truncated sequential probability ratio test boundary and a boundary proposed by Besag and Clifford (1991). It gives valid p-values and confidence intervals on p-values. *speff2trial* performs estimation and testing of treatment effect in a 2-group randomized clinical trial with a quantitative or dichotomous endpoint.

Other packages are available including those for meta-analyses and other analyses in general.

1.4   A Simple Simulated Clinical Trial

To demonstrate basic application of R and its functionality, we simulate a simple two-arm clinical trial to compare a new drug to placebo on reducing diastolic blood pressure in hypertensive adult men.

Let's assume an appropriate power analysis indicated the sample size required to detect a specified treatment difference is $n = 100$ for both treatment groups (i.e., *drug* vs. *placebo*). For these n participants, we record their age and measure baseline diastolic blood pressure just before randomization; note that *age* is an important risk factor linked to blood pressure.

The new drug and placebo are administered and blood pressure is measured and recorded periodically thereafter, including at the end of the trial. Then the change in blood pressure between the endpoint and baseline may be calculated and analyzed as an index of the antihypertensive efficacy of the new drug.

We illustrate simulation of the data, data manipulation and analysis with appropriate statistical graphics. Since this is the very first introduction to R, we intentionally use the basic R command so that readers can follow the logic without difficulty.

1.4.1   Data Simulation

1.4.1.1   R Functions

R has a wide range of functions to handle probability distributions and data simulation. For example, for the commonly used normal distribution, its *Density, cumulative distribution function, quantile function* and *random generation* with mean equal to *mean* and standard deviation equal to *sd* can be generated using the following R functions:

```
dnorm(x, mean = 0, sd = 1, log = FALSE)
pnorm(q, mean = 0, sd = 1, lower.tail = TRUE, log.p = FALSE)
qnorm(p, mean = 0, sd = 1, lower.tail = TRUE, log.p = FALSE)
rnorm(n, mean = 0, sd = 1)
```

where

x, q	*is*	vector of quantiles
p	*is*	vector of probabilities
n	*is*	number of observations
mean	*is*	vector of means
sd	*is*	vector of standard deviations.

The above specification can be found using the *Help* function as follows:

```
> help(rnorm)
```

There are similar sets of *d, p, q, r* functions for *Poisson, binomial, t, F, hypergeometric,* χ^2, *Beta,* etc. Also there is a *sample* function for sampling from a vector *replicate* for repeating a computation.

1.4.1.2   Data Generation and Manipulation

With this introduction, we now simulate the clinical trial data assuming that the baseline diastolic blood pressures for these 200 ($n = 100$ for each treatment) recruited participants are normally distributed with mean (mu) = 100 (mmHg) and standard deviation $sd = 10$ (mmHg). The *age* for these 200 middle-age men is assumed to be normally distributed with mean age *age.mu* = 50 (year old) and standard deviation *age.sd* = 10 (year). In addition, we assume the new drug will decrease diastolic blood pressure by *mu.d* = 20 (mmHg).

These input values for this simulation can be specified in R as follows:

```
> # simulated input values
> n       = 100
> mu      = 100
> sd      = 10
> mu.d    = 20
> age.mu = 50
> age.sd = 10
```

We first simulate data for the *n placebo* participants with *age*, baseline blood pressure (denoted by *bp.base*), endpoint blood pressure (denoted by *bp.end*) and change in blood pressure from baseline to endpoint (denoted by *bp.diff=bp.end-bp.base*) with following R code chunk:

```
> # fix the seed for random number generation
> set.seed(123)
> # use "rnorm" to generate random normal
> age        = rnorm(n, age.mu, age.sd)
> bp.base     = rnorm(n,mu,sd)
> bp.end      = rnorm(n,mu,sd)
> # take the difference between endpoint and baseline
> bp.diff     = bp.end-bp.base
> # put the data together using "cbind" to column-bind
> dat4placebo = round(cbind(age,bp.base,bp.end,bp.diff))
```

Note that the simulation seed is set at 123 so that simulation can be reproduced, which is done by `set.seed(123)`. Otherwise, results can be different from each simulation.

We can manipulate the data using column bind (R command `cbind`) to combine all the simulated data together and round the data into the nearest

whole number (R command **round**) to produce a dataset and give the data
matrix a name: *dat4placebo*. The first few observations may be viewed using
the following R code:

```
> head(dat4placebo)
```

	age	bp.base	bp.end	bp.diff
[1,]	44	93	122	29
[2,]	48	103	113	11
[3,]	66	98	97	0
[4,]	51	97	105	9
[5,]	51	90	96	5
[6,]	67	100	95	-4

Similarly, we can simulate data for the *new drug*. We use the same variable
names here, but give a different name to the final dataset: *dat4drug*. Note that
the *mean* for the *bp.end* is now *mu-mu.d* to simulate the decrease in mean
value:

```
> age       = rnorm(n, age.mu, age.sd)
> bp.base   = rnorm(n,mu,sd)
> bp.end    = rnorm(n,mu-mu.d,sd)
> bp.diff   = bp.end-bp.base
> dat4drug = round(cbind(age,bp.base,bp.end,bp.diff))
```

We do not print the observations at this time. To further manipulate the
data, we stack the two datasets from *placebo* and *new drug* using R command
rbind to produce a data frame using R command **data.frame**. We also create
a column *trt* with two factors of *Placebo* and *Drug* to indicate there are two
treatments in this dataset and finally name this data *dat*:

```
> # make a dataframe to hold all data
> dat      = data.frame(rbind(dat4placebo,dat4drug))
> # make "trt" as a factor for treatment.
> dat$trt = as.factor(rep(c("Placebo", "Drug"), each=n))
```

With these manipulations, the data frame *dat* should have 200 observations
with 100 from *Placebo* and 100 from *Drug*. Also this dataframe should have 5
age, bp.base, bp.end, bp.diff,trt as columns. We can check it using following R
code chunk:

```
> # check the data dimension
> dim(dat)
```

```
[1] 200    5
```

```
> # print the first 6 obervations to see the variable names
> head(dat)
```

	age	bp.base	bp.end	bp.diff	trt
1	44	93	122	29	Placebo
2	48	103	113	11	Placebo
3	66	98	97	0	Placebo
4	51	97	105	9	Placebo
5	51	90	96	5	Placebo
6	67	100	95	-4	Placebo

1.4.1.3   Basic R Graphics

R is well-known for its graphics capabilities. We can display the distributions for the data just generated to view whether they appear to be normally distributed using the R command `boxplot` as follows:

```
> # call boxplot
> boxplot(dat4placebo, las=1, main="Placebo")
```

This will generate Figure 1.1 from which one can see that the data appear to be normally distributed except for one outlier from the baseline data.

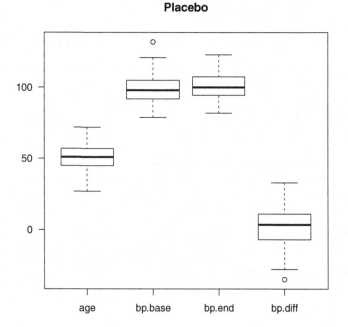

FIGURE 1.1: Distributions for Data Generated for "Placebo"

Similarly we can produce the distribution for *Drug* using following R code chunk:

```
> boxplot(dat4drug, las=1, main="Drug")
```

This will produce Figure 1.2 to show that the data are in fact normally distributed. The boxplot for endpoint is 20 mmHG lower than the baseline blood pressure.

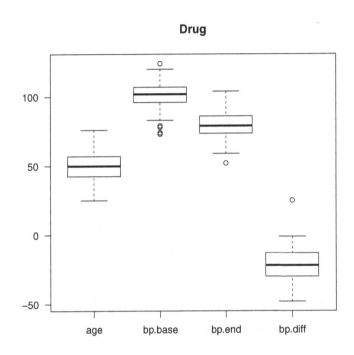

FIGURE 1.2: Distributions for Data Generated for "Drug"

Before performing any statistical analysis of the clinical trial data, we recommend exploring the data using appropriate plots to assess whether distributional or other relevant assumptions required for the validity of the analysis methods hold for the data. There is another suite of advanced R graphics to use for this purpose, i.e., the package *lattice* with implementation of Trellis Graphics.

This package is maintained by Deepayan Sarkar (Sarkar (2008)) and can be downloaded from

http://r-forge.r-project.org/projects/lattice/

or simply from RGUI. We first load the package into R by `library(lattice)` and display the relationship between the blood pressure difference as a function of *age* for each treatment to assess whether there exists a statistically significant relationship in addition to a treatment difference. This can be done with the following R code chunk:

```
> #load the lattice library
> library(lattice)
> # call xyplot function and print it
> print(xyplot(bp.diff~age|trt, data=dat,xlab="Age",
 strip=strip.custom(bg="white"),
 ylab="Blood Pressure Difference",lwd=3,cex=1.3,pch=20,
 type=c("p", "r")))
```

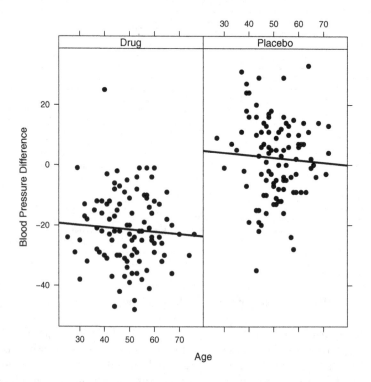

FIGURE 1.3: Data with Regression Line for Each Treatment

This produces Figure 1.3 from which we conclude that the relationship between the blood pressure decrease and age is not significant, but that the new drug did reduce blood pressure.

1.4.2 Data Analysis

With these preliminary graphical illustrations, we comfortably proceed to data analysis. The general statistical model we start with is

$$y = \beta_0 + \beta_1 \times trt + \beta_2 \times age + \beta_3 age \times trt + \epsilon \qquad (1.1)$$

where y denotes the change in blood pressure and β's are the parameters. ϵ is the error term which is assumed to be independently identically distributed (*i.i.d.*) with normal distribution with standard deviation σ. Note that we start with the *age* and *trt* interaction.

The fitting of this linear model (1.1) is accomplished in one line of R code using lm as:

```
> lm1 = lm(bp.diff~trt*age, data=dat)
> summary(lm1)

Call:
lm(formula = bp.diff ~ trt * age, data = dat)

Residuals:
    Min     1Q Median     3Q    Max
 -37.97  -8.88   0.04   8.49  45.68

Coefficients:
                Estimate Std. Error t value Pr(>|t|)
(Intercept)     -17.62709    6.24247   -2.82   0.0052 **
trtPlacebo       24.15364    9.58693    2.52   0.0126 *
age              -0.07628    0.12321   -0.62   0.5365
trtPlacebo:age   -0.00631    0.18697   -0.03   0.9731
---
Signif. codes:
0 *** 0.001 ** 0.01 * 0.05 .

Residual standard error: 12.8 on 196 degrees of freedom
Multiple R-squared:  0.468,          Adjusted R-squared:  0.46
F-statistic: 57.6 on 3 and 196 DF,   p-value: <2e-16
```

The summary prints a summary of the model fitting including the analysis of variance (ANOVA) table, R^2 and p-values, etc. A prettier table can be generated from the R package *xtable* on tests for significance of the coefficients which are shown in Table 1.1; this confirms the conclusion from Figure 1.3 that the new drug reduced blood pressure in a statistically significant manner.

```
> # load the xtable library
> library(xtable)
> # call xtable to make the table
```

```
> print(xtable(lm1, caption="ANOVA Table for Simulated
  Clinical Trial Data", label = "tab4RI.coef"),
  table.placement = "htbp",caption.placement = "top")
```

TABLE 1.1: ANOVA Table for Simulated Clinical Trial Data

	Estimate	Std. Error	t value	Pr($>$|t|)
(Intercept)	-17.6271	6.2425	-2.82	0.0052
trtPlacebo	24.1536	9.5869	2.52	0.0126
age	-0.0763	0.1232	-0.62	0.5365
trtPlacebo:age	-0.0063	0.1870	-0.03	0.9731

The diagnostics for model assumptions may be illustrated in simple R code to generate the residual plot, QQ-plot and the associated plot for outlier and leverages as in Figure 1.4.

```
> plot(lm1)
```

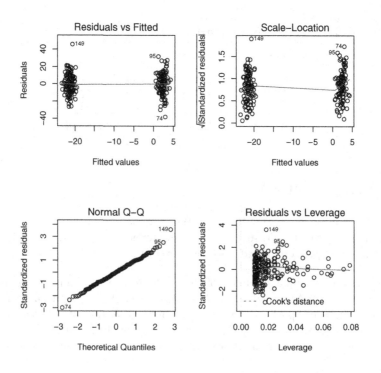

FIGURE 1.4: Diagnostics Plot

1.5 Summary and Recommendations for Further Reading

In this chapter, we introduced the reader to the R system, its installation, and its related packages. We illustrated the use of R for data simulation and manipulation, statistical graphics and statistical modeling by simulating data for a simple clinical trial.

For further reading to gain more familiarity with the R system, we recommend:

- **R fundamentals to *S* languages**: Two books from John Chambers (Chambers (1998) and Chambers (2008)) are excellent references to understand the R language and its programming structures.

- **R graphics:** Besides Sarkar's book (Sarkar (2008)) on *lattice*, we also recommend Paul Murrell's book (Murrell (2005)).

- **Statistical data analysis using R:** We recommend Faraway's two books published in 2004 (Faraway (2004)) and 2006 (Faraway (2006)), which are two excellent books in using R for statistical modelling. Everitt and Hothorn's book (Everitt and Hothorn (2006)) on statistical data analysis using R is another excellent book we have used in the classroom which students found interesting.

- **Statistical computing:** Maria Rizzo's book on "Statistical Computing with R" (Rizzo (2008)) is an excellent book.

- **R online documentations:** We emphasize again that there are many free online books, manuals, journals and others to be downloaded from R homepage at "Documentation".

1.6 Appendix: SAS Programs

The SAS program below corresponds to the R program in Section 1.4. Note that the data are randomly generated, the values are different.

```
/***********************************
   Section 1.4.1.2: Data Generation
**********************************/
/* simulate the "Placebo"  */
data dat4placebo(keep =age bp4base bp4end bp4diff trt);
```

```
trt = "Placebo";
n=100;mu=100;sd=10;mud =20;agemu=50;agesd=10;
do i =1 to n;
age      = agemu+agesd*rand("Normal");
bp4base = mu+sd*rand("Normal");
bp4end  = mu+sd*rand("Normal");
bp4diff = bp4end-bp4base;
output;
end;
run;
/* simulate the "drug"  */
data dat4drug(keep =age bp4base bp4end bp4diff trt);
trt = "Drug";
n=100;mu=100;sd=10;mud =20;agemu=50;agesd=10;
do i =1 to n;
age      = agemu+agesd*rand("Normal");
bp4base = mu-mud+sd*rand("Normal");
bp4end  = mu+sd*rand("Normal");
bp4diff = bp4end-bp4base;
output;
end;
run;
/* combine these two datasets into "dat"*/
data dat;
set dat4placebo dat4drug;
run;

proc print data=dat;
run;


/**********************************************
  Section 1.4.2 Data analysis
**********************************************/
ods graphics on;
proc glm data=dat;
class trt(ref="Placebo");
model bp4diff = age trt trt*age/solution;
run;
ods graphics off;
```

Chapter 2

Overview of Clinical Trials

2.1 Introduction

A clinical trial is a research study conducted to assess the utility of an intervention in volunteers. Interventions may be diagnostic, preventative or treatment in nature and may include drugs, biologics, medical devices or methods of screening. Interventions may also include procedures whose aim is to improve quality of life or to better understand how the intervention works in volunteers.

Quality clinical research must be well planned, closely and carefully monitored and conducted, and appropriately analyzed and reported. Greater attentiveness to detail at the design stage argues for greater efficiency at the analysis and reporting stages. This is important on a per protocol basis as well as across the entire clinical development plan to support regulatory filing.

2.2 Phases of Clinical Trials and Objectives

It is well known that evidence to support regulatory approval of a new drug derives from clinical trials. Such trials are categorized as Phase 0 (although not conducted for all drugs) Phase I, Phase II, or Phase III. Although these categories may not be mutually exclusive (nor in some cases mutually exhaustive), there is general agreement as to what types of clinical studies comprise the bulk of the trials within each phase.

2.2.1 Phase 0 Trials

For some drugs, drug companies may carry out Phase 0 studies on drug candidates in order to decide which has the best pharmacokinetic profile in humans before elevating to further development. Such trials are conducted at a very low dose and provide no efficacy or safety information but the information on pharmacokinetics may help to design Phase I trials.

2.2.2   Phase I Trials

Phase I trials may consist of "early Phase I" trials, early dose ranging trials, bioavailability or pharmacokinetic trials, or mechanism of action studies. Early Phase I trials represent the initial introduction of the drug in humans, in order to characterize the acute pharmacological effect. For most classes of drugs, healthy subjects are enrolled, in an attempt to reduce the risk of serious toxicity and to avoid confounding pharmacological and disease effects. The idea is to introduce the drug to humans and escalate the dose without inducing acute toxicity.

Early dose ranging trials, often called "dose tolerance" or "dose titration trials", are also most often conducted in healthy subjects. Both the effects of single dosing and multiple dosing schemes are studied. The objective of these trials is to determine a "tolerable" dose range, such that as long as future dosing remains in this range, no intolerable side effects of toxicities would be expected to be seen.

Early Phase I trials and early dose ranging trials do not establish nor quantitate efficacy characteristics of a drug. These studies have to be conducted first, so that acute pharmacological effects may be described, and a range of tolerable doses determined, which guide clinical use of the drug for later studies.

The primary objectives of Phase I bioavailability and pharmacokinetic trials are to characterize what happens to the drug once it is injected into the human body. That is, properties such as absorption, distribution, metabolism, elimination, clearance, and half-life need to be described. These trials also usually enroll healthy subjects and are often called "blood level trials".

Mechanism of action trials attempt to identify how the drug induces its effects. An example is the class of H2-receptor antagonists, such as cimetidine, ranitidine, famotidine and zanatidine, which by blocking the H2-receptor reduce the secretion of gastrin which in turn leads to a reduction of gastric acid production. Another example is the H1-receptor antagonist, seldane, which by blocking the H1-receptor reduces histamine release. Other examples are the ACE (angiotensin-converting-enzyme) inhibitors (e.g., captopril, enalapril, quinapril) which are competitive inhibitors of ACE. ACE inhibitors block the formation of the chemical: angiotensin II (AT-II) which causes muscles surrounding blood vessels to contract. Blocking the formation of AT-II leads to reduced vasoconstriction, increased vasodilation, and reduced blood pressure.

Bioavailability or pharmacokinetic studies and mechanism of action studies provide additional information so that the drug may be clinically used more effectively and safer in future studies.

2.2.3   Phase II Trials

Phase II trials represent the earliest trials of a drug in patients. Patients should have the disease under investigation. Patients who enter such trials represent a relatively restricted yet homogeneous population. In some areas of drug development, such as oncology, Phase II trials are categorized as Phase IIA and Phase IIB.

Phase IIA trials may include clinical pharmacology studies in patients, and more extensive or detailed pharmacokinetic and pharmacodynamic studies in patients. Phase IIB trials are controlled and represent the initial demonstration of efficacy and safety of a drug at the doses from the clinical pharmacology studies. Also of interest is to estimate the effective dose range, to characterize the dose response curve, and to estimate the minimally effective dose. Often it is difficult to distinguish between Phase IIB trials and Phase III trials, particularly in terms of objectives. The primary differences are the inclusion/exclusion criteria and the sample size.

2.2.4 Phase III Trials

Phase III trials may be viewed as extensions of Phase IIB trials. They are larger and the inclusion/exclusion criteria may be less restrictive than those of Phase IIB trials. For a drug to proceed to the Phase III portion of the development program, it must be deemed effective from the Phase IIB program. At this stage, effectiveness has been indicated, but not confirmed.

The primary objectives of the Phase III program are to confirm the effectiveness of the drug in a more heterogeneous population, and to collect more and longer term safety data. Information from Phase IIB provides pilot data for the purpose of sample size determination in Phase III.

For the purpose of obtaining more safety data under conditions which better approximate the anticipated clinical use of the drug, relatively large, uncontrolled, non-comparative trials may also be conducted in Phase III. Since if the drug is given approval to be marketed, it may be used in the elderly, in the renally impaired, etc., and since such patients are usually excluded from other trials, studies in special populations may also be conducted in Phase III.

2.2.5 Phase IV Trials

Phase IV trials are conducted after the FDA has approved the new drug. These trials are conducted for the purpose of gathering pharmacovigilance and post-marketing surveillance data–particularly adverse events in a population reflecting more general use of the drug as it is prescribed to patients by physicians.

2.3   The Clinical Development Plan

The clinical development plan for a new drug includes Phase I, Phase II, and Phase III trials. In viewing the types of trials within each phase of clinical development, it is obvious that the objectives of the trials describe characteristics of a drug which should be known before proceeding sequentially with subsequent clinical use. Further upon the successful completion of the trials through Phase III, sufficient information should exist for the drug to be approved to be marketed.

The drug sponsor may wish to include other trials in the clinical development plan particularly to provide a marketing "hook" for launch. Prior to finalizing the clinical development plan, the drug sponsor should formulate draft labeling. The draft labeling should accommodate what is required to be said and what is desired to be said about the compound in the package insert of the marketed product. The clinical development plan then serves as a blueprint for labeling.

Basically, the labeling should communicate characteristics of the drug and give instructions for its use. Usually, the objectives of the trials described in Phase I, Phase II, and Phase III, if met in carrying out the attendant investigations, provide sufficient information to communicate the characteristics of the drug. However, since the population studied pre-market approval is likely to be more homogeneous than the user population post-market approval, and since inferences are based upon group averages, there may be insufficient information from the usual Phase I, Phase II, and Phase III program as to optimal clinical use of the drug, particularly in individual patients.

Therefore, drug sponsors may consider implementing a "Phase III 1/2" program directed more toward clinical use than toward establishing efficacy as a characteristic of the drug – which in our mind is what the typical pivotal proof of efficacy trials in Phase III do. Such a targeted program may be unnecessary if more efficient and more optimal designs and methods, such as response surface methodology, and evolutionary operations procedures are incorporated into the clinical development program as early as Phase II. In addition, being proactive in developing an integrated data base consisting of all data collected on a compound, so that meta-analysis and other techniques may be used, should enable the drug sponsor to do a better job at labeling.

2.4   Biostatistical Aspects of a Protocol

A protocol has to be developed for each clinical trial. An important responsibility of the statistician or biostatistician assigned to the protocol is to provide its statistical content. This includes ensuring that the objectives are clear; recommending the most appropriate design (experimental design and determination of sample size) for the condition being studied; assessing the adequacy of endpoints to address study objectives; assigning participants to protocol interventions to minimize bias; and developing the statistical analysis section. In addition, it is imperative that the biostatistician provides a review of the protocol for completeness and consistency.

The next four subsections: Background or Rationale, Objective, Plan of Study, and Statistical Analysis Section provide an overview of their counterparts in a clinical trial protocol. Biostatistical input to these subsections is discussed.

2.4.1 Background or Rationale

Sufficient information should be given in this section to set the stage for the clinical trial for which the protocol is being developed. This requires integrating the results (with references) of previous studies that have bearing on the current protocol. The section should end with a paragraph explaining why the current protocol is needed or why it is being developed.

2.4.2 Objective

The objective or research question of the protocol should be defined so that it is unambiguous. For example, in an investigation about the antihypertensive efficacy of drug D in some defined population, the statement: *"The objective of this investigation is to assess the efficacy of drug D"* is ambiguous. It provides only general information as to the question ("Is D efficacious?"). The statement: *"The objective of this investigation is to assess whether drug D is superior to placebo P in the treatment of hypertensive patients with diastolic blood pressure (DBP) between 90 and 105 mmHg for six months"* is better, as the hypertensive population to be treated and what is meant by efficacious in a comparative sense are specified.

However, the data or endpoint(s) upon which antihypertensive efficacy will be based is (are) not specified. DBP is stated, but how will it be measured? – Using a sphygmomanometer or a digital monitor? Will DBP be measured in the sitting, standing or supine position? Further, what function of the DBP will be used? - The change from baseline to the end of the treatment period? Or whether the patient achieves a therapeutic goal of normotension (DBP $\leq$ 80 mmHg) by the end of the treatment period?

If there is more than one question or objective, one should identify which is primary versus which is secondary.

2.4.3   Plan of Study

The plan of study entails all that is to be done in order to enroll and treat patients, monitor the study, ensure patient safety, and collect valid data. The study population has to be specified. Design aspects of the study, including all procedures to be used in the diagnoses, treatment or management of patients must be delineated.

2.4.3.1   Study Population

Characteristics of the population of patients to be entered into the protocol must be specified. This is typically accomplished by specifying inclusion and exclusion criteria appropriate for the disease and drug under study. In specifying these criteria, one has to be cognizant that patients entered must have the disease under study, that the condition of the patient must not compromise patient safety by participating in the protocol, and that the patients entered should enable the efficacy of the drug under study to be determined (absence of masking or confounding factors).

The inclusion criteria specify the demography of the patient population, their disease characteristics, acceptable vital signs ranges, acceptable clinical laboratory tests ranges, etc. Exclusion criteria are generally the complement of the inclusion criteria, with delineation of a subset that specifically excludes patients from entry. For example, non-menopausal females who are pregnant or who do not agree to practice an acceptable form of birth control during the intervention period are excluded; as are patients who do not agree to abstain from using concomitant medications that may mask or interfere with the activity of the drug under study. Inclusion/exclusion criteria essentially define the population to be studied. Therefore, they provide general descriptors of the population to which inferences from analyses of the data collected pertain.

2.4.3.2   Study Design

The study design subsection should identify the type of study; the treatment or intervention groups and how patients who qualify for the protocol will be assigned to treatment groups; what measures will be taken to ensure the absence of bias; requirements relative to patients taking medications other than those constituting the assigned intervention; and all procedures that are required by the protocol in order to diagnose, treat, ensure patient safety, and collect data.

1. **Type of Study**. The type of study should be described. Is the study prospective? What type of control (placebo, positive, historical, etc.) will be used? Is it single or multi-center? Is the study parallel, crossover, stratified, or some other type?

2. **Treatment Group Specification and Assignment**. The treatment groups and the interventions (drug, dose, etc.) that patients in the groups

will receive should be specified. Then, how patients will be assigned to the treatment groups to remove assignment bias should be articulated. The gold standard is to randomly assign patients to the groups in balanced fashion. Minor departures from balance are acceptable and may be more ethical. For example, for a placebo control trial of a new drug, our preference is to recommend that twice as many patients be randomly assigned to the drug than to placebo. This reduces the number of patients assigned to placebo by 1/6 and ensures that twice as many patients are assigned to the drug group as to the placebo group. A 2-to-1 departure from balance has a relatively small impact on power.

3. **Packaging to Achieve Blinding**. Intervention group medications should be packaged so that neither the patient nor personnel (physician, research nurse or assistant) who will either treat, assign medication, draw blood, administer procedures, or collect data knows the identity of the interventions. This requires interaction between the protocol biostatistician (who will generate the randomization schedule) and the formulation or packaging chemists (who will package the medication). Both have to thoroughly know the protocol, particularly the drug, dose and frequency of dosing of intervention medications, when patients are at the clinic for medication dispensing, and how many days are between visits.

4. **Concomitant Medication**. The protocol should indicate whether any medications other than those comprising the treatment or intervention groups are permitted while the patient is participating in the protocol. Generally, any medication, prescription or over-the-counter (OTC), that would mask, cloud or otherwise interfere with the effect of the intervention medications should be excluded.

5. **Procedures**. All procedures required for enrolling, diagnosing, treating, or medically monitoring patients should be clearly identified and described. This applies to all phases: pre-treatment, during treatment, or post-treatment, of the protocol. Providing a study schema at the end of the protocol that identifies procedures to be administered by day of study is helpful.

   Observers (personnel who see patients that result in data collection and recording) should be specified. The assignment of observers to patients should be made to try to eliminate or minimize the introduction of observer variability into the trial. For example, in hypertension studies, different observers for different patients are permitted; but each patient should have the same observer throughout the trial.

   Procedures for recording the data to be collected in the trial should be specified. Whether data are to be recorded on paper data collection forms (DCFs) or electronically requires protocol sponsor personnel to interact with site personnel to ensure proper and valid recording of data.

2.4.3.3   Problem Management

In this subsection of the protocol, criteria for dealing with problems related to patient safety, or that may compromise study objectives if left unattended, should be specified. For example, clinically significant changes in clinical laboratory parameters; criteria for discontinuing study drug including severe adverse events; actions to be taken for protocol deviations or violations, including taking prohibited drugs, missed visits, dropouts, etc. should be specified. Contact information from the investigational sites to the protocol sponsor for problem management should be clearly delineated.

2.4.4   Statistical Analysis Section

There are many ways to organize the content of the statistical analysis section. One organization is to have six sections or paragraphs: Study Objectives as Statistical Hypotheses; Endpoints; Statistical Methods; Statistical Monitoring Procedures; Statistical Design Considerations; and Subset Analyses.

2.4.4.1   Study Objectives as Statistical Hypotheses

It is important to classify study objectives according to those that reflect primary efficacy, those that reflect secondary efficacy, those that reflect safety, and those that reflect other questions of interest (e.g., quality of life). Then the objectives within each classification should be translated into statistical questions.

If inferential decisions regarding the questions are to be made on the basis of hypothesis or significance testing, the questions should be translated into statistical hypotheses. It is desirable from a statistical viewpoint, for the alternative hypothesis (H_a) to embody the research question, both in substance and direction. For placebo controlled studies or for studies in which superior efficacy is the objective, this is routinely the case. For studies in which clinical equivalence (or non-inferiority) is the objective, the usual framing of the objective translates it as the null hypothesis (H_0). In this framework, failure to reject H_0 does not permit a conclusion of equivalence or non-inferiority. This will depend on a specification of how much the treatment regimens may truly differ in terms of therapeutic endpoints, yet still be considered clinically equivalent or non-inferior (refer to FDA draft guideline in March 2010 available from `http://www.fda.gov/downloads/Drugs/ GuidanceComplianceRegulatoryInformation/Guidances/UCM202140.pdf`), and the power of the test to detect such a difference.

Separate univariate, null and alternative hypotheses should be specified for each question. The reasons for separate specifications are primarily clarity and insight: clarity because the questions have been clearly elucidated and framed as statistical hypotheses. This sets the stage for appropriate statistical analyses when the data become available. When analyses directed toward the questions occur, it should be clear whether the statistical evidence is sufficient to answer them. Insight is gained from the univariate specifications, as to the significance level at which the tests should be performed. This is true even though the study objective may represent a composite hypothesis.

Secondary efficacy objectives should not invoke a penalty on the Type-I error associated with the primary efficacy objectives. It may be argued that each secondary objective can be addressed using a Type-I error of 5%, providing inference via significance testing is preferred. Ninety-five percent confidence intervals represent a more informative alternative. Since the use of confidence intervals implies interest in estimates of true treatment differences, rather than interest in being able to decide whether true treatment differences are some pre-specified values, confidence intervals are more consistent with a classification of secondary.

Safety objectives, unless they are the primary objectives, should not invoke a penalty on the Type-I error associated with the primary efficacy objectives. It is uncommon that a study conducted prior to market approval of a new drug would have safety objectives that are primary. This does not mean that safety is not important. The safety of a drug, in the individual patient, and in groups of patients, is of utmost importance.

2.4.4.2   Endpoints

Data collected in the protocol reflecting primary efficacy, secondary efficacy, safety or other objectives should be identified. Then endpoints to be statistically analyzed to address protocol objectives should be defined. An endpoint may be the actual data collected or a function of the data collected. Endpoints are the analysis units on each individual patient that will be statistically analyzed to address study objectives. In an antihypertensive study, actual data reflecting potential efficacy are supine diastolic blood pressure measurements. Whereas it is informative to describe these data at baseline and at follow-up visits during the treatment period, inferential statistical analyses are usually based upon the endpoint: change from baseline in supine diastolic blood pressure. The reason for this is that change from baseline within each treatment group is an indicator of the extent to which the drug received in each group is effective.

Another endpoint of clinical interest is whether a patient experienced a clinically significant reduction in supine diastolic blood pressure from baseline to the end of the treatment period. Clinically significant is usually defined as a decrease from baseline of at least 10 mmHg or becoming normotensive (DBP $\leq$ 80 mgHg). This definition of an endpoint essentially dichotomizes DBP at the end of treatment.

2.4.4.3   Statistical Methods

Statistical methods that will be used to analyze the data collected and the endpoints should be described. The methods chosen should be appropriate for the type of data or endpoint; e.g., parametric procedures such as analysis of variance techniques for continuous endpoints, and nonparametric procedures such as categorical data methods for discrete endpoints. Analysis methods should also be appropriate for the study design. For example, if the design has blocking factors, then statistical procedures should account for these factors. It is prudent to indicate that the methods stipulated will be used to analyze study data and endpoints, subject to actual data verification that any assumptions underlying the methods reasonably hold. Otherwise alternative methods will be considered.

The use of significance tests may be restricted to the primary efficacy questions. Otherwise, confidence intervals should be used. The method for constructing confidence intervals, particularly how the variance estimate will be determined, should be indicated.

Unless there are specific safety questions as part of the study objectives, for which sample sizes with reasonable power to address them have been determined, it may be sufficient to use descriptive procedures for summarizing safety data. Many statisticians routinely provide p-values for treatment group comparisons in the analysis of safety data. There are many opportunities for false positive (from the multiplicity of testing) and false negative (from being underpowered) conclusions in doing this. Small p-values may be helpful in identifying events of possible clinical importance, which require clinical review along with the proper statistical context.

The last portion of the statistical methods subsection should identify methods to be used to address generalizability of results across design blocking factors or across demographic or prognostic subgroups. Methods for generalizability include descriptive presentations of treatment effects across blocks or subgroups, a graphical presentation of confidence intervals on treatment differences across blocks or subgroups, and analysis of variance models that include terms for interaction between treatment and blocks or subgroups.

2.4.4.4   Statistical Monitoring Procedures

Most clinical trials of new drugs are designed to provide answers to questions of efficacy; this is particularly true for Phase III trials, as they are typically the pivotal proof of efficacy trials. Therefore, monitoring for efficacy while the study is in progress, particularly in an unplanned, ad hoc manner, will almost always be seen to compromise the integrity of such trials. If it is anticipated that the efficacy data will be summarized or statistically analyzed prior to study termination, for whatever reason, it is wise to include an appropriate plan for doing this in the protocol. The plan should address Type-I error penalty considerations, what steps will be taken to minimize bias, and permit early termination.

The early termination procedure of O'Brien and Fleming (1979) is usually reasonable. It allows periodic interim analyses of the data while the study is in progress, while preserving most of nominal Type-I error for the final analysis upon scheduled study completion - providing there was insufficient evidence to terminate the study after an interim analysis. Other procedures such as Pocock's (Pocock (1977)), or Lan and DeMets (Lan and DeMets (1983)) may also be used, as well as publications by numerous authors. The paper (PMA (1993)) by the PMA Working Group addressing the topic of interim analyses provides a good summary of the concerns about, and procedures for, interim analyses. The sample sizes for early termination, group sequential procedures, such as O'Brien and Fleming's, are determined as per fixed sample size procedures, and then this sample size is spread across sequential groups. Safety data, particularly serious adverse events should be monitored for all trials as the data accumulate. A comprehensive discussion can be found in Herson (2009), Piantadosi (2005) and Proschan et al. (2006). The group sequential procedures referenced above may be used for these purposes. However, unless the trial has been designed to provide statistical evidence regarding some safety objective, it is unclear that a pre-specified overall Type-I error rate should be preserved as discussed in Peace (1987). The idea is to be alerted as early as possible about any events that may reflect possible safety concerns so that appropriate intervention may be taken. Often, the repeated confidence interval method of Jennison and Turnbull is helpful (Jennison and Turnbull (1984)).

The subsection on statistical monitoring procedures should begin with a paragraph that specifies what data and endpoints will be sequentially monitored (analyzed); when such monitoring will occur (calendar time or cumulative number of patients at each planned analysis); how the data will be quality assured; and specification of procedures to be followed to minimize bias or otherwise jeopardizing the integrity of the study.

2.4.5 Statistical Design Considerations

The statistical, experimental design for the study should be described. Is the experimental design parallel using a completely randomized design (CRD)? Or is the design parallel using a completely randomized block design (CRBD)? Or is the design a two-sequence, two-period, two-treatment crossover design (2 by 2 by 2)? Or is a balanced incomplete block design (BIBD) used? What are the stratification variables, if any? What type of control (placebo, positive, historical, etc.) will be used? Is it single or multicenter? The type of experimental design used in the trial impacts the type of statistical methods that will be used to analyze data collected.

Once the design is known, the number of clinical trial participants necessary to provide valid inferences to protocol objectives may be determined. This requires one to know what the objectives are in terms of statistical questions; i.e., what is the δ in each separate alternative hypothesis? Specifying δ requires collaboration between the biostatistician and the clinician.

The specification of δ is the responsibility of the clinician or medical director, and requires careful thinking and exploration by both the biostatistician and the medical expert. A δ too large may lead to failure to answer the question due to too small a sample. A δ too small would increase costs of conducting the investigation and may not be accepted as clinically meaningful.

Once δ is specified, the magnitude of the Type-I error α, and the statistical power $1 - \beta$ or degree of certainty required to detect δ must be specified. Then an estimate of variability σ^2 of the data or endpoint reflecting the question is needed. When the biostatistician has the inputs: δ, α, $1 - \beta$, and an estimate of σ^2, the sample size may be computed using well-known sample size formulae, sample size computational software programs, or using simulation techniques.

2.4.6   Subset Analyses

The last subsection of the statistical or data analysis section should identify what subsets or subpopulations among trial participants will be investigated or subjected to statistical analyses. Both the Gender Rule and the Demographic Rule US FDA Regulatory Guidelines identify subpopulations indexed by age, gender and race or ethnicity. But other subpopulations may be of interest; e.g., levels of disease severity. In addition, methods to be used for investigating subsets or performing analyses of subsets should be specified. How one views the objective of subset investigation will dictate the type of analyses (Peace (1995)).

If the objective is to provide valid inferences of treatment effects within subpopulations, then one could stratify the protocol by subpopulation and design the trial to have sufficient power and numbers of participants to assess the effectiveness of treatment in each subpopulation. This would seldom be required if ever. Few if any drug sponsors could afford to conduct such clinical trials. Alternatively, step down procedures may be helpful in providing valid inferences with subpopulations. The article by Alosh and Huque (2009) provides an alternative method.

What is of interest is to assess whether the treatment effects in the total population are generalizable across subpopulations. This can be assessed by introducing subpopulation and treatment-by-subpopulation as fixed effects into the analysis model and noting the size of the p-value for the interaction term. Large p-values are consistent with an interpretation of treatment effects being generalizable across subpopulations, whereas small p-values provide evidence that treatment effects differ across some subpopulations. Since clinical trials are not usually designed to have large power to detect significant interactions, many biostatisticians use a p-value of less than or equal to 0.10 to quantify small. Some suggest that the protocol should be stratified by subpopulation to ensure balance across treatment groups in terms of subpopulations.

In addition to interaction tests to address generalizability of treatment effects across subpopulations, descriptive tables of treatment effects and graphical presentations of confidence intervals on treatment effects by subpopulation are helpful. In such graphical presentations, the centers of the confidence intervals representing random variation about a horizontal line are indicative of generalizability of treatment effects. Lack of generalizability requires the biostatistician to identify what subpopulations are discrepant, and then through collaboration with the clinician and/or monitoring or investigational site, assess whether there are explanations for the discrepancies.

After the statistical analysis section has been finalized and the protocol approved, the project biostatistician should develop the statistical analysis plan (SAP). The SAP should follow the data analysis section but would contain greater specificity. The SAP serves as a blue print for biostatistical analyses of the data and endpoints. It should be developed so that if the project biostatistician has to be replaced, the new biostatistician would not require much time to become fully engaged with analyses. An example of a statistical analysis plan for a protocol is presented in Chapter 7 of Peace and Chen (2010).

2.5 Concluding Remarks

Quality clinical research must be well planned, closely and carefully monitored, utilize procedures that ensure quality collection and management of data, use appropriate statistical analysis procedures, and properly interpret the results so that inferences are valid and without bias. The first step in this process is to develop a quality protocol for every clinical trial.

Chapter 3

Treatment Comparisons in Clinical Trials

Although clinical trials are conducted with multiple treatment groups, questions of interest are often expressed as pairwise comparisons among the groups. For example, a clinical trial of two dose (D_1 and D_2) groups and placebo (P) may have as its objective the effectiveness of each dose, and whether the doses differ in their effectiveness. That objective may be formulated in terms of the three pairwise comparisons: $D_1 - P$, $D_2 - P$, and $D_2 - D_1$. Other contrasts among the groups may be of interest; e.g., the average of the doses versus placebo. Of course if a trial consists of only two treatment groups, the objective would be formulated as a single comparison of the two groups.

In this chapter, we present statistical methods for comparing treatment groups in clinical trials using the R and SAS systems. Specifically, we present two datasets from clinical trials in Section 3.1 with the first dataset for continuous outcome and the second for categorical outcome. In Section 3.2, we introduce the associated statistical models for these types of data which include the t-test, the one-way and two-way analysis of variances (ANOVA) for univariate outcome (i.e., change from baseline to the last post-baseline measurement) as well as multivariate analysis of variance (MANOVA) for the multiple changes from baseline to the four post-baseline measurements to incorporate the correlations among these four multiple outcomes. We conclude this chapter with discussion in Section 3.3.

3.1 Data from Clinical Trials

3.1.1 Diastolic Blood Pressure

The first dataset appears in Table 3.1. This dataset is typical of diastolic blood pressure data measured in small clinical trials in hypertension from the mid-to-late 1960s and for approximately a decade thereafter. During this time, hypertension was more severe, the number of effective treatments was relatively small, and the definition (DBP > 95 mmHg) of essential hypertension was not as stringent as it is now (DBP > 80 mmHg) - as seen in the

1967 report from the Veterans Administration Cooperative Study Group on Antihypertensive Agents (VA Study Group (1967)).

TABLE 3.1: Diastolic Blood Pressure Trial Data

Subject	TRT	DBP1	DBP2	DBP3	DBP4	DBP5	Age	Sex
1	A	114	115	113	109	105	43	F
2	A	116	113	112	103	101	51	M
3	A	119	115	113	104	98	48	F
4	A	115	113	112	109	101	42	F
5	A	116	112	107	104	105	49	M
6	A	117	112	113	104	102	47	M
7	A	118	111	100	109	99	50	F
8	A	120	115	113	102	102	61	M
9	A	114	112	113	109	103	43	M
10	A	115	113	108	106	97	51	M
11	A	117	112	110	109	101	47	F
12	A	116	115	113	109	102	45	M
13	A	119	117	110	106	104	54	F
14	A	118	115	113	102	99	52	M
15	A	115	112	108	105	102	42	M
16	A	114	111	111	107	100	44	F
17	A	117	114	110	108	102	48	M
18	A	120	115	113	107	103	63	F
19	A	114	113	109	104	100	41	M
20	A	117	115	113	109	101	51	M
21	B	114	115	113	111	113	39	M
22	B	116	114	114	109	110	40	F
23	B	114	115	113	111	109	39	F
24	B	114	115	113	114	115	38	M
25	B	116	113	113	109	109	39	F
26	B	114	115	114	111	110	41	M
27	B	119	118	118	117	115	56	F
28	B	118	117	117	116	112	56	M
29	B	114	113	113	109	108	38	M
30	B	120	115	113	113	113	57	M
31	B	117	115	113	114	115	47	F
32	B	118	114	112	109	110	48	M
33	B	121	119	117	114	115	61	F
34	B	116	115	116	114	111	49	M
35	B	118	118	113	113	112	52	M
36	B	119	115	115	114	111	55	F
37	B	116	114	113	109	109	45	F
38	B	116	115	114	114	112	42	M
39	B	117	115	113	114	115	49	F
40	B	118	114	114	114	115	50	F

In Table 3.1, diastolic blood pressure (DBP) was measured (mmHg) in the supine position at baseline (i.e., "DBP1") before randomization and monthly thereafter up to 4 months as indicated by "DBP2", "DBP3", "DBP4" and "DBP5". Patients' age and sex were recorded at baseline and represent potential covariates. The primary objective in this chapter in the analysis of this dataset is to test whether treatment A (new drug) may be effective in lowering DBP as compared to B (placebo) and to describe changes in DBP across the times at which it was measured. Additional analysis may be found in Chapter 6.

3.1.2 Clinical Trial on Duodenal Ulcer Healing

Duodenal ulcers occur in the duodenum–the upper portion of the small intestine as it leaves the stomach. A duodenal ulcer is characterized by the presence of a well-demarcated break (ulcer crater) in the mucosa that may extend into the muscularis propria. Cimetidine was the first H2-Receptor Antagonist to receive regulatory approval (in the late 1970s) for the treatment of duodenal ulcers. The first Cimetidine regimen approved for the treatment of duodenal ulcers in the United Kingdom was 1000 mg per day, given as 200 mg at breakfast, lunch and dinner, and 400 mg at bed time, for up to 4 weeks. The first regimen approved in the United States for this indication was 1200 mg per day, given as 300 mg q.i.d. for up to 4 weeks.

In the mid 1980s, based upon acid suppression data from gastric acid antisecretory studies at various doses and frequencies of dosing, there was reason to believe that a single nighttime (h.s.) dose of 800 mg of Cimetidine (C) for up to 4 weeks would be the clinically optimal way to treat patients with duodenal ulcers. A large dose comparison clinical trial was undertaken to confirm the effectiveness of 800 C mg h.s. in the treatment of duodenal ulcers for up to four weeks. The trial was multi-center, stratified by smoking status, randomized, double-blind and placebo controlled. After endoscopic confirmation of a duodenal ulcer at baseline, patients were randomized to the four double-blinded treatment groups:

1. **0 mg C Group**: Four 400-mg Placebo tablets

2. **400 mg C Group**: One Cimetidine 400-mg tablet + three 400-mg Placebo tablets

3. **800 mg C Group**: Two Cimetidine 400-mg tablets + two 400-mg Placebo tablets

4. **1600 mg C Group**: Four Cimetidine 400-mg tablets.

Details of this clinical trial may be found in Peace and Chen (2010). In summary at the end of clinical trial, 168, 182, 165 and 188 patients were efficacy evaluatable, in the 0 mg C Group (Placebo), 400 mg C, 800 mg C and 1600 mg C groups, respectively. The cumulative duodenal ulcer healing rates were: 17%, 16%, 15% and 21% at week 1; 30%, 40%, 42% and 48% at week 2; and 41%, 62%, 73% and 77% at week 4; for the Placebo, 400 mg C, 800 mg C and 1600 mg C groups, respectively. At week 4: 800 mg C was effective (p-value $< 10^{-8}$) as compared to Placebo; 800 mg C was superior to 400 mg C (p-value < 0.05); and 1600 mg C provided no clinically significant greater benefit than did 800 mg C (p-value $= 0.41$ with 95% CI) (-0.14, 0.05). Therefore, the study demonstrated that 800 mg C was clinically optimal. In this chapter, the final data were re-created in Table 3.2 to illustrate the application of treatment comparisons for categorical data using the R system.

TABLE 3.2: Duodenal Ulcer Trial Data

	Placebo	400 mg C	800 mg C	1600 mg C
Total	168	182	165	188
Week 1 (n_1)	29	29	25	39
Week 2 (n_2)	50	73	69	90
Week 4 (n_4)	69	113	120	145
Week 1 (p_1)	17%	16%	15%	21%
Week 2 (p_2)	30%	40%	42%	48%
Week 4 (p_4)	41%	62%	73%	77%

3.2 Statistical Models for Treatment Comparisons

3.2.1 Models for Continuous Endpoints

We begin with comparison of two treatments based on the well-known t-test and then extend the concepts to multiple treatment comparisons for the analysis of variance approach.

3.2.1.1 Student's t-Tests

The Student t-test is used to compare two treatment group means assuming that the clinical trial endpoints are continuous and follow a normal distribution. To reflect this situation, a clinical trial of two treatment groups is conducted with the numbers of patients entered in the two groups denoted as n_1 and n_2. At the end of trial we observe clinical endpoints x_{1i} and x_{2i} on patients from each treatment group, where $i = 1, \cdots, n_i$. We test the null hypothesis that the means of the two treatment groups are the same:

$$H_0 : \mu_1 = \mu_2 \tag{3.1}$$

and the alternative could be two-sided as $H_a : \mu_1 \neq \mu_2$ or one-sided as $H_a : \mu_1 > ($ or $<)\mu_2$ depending on the trial objective.

The test statistic is constructed as:

$$t = \frac{\bar{y}_1 - \bar{y}_2}{s\sqrt{1/n_1 + 1/n_2}}, \tag{3.2}$$

where $\bar{y}_i = \frac{\sum_{j=1}^{n_i} y_{ij}}{n_i}$ are the ith treatment group means of the observed data, and s is the pooled standard error calculated as:

$$s = \sqrt{\frac{(n_1 - 1)s_1^2 + (n_2 - 1)s_2^2}{n_1 + n_2 - 2}},$$

where s_1 and s_2 are the sample standard deviations of the two treatment groups. It is noted that the t-statistic in Equation (3.2) is essentially the standardized difference of the two treatment group means.

Under the null hypothesis, this t-statistic has a Student's t-distribution with $n_1 + n_2 - 2$ degrees of freedom. The null hypothesis is not rejected if $|t| < t_{\alpha/2, n_1 + n_2 - 2}$ with $100(1 - \alpha)\%$ confidence coefficient (for a two-sided test).

Alternatively, a $100(1 - \alpha)\%$ confidence interval (CI) may be constructed on the true difference in treatment group means and used as the basis of statistical inference. The CI is constructed as:

$$\bar{y}_1 - \bar{y}_2 \pm t_{\alpha/2, n_1 + n_2 - 2} s \sqrt{n_1^{-1} + n_2^{-1}}$$

where $t_{\alpha/2, n_1 + n_2 - 2}$ is the $\alpha/2$-percentile.

The CI including zero is consistent with insufficient evidence to contradict or reject the null hypothesis.

The underlying assumptions for a valid t-test are that the observed clinical endpoints of x_1 and x_2 are independent and normally distributed with common variance σ^2. If any of these assumptions is violated, there are remedies:

1. *Unequal variances:* If the two treatment groups have different variances, the t-statistic in Equation (3.2) may be modified as:

$$t = \frac{\bar{y}_1 - \bar{y}_2}{\sqrt{s_1^2/n_1 + s_2^2/n_2}} \tag{3.3}$$

with ν degrees of freedom calculated as

$$\nu = \left[\frac{c^2}{n_1 - 1} + \frac{(1 - c)^2}{n_2 - 1} \right]^{-1}$$

with

$$c = \frac{s_1^2/n_1}{s_1^2/n_1 + s_2^2/n_2}$$

This test statistic t has a Student's t-distribution, is known as the Welch test as in Welch (1947), and is implemented in R as t.test.

2. *Non-normal data:* The t-test is usually quite robust against departures from normality. However, when the departure is extreme, the recommended remedy is to use the Mann-Whitney-Wilcoxon (MWW) U-test (also called Wilcoxon rank-sum test, or Wilcoxon-Mann-Whitney test). This is a non-parametric test for assessing whether two independent samples of observations come from the same distribution. It is one of the most widely used non-parametric significance tests. It was proposed initially by Wilcoxon (1945), for equal sample sizes, and extended to arbitrary sample sizes and in other ways by Mann and Whitney (1947). MWW is virtually identical to performing an ordinary parametric two-sample t-test on the ranks of the data after ranking over the combined samples. This U-test is implemented in R system as `wilcox.test`.

3. *Bootstrap resampling:* When any of the assumptions underlying the validity of the t-test do not hold for the data being analyzed, bootstrapping provides a viable alternative. The bootstrap method involves iteratively resampling the data with replacement, calculating the value of the statistic for each sample obtained, and generating the resampling distribution. Percentile points corresponding to the Type-I error level and the sidedness of the alternative hypothesis of the resampling distribution are then used in the assessment of statistical significance. We illustrate the bootstrapping approach using the R function `bootstrap`.

3.2.1.2   One-Way Analysis of Variance (ANOVA)

For comparisons involving more than two treatment groups, F-tests deriving from a one-way analysis of variance (ANOVA) model are used. The fundamental idea for ANOVA is to partition the overall variance in clinical response into a component reflecting variation among treatment groups (factor levels) and variation due to measurement error (residual or variation within treatment groups). For a factor α occurring at $i = 1, \cdots, I$ levels, with $j = 1, \cdots, n_i$ observations per level, the typical one-way ANOVA model may be expressed as:

$$y_{ij} = \mu + \alpha_i + \epsilon_{ij} \qquad (3.4)$$

The above model is over-parameterized and not all the parameters are identifiable. The common constraints are:

1. Set $\mu = 0$ and use I different dummy variables to estimate α_i for $i = 1, \cdots, I$.

2. Set $\alpha_1 = 0$, μ represents the expected mean response for level one and α_i for $i \neq 1$ represents the difference between level i and level one. Level one is then called "the reference level" or "baseline level". This corresponds to "treatment contrasts" as commonly outputted in R output.

Treatment effects (differences among specified treatments) are commonly estimated using least squares. Inference on the statistical significance of a treatment difference may be constructed as:

$$H_0 : \alpha_i = 0, i = 1, \cdots, I$$
$$H_1 : \text{at least one of the } \alpha_i \text{ is not zero}$$

If the null hypothesis fails to be rejected, the analysis ends and it is concluded that there is insufficient evidence to conclude that the treatment group means differ. However, if the null hypothesis is rejected, the next logical step is to investigate which levels differ by using the so-called `multiple comparisons`.

We warn readers that the t-test from the above section applied individually to all pairwise comparisons is not the solution since it will inflate the type-I error rate. Therefore, procedures that adjust for multiple comparisons are used. Tukey's honest significant difference (HSD) procedure is commonly used for adjustment in the literature and it is easy to understand. Tukey's HSD procedure is based on the distribution of the studentized range with quantile of q_{α, df_1, df_2} where $df_1 = I$ and $df_2 = \sum_{i=1}^{I} n_i - I$ as:

$$\hat{\alpha}_i - \hat{\alpha}_j \pm \frac{q_{\alpha, df_1, df_2}}{\sqrt{2}} se(\hat{\alpha}_i - \hat{\alpha}_j) \tag{3.5}$$

The ANOVA procedure is implemented in the R system as `aov` and Tukey's HSD procedure as `TukeyHSD`.

3.2.1.3   Multi-Way ANOVA: Factorial Design

The R system permits extending the one-way ANOVA in Section 3.2.1.2 to ANOVA accounting for several factors (multi-way ANOVA). We describe the two-way ANOVA corresponding to a two-factor design and illustrate this procedure in analyzing the DBP data in Section 3.1.

Suppose we have two factors, α (e.g., treatment groups) at I levels and β (e.g., time at which DBP is measured; time $= 1,..., 5$) at J levels. Let n_{ij} be the number of observations at level i of α and level j of β, and denote those observations by $y_{ijk}, k = 1, \cdots, n_{ij}$. The full ANOVA model with fixed effects is:

$$y_{ijk} = \mu + \alpha_i + \beta_j + (\alpha\beta)_{ij} + \epsilon_{ijk} \tag{3.6}$$

where α_i and β_j are the main effects. The term $(\alpha\beta)_{ij}$ is the interaction effect between the two factors α and β, which may be interpreted as that part of the main effects not explained by the additive effects of α and β.

A significant interaction means the main effect of α cannot be assessed independent of β. A comparison of the levels of α is dependent on the level of β.

The interaction effect may be tested using the F-test from the ANOVA, which is implemented in R system with the `aov`. If the interaction is found to be significant, further investigation is needed for inference about main effects of interest.

If the interaction is found to be insignificant, then main effects may be tested from the ANOVA table corresponding to the reduced model without interaction:

$$y_{ijk} = \mu + \alpha_i + \beta_j + \epsilon_{ijk} \tag{3.7}$$

3.2.1.4   Multivariate Analysis of Variance (MANOVA)

Multivariate analysis of variance (MANOVA) is simply an ANOVA described in Section 3.2.1.2 with multiple dependent variables such as in the Table 3.1 for diastolic blood pressure (DBP) measures of "DBP1", "DBP2", "DBP3", "DBP4" and "DBP5". As seen in Section 3.2.1.2, ANOVA tests for the difference in means between two or more groups. Therefore, MANOVA extends the ANOVA for univariate to test the difference in two or more vectors of means from these multivariate dependent variables with special consideration of the dependence where a "covariance" structure is included in the MANOVA. MANOVA can then take these correlations into account when performing the significance test. Testing the multiple dependent variables is accomplished by creating new dependent variables that maximize group differences. These artificial dependent variables are linear combinations of the measured dependent variables. For more complete description of MANOVA, readers can refer to Hand and Taylor (1987), Krzanowski (1998) and Anderson (1994).

Similar to the univariate F-test used in ANOVA, a multivariate F-value can be formulated based on a comparison of the error variance/covariance matrix and the effect variance/covariance matrix, such as Wilks'-λ, Hotelling-Lawley's trace, Pillai-Bartlett's criterion and Roy's greatest root. The Wilks'-statistic is most popular in the literature, but the default Pillai-Bartlett statistic is recommended by Hand and Taylor (1987).

3.2.2   Models for Categorical Endpoints: Pearson's χ^2-test

There are many methods for categorical data analyses. Readers are referred to Agresti (2002) for a comprehensive treatise. We introduce Pearson's chi-square test in this chapter to draw comparisons with other methods of analyses of the clinical trial on duodenal ulcer healing. In addition, Pearson's χ^2 test is probably the most commonly used statistical method for analyses of categorical or contingency table data.

The first step in the chi-square test is to calculate the value of the chi-square statistic. It is obtained by (1) forming the difference between the observed number of frequencies and the expected (under the null hypothesis of no difference among the groups being compared) number of frequencies in each cell of the contingency table, (2) squaring each difference, (3) dividing each squared difference by the expected number of frequencies, and (4) summing the results. The second step is to determine the degrees of freedom of the test, which is essentially the total number of observed frequencies adjusted for the impact of using some of the observations to compute the "expected frequencies".

The value of the test-statistic is:

$$\chi^2 = \sum_i \frac{(O_i - E_i)^2}{E_i} \tag{3.8}$$

where O_i is the observed frequency, and E_i is the expected (theoretical) frequency under the null hypothesis.

Asymptotically, the distribution of the test statistic χ^2 is a chi-square distribution. The "asymptotical" approximation to the chi-square distribution breaks down if expected frequencies are too low. In this case, a better approximation is obtained by using Yates' correction for lack of continuity. This is accomplished by reducing the absolute value of each difference between observed and expected frequencies by 0.5 before squaring. This Pearson χ^2-test is implemented in R as `prop.test`.

3.3 Data Analysis in R

3.3.1 Analysis of the DBP Trial

3.3.1.1 Preliminary Data analysis

We first read the data into R using function `read.csv` and create a new variable "diff", which represents changes in DBP from baseline to the last post-baseline time (visit):

```
> # read the data into R
> dat  = read.csv("DBP.csv",header=T)
> # create the difference
> dat$diff = dat$DBP5-dat$DBP1
> # print the first a few observation
> head(dat)
```

	Subject	TRT	DBP1	DBP2	DBP3	DBP4	DBP5	Age	Sex	diff
1	1	A	114	115	113	109	105	43	F	-9
2	2	A	116	113	112	103	101	51	M	-15
3	3	A	119	115	113	104	98	48	F	-21
4	4	A	115	113	112	109	101	42	F	-14
5	5	A	116	112	107	104	105	49	M	-11
6	6	A	117	112	113	104	102	47	M	-15

As the first step in the data analysis, we gain a better understanding of the data by displaying treatment group differences in a boxplot as seen in Figure

3.1. From this boxplot, we make some preliminary observations. Firstly, the data appear symmetric from both boxes implying that there are no obvious outliers. Secondly, the new drug treatment "A" seems to be more effective than the "Placebo" treatment "B", since on average, the DBP decrease for drug A is about 15 mmHg as compared to a decrease of 5 mmHg for the "Placebo" treatment "B". This difference needs to be formally tested to assess whether it is statistically significant.

```
> # call R function "boxplot" for distribution plot
> boxplot(diff~TRT, dat, xlab="Treatment",
        ylab="DBP Changes", las=1)
```

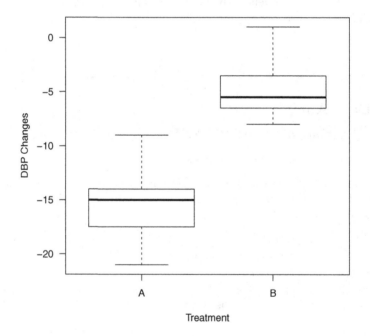

FIGURE 3.1: Boxplot for Two Treatments

3.3.1.2   *t*-test

For statistical significance, we use the *t*-test in Section 3.2.1.1. First, we assume *equal variances* as follows:

```
> # call t-test with equal variance
> t.test(diff~TRT, dat, var.equal=T)
```

Two Sample t-test

```
data:  diff by TRT
t = -10, df = 40, p-value = 1e-14
alternative hypothesis: true difference in means is not equal to 0
95 percent confidence interval:
 -12.13  -8.67
sample estimates:
mean in group A mean in group B
          -15.2            -4.8
```

From the output, we note that the t-statistic = -12.15 with 38 degrees of freedom, which gives a p-value of 1.169e-14, indicating that the difference (10.4 = -4.8-(-15.2)) between the new treatment "A" and the placebo "B" in terms of decreases in DBP is strongly statistically significant.

We may question the assumption of equal variances in the above test. If this is not the case, we can use the Welch t-test as:

```
> t.test(diff~TRT, dat, var.equal=F)
```

Welch Two Sample t-test

```
data:  diff by TRT
t = -10, df = 40, p-value = 2e-14
alternative hypothesis: true difference in means is not equal to 0
95 percent confidence interval:
 -12.14  -8.66
sample estimates:
mean in group A mean in group B
          -15.2            -4.8
```

We note that the t-statistic is -12.15, with 36.522 degrees of freedom, which gives a p-value = 2.149e-14. Note that the degree of freedom is no longer an integer based on the calculation in Equation (3.3). However, it is close to the degrees of freedom (38) in the previous test. This suggests that the assumption of equal variances is not really violated for this dataset. We may statistically test the null hypothesis of equal variances using the so-called F-test for variances as:

```
> var.test(diff~TRT, dat)
```

F test to compare two variances

```
data:  diff by TRT
F = 2, num df = 20, denom df = 20, p-value =
0.4
alternative hypothesis: true ratio of variances is not equal to 1
```

```
95 percent confidence interval:
 0.595 3.799
sample estimates:
ratio of variances
              1.5
```

The value of the statistic F is 1.5036 with degrees of freedom of 19 and 19, which gives p-value $= 0.3819$. This means that there is insufficient evidence to reject the null hypothesis of equal variances even though the observed variance ratio $= 1.504$. We caution readers to always test the assumption of equality of variances before performing the standard t-test.

If the assumptions of normality and equal variances are violated, we may use the nonparametric version of the t-test (Wilcoxon rank-sum test) as follows:

```
> wilcox.test(diff~TRT, dat)

        Wilcoxon rank sum test with continuity
        correction

data:   diff by TRT
W = 0, p-value = 6e-08
alternative hypothesis: true location shift is not equal to 0
```

Again the Wilcoxon rank-sum test gives the same conclusion. Since "B" is a Placebo, the one-sided t-test may be more appropriate to test the treatment effect, which can be done in R as:

```
> # data from treatment A
> diff.A = dat[dat$TRT=="A",]$diff
> # data from treatment B
> diff.B = dat[dat$TRT=="B",]$diff
> # call t.test for one-sided test
> t.test(diff.A, diff.B,alternative="less")

        Welch Two Sample t-test

data:   diff.A and diff.B
t = -10, df = 40, p-value = 1e-14
alternative hypothesis: true difference in means is less than 0
95 percent confidence interval:
  -Inf -8.96
sample estimates:
mean of x mean of y
    -15.2      -4.8
```

This shows that t-statistic $= -12.15$ with $df = 36.522$ which gives p-value $= 1.074e\text{-}14$ indicating again the greater reduction in DBP of treatment "A" as compared to the placebo control "B" is highly statistically significant. The 95% one-sided CI (-∞, -8.955) which again leads to the conclusion that "B" and "A" are statistically significantly different; i.e., there is evidence that "A" is more effective.

3.3.1.3 Bootstrapping Method

Bootstrapping is a resampling procedure extensively used in statistics. In this situation, we repeatedly draw samples with replacement from the data, compute the statistic of interest and generate the sampling distribution of the statistic. Bootstrapping is easily programmed in R, but in this section, we illustrate the procedure using the built-in function `bootstrap` to test the significance of the difference in DBP treatment means.

To use `bootstrap`, first load the library and define a function to calculate the difference in treatment group means as follows:

```
> # load the library "bootstrap"
> library(bootstrap)
> # define a function to calculate the mean difference
> #         between treatment groups A to B:
> mean.diff = function(bn,dat)
   diff(tapply(dat[bn,]$diff, dat[bn,]$TRT,mean))
```

Now generate `nboot`=1,000 bootstrap samples using the `bootstrap` function as follows:

```
> # number of bootstrap
> nboot     = 1000
> # call "bootstrap" function
> boot.mean = bootstrap(1:dim(dat)[1], nboot, mean.diff,dat)
```

The "boot.mean" will have 1000 values representing the DBP mean difference between treatment groups A and B. The bootstrap sampling distribution may be displayed as in Figure 3.2 using following R code chunk:

```
> # extract the mean differences
> x = boot.mean$thetastar
> # calculate the bootstrap quantiles
> x.quantile = quantile(x, c(0.025,0.5, 0.975))
> # show the quantiles
> print(x.quantile)

 2.5%   50% 97.5%
 8.8  10.4  12.1

> # make a histogram
> hist(boot.mean$thetastar, xlab="Mean Differences", main="")
> # add the vertical lines for the quantiles
> abline(v=x.quantile,lwd=2, lty=c(4,1,4))
```

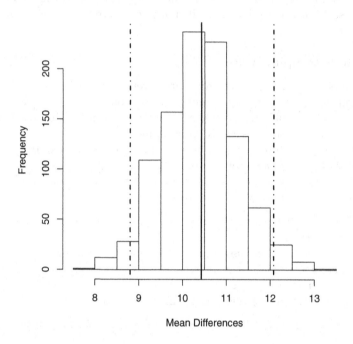

FIGURE 3.2: Bootstrap Distribution of Mean Differences

In Figure 3.2, the solid vertical line in the middle is the 50% quantile, which equals -10.4 mmHg corresponding to the mean difference between treatment group "A" and "B". The two dashed vertical lines on both sides are the 95% confidence limits which are -12.09 and -8.69 mmHg. Since this 95% bootstrap CI does not cover zero, we conclude that the mean difference between treatment groups "A" and "B" is statistically significant (at the two-sided Type-I error level of 5%).

3.3.1.4   One-Way ANOVA for Time Changes

The treatment period in DBP trial was four months with DBP measured at months 1, 2, 3, and 4 post-baseline. To see the mean changes the months following baseline, we extract the means by treatment group using the R function **aggregate** as follows:

```
> aggregate(dat[,3:7], list(TRT=dat$TRT), mean)

  TRT DBP1 DBP2 DBP3 DBP4 DBP5
1   A  117  114  111  106  101
2   B  117  115  114  112  112
```

We note that mean DBP at baseline and at each month of followup are 116.55, 113.5, 110.70, 106.25 and 101.35 mmHg, for the new drug treatment "A", and are 116.75, 115.2, 114.05, 112.45 and 111.95 mmHg, for the Placebo "B". The corresponding mean changes from baseline at each month of followup are -3.05, -5.85, -10.30, -15.20 mmHg, for treatment "A", and -1.55, -2.70, -4.30, -4.80 mmHg, for treatment "B", which illustrates that mean DBP changes from baseline for the new drug "A" are greater than those for the Placebo "B". We may employ the one-way ANOVA to test the change over time.

We first re-arrange the dataframe `dat` into a "long" format using `reshape` to re-shape the data as:

```
> # call reshape
> Dat = reshape(dat, direction="long",
  varying=c("DBP1","DBP2","DBP3","DBP4","DBP5"),
   idvar = c("Subject","TRT","Age","Sex","diff"),sep="")
> colnames(Dat) = c("Subject","TRT","Age","Sex","diff","Time","DBP")
> Dat$Time = as.factor(Dat$Time)
> # show the first 6 observations
> head(Dat)

              Subject TRT Age Sex diff Time DBP
1.A.43.F.-9.1       1   A  43   F   -9    1 114
2.A.51.M.-15.1      2   A  51   M  -15    1 116
3.A.48.F.-21.1      3   A  48   F  -21    1 119
4.A.42.F.-14.1      4   A  42   F  -14    1 115
5.A.49.M.-11.1      5   A  49   M  -11    1 116
6.A.47.M.-15.1      6   A  47   M  -15    1 117
```

We then use the one-way ANOVA in Section 3.2.1.2 to test the null hypotheses that the means of DBP at all five times of measurement are equal for each treatment, i.e.,

$$H_0 : \mu_1 = \mu_2 = \mu_3 = \mu_4 = \mu_5$$
$$H_a : \text{Not all means are equal}$$

We use the R function `aov` as follows:

```
> # test treatment "A"
> datA   = Dat[Dat$TRT=="A",]
> test.A = aov(DBP~Time, datA)
> summary(test.A)

            Df Sum Sq Mean Sq F value Pr(>F)
Time         4   2880     720     127 <2e-16 ***
Residuals   95    538       6

> # test treatment "B"
> datB   = Dat[Dat$TRT=="B",]
```

```
> test.B = aov(DBP~Time, datB)
> summary(test.B)

            Df Sum Sq Mean Sq F value  Pr(>F)
Time         4    312    77.9    17.6 7.5e-11 ***
Residuals   95    420     4.4
```

From the small p-values, we note that both tests lead to rejection of the null hypotheses of equal means at baseline and across months of followup. The next logical step is to use multiple testing to determine the times at which DBP means are statistically significantly different. We call the R function TukeyHSD for this purpose:

```
> TukeyHSD(test.A)

  Tukey multiple comparisons of means
    95% family-wise confidence level

Fit: aov(formula = DBP ~ Time, data = datA)

$Time
        diff      lwr      upr p adj
2-1   -3.05   -5.14   -0.956 0.001
3-1   -5.85   -7.94   -3.756 0.000
4-1  -10.30  -12.39   -8.206 0.000
5-1  -15.20  -17.29  -13.106 0.000
3-2   -2.80   -4.89   -0.706 0.003
4-2   -7.25   -9.34   -5.156 0.000
5-2  -12.15  -14.24  -10.056 0.000
4-3   -4.45   -6.54   -2.356 0.000
5-3   -9.35  -11.44   -7.256 0.000
5-4   -4.90   -6.99   -2.806 0.000

> TukeyHSD(test.B)

  Tukey multiple comparisons of means
    95% family-wise confidence level

Fit: aov(formula = DBP ~ Time, data = datB)
$Time
       diff   lwr    upr p adj
2-1  -1.55 -3.40  0.299 0.144
3-1  -2.70 -4.55 -0.851 0.001
4-1  -4.30 -6.15 -2.451 0.000
5-1  -4.80 -6.65 -2.951 0.000
3-2  -1.15 -3.00  0.699 0.421
4-2  -2.75 -4.60 -0.901 0.001
```

```
5-2 -3.25 -5.10 -1.401 0.000
4-3 -1.60 -3.45  0.249 0.122
5-3 -2.10 -3.95 -0.251 0.018
5-4 -0.50 -2.35  1.349 0.943
```

We note that all pairwise comparisons for treatment "A" are statistically significant. But for treatment "B", the pairwise comparisons of Time 2 v.s. Time 1, Time 3 v.s. Time 2, Time 4 v.s. Time 3, and Time 5 v.s. Time 4 are not statistically significantly different. Again this indicates that the new drug treatment is more effective reducing DBP.

It should be noted that the data are correlated across time. The HSD procedure used above from R does not recognize the correlation, and is presented here for illustration. For correlated observations, the reader may wish to program in R using the methodology in Duncan (1957).

3.3.1.5   Two-Way ANOVA for Interaction

The DBP trial has two factors: treatment and Time. Whenever there is more than one factor, the one-way ANOVA (within treatment groups across Time) in previous sections cannot capture the interaction between these factors. A two-way or multi-way ANOVA is needed to analyze the interaction before making statistical inferences about the main effects as shown in Model (3.7).

For the DBP trial, we use the R function aov to test the significance of the interaction as:

```
> mod2 = aov(DBP~ TRT*Time, Dat)
> summary(mod2)

            Df Sum Sq Mean Sq F value Pr(>F)
TRT          1    972     972   192.8 <2e-16 ***
Time         4   2514     629   124.6 <2e-16 ***
TRT:Time     4    677     169    33.6 <2e-16 ***
Residuals  190    958       5
```

We note that the p-value associated with the interaction is $< 2.2e\text{-}16$, which is highly statistically significant. Since "A" is a new drug and "B" is a Placebo and the groups were comparable at baseline in terms of DBP, the statistical significance of the interaction provides evidence of effectiveness of "A", but the magnitude of the treatment difference ("A - B") depends on the time of measuring DBP. We plot the interactions between "TRT" and "Time" using the R function interaction.plot as follows, which produces Figure 3.3:

```
> par(mfrow=c(2,1),mar=c(5,3,1,1))
> with(Dat,interaction.plot(Time,TRT,DBP,las=1,legend=T))
> with(Dat,interaction.plot(TRT,Time,DBP,las=1,legend=T))
```

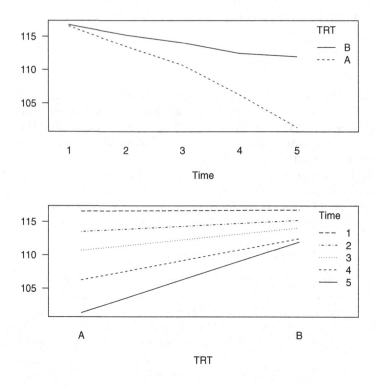

FIGURE 3.3: Interaction Plots for DBP Trial

In the upper panel of Figure 3.3, both treatments "A" and "B" started with similar means at baseline, and both reflected decreases in DBP over the months of followup. However, decreases in mean DBP for the new drug treatment "A" are greater than those for the Placebo treatment "B". At the end of trial, mean DBP for new drug treatment "A" decreased from 116.55 to 101.35 mmHg whereas mean DBP decreased from 116.75 to 111.95 mmHg for the Placebo treatment "B". This is also reflected in the lower panel in Figure 3.3. This means that the decline in DBP for both treatment groups varies across the times of DBP measurement.

Therefore, any statistical significance tests for main effects are entangled with the interactions. We may use a multiple comparison approach for testing main effects. For example Tukey's HSD procedure TukeyHSD is invoked as:

```
> TukeyHSD(aov(DBP ~ TRT*Time,Dat))

  Tukey multiple comparisons of means
    95% family-wise confidence level

Fit: aov(formula = DBP ~ TRT * Time, data = Dat)
```

```
$TRT
    diff  lwr  upr p adj
B-A 4.41 3.78 5.04     0
```

```
$Time
      diff     lwr     upr p adj
2-1  -2.30  -3.68  -0.917 0.000
3-1  -4.28  -5.66  -2.892 0.000
4-1  -7.30  -8.68  -5.917 0.000
5-1 -10.00 -11.38  -8.617 0.000
3-2  -1.97  -3.36  -0.592 0.001
4-2  -5.00  -6.38  -3.617 0.000
5-2  -7.70  -9.08  -6.317 0.000
4-3  -3.03  -4.41  -1.642 0.000
5-3  -5.72  -7.11  -4.342 0.000
5-4  -2.70  -4.08  -1.317 0.000
```

```
$`TRT:Time`
             diff     lwr     upr p adj
B:1-A:1      0.20  -2.074   2.474 1.000
A:2-A:1     -3.05  -5.324  -0.776 0.001
B:2-A:1     -1.35  -3.624   0.924 0.668
A:3-A:1     -5.85  -8.124  -3.576 0.000
B:3-A:1     -2.50  -4.774  -0.226 0.019
A:4-A:1    -10.30 -12.574  -8.026 0.000
B:4-A:1     -4.10  -6.374  -1.826 0.000
A:5-A:1    -15.20 -17.474 -12.926 0.000
B:5-A:1     -4.60  -6.874  -2.326 0.000
A:2-B:1     -3.25  -5.524  -0.976 0.000
B:2-B:1     -1.55  -3.824   0.724 0.472
A:3-B:1     -6.05  -8.324  -3.776 0.000
B:3-B:1     -2.70  -4.974  -0.426 0.007
A:4-B:1    -10.50 -12.774  -8.226 0.000
B:4-B:1     -4.30  -6.574  -2.026 0.000
A:5-B:1    -15.40 -17.674 -13.126 0.000
B:5-B:1     -4.80  -7.074  -2.526 0.000
B:2-A:2      1.70  -0.574   3.974 0.336
A:3-A:2     -2.80  -5.074  -0.526 0.004
B:3-A:2      0.55  -1.724   2.824 0.999
A:4-A:2     -7.25  -9.524  -4.976 0.000
B:4-A:2     -1.05  -3.324   1.224 0.899
A:5-A:2    -12.15 -14.424  -9.876 0.000
B:5-A:2     -1.55  -3.824   0.724 0.472
A:3-B:2     -4.50  -6.774  -2.226 0.000
```

```
B:3-B:2   -1.15   -3.424    1.124 0.837
A:4-B:2   -8.95  -11.224   -6.676 0.000
B:4-B:2   -2.75   -5.024   -0.476 0.006
A:5-B:2  -13.85  -16.124  -11.576 0.000
B:5-B:2   -3.25   -5.524   -0.976 0.000
B:3-A:3    3.35    1.076    5.624 0.000
A:4-A:3   -4.45   -6.724   -2.176 0.000
B:4-A:3    1.75   -0.524    4.024 0.295
A:5-A:3   -9.35  -11.624   -7.076 0.000
B:5-A:3    1.25   -1.024    3.524 0.759
A:4-B:3   -7.80  -10.074   -5.526 0.000
B:4-B:3   -1.60   -3.874    0.674 0.425
A:5-B:3  -12.70  -14.974  -10.426 0.000
B:5-B:3   -2.10   -4.374    0.174 0.098
B:4-A:4    6.20    3.926    8.474 0.000
A:5-A:4   -4.90   -7.174   -2.626 0.000
B:5-A:4    5.70    3.426    7.974 0.000
A:5-B:4  -11.10  -13.374   -8.826 0.000
B:5-B:4   -0.50   -2.774    1.774 0.999
B:5-A:5   10.60    8.326   12.874 0.000
```

It is noted that the data are correlated. Again, the reader may wish to refer to the methodology in Duncan (1957).

From the output, we can see that the following pairwise comparisons are not statistically significant:

1. For Treatment "A" at Time 1 (i.e., A1), the "Placebo" at Time points 1 and 2 (i.e., B1, B2);

2. For Treatment "A" at Time 2 (i.e., A2), the "Placebo" at Time points 2, 3, 4 and 5 (i.e., B2, B3, B4 and B5);

3. For Treatment "A" at Time 3 (i.e., A3), the "Placebo" at Time points 4 and 5 (i.e., B4 and B5);

4. For Placebo "B" at Time 1 (i.e., B1), the "Placebo" at Time point 2 (i.e., B2);

5. For Placebo "B" at Time 2 (i.e., B2), the "Placebo" at Time point 3 (i.e., B3);

6. For Placebo "B" at Time 3 (i.e., B3), the "Placebo" at Time points 4 and 5 (i.e., B4 and B5);

7. For Placebo "B" at Time 4 (i.e., B4), the "Placebo" at Time point 5 (i.e., B5);

This corresponds to the results from Figure 3.3 and the reader may wish to reproduce this result.

3.3.1.6 MANOVA for Treatment Difference

To test treatment difference for the changes from baseline, we first create the changes from baseline at the four time points using the following R code chunk:

```
> # attached the data into this R session
> attach(dat)
> # create the changes from baseline
> diff2to1 = DBP2-DBP1
> diff3to1 = DBP3-DBP1
> diff4to1 = DBP4-DBP1
> diff5to1 = DBP5-DBP1
```

The correlations among these DBP changes can be calculated as follows:

```
> # calculate the correlations
> cor(cbind(diff2to1,diff3to1,diff4to1,diff5to1))
```

```
         diff2to1 diff3to1 diff4to1 diff5to1
diff2to1    1.000    0.736    0.623    0.579
diff3to1    0.736    1.000    0.578    0.599
diff4to1    0.623    0.578    1.000    0.835
diff5to1    0.579    0.599    0.835    1.000
```

It can be seen that they are highly correlated from the lowest correlation of 57.8% to the highest correlation of 83.5%. Their mean changes can be also calculated as follows:

```
> # calculate the mean changes
> MCh =aggregate(cbind(diff2to1,diff3to1,diff4to1,diff5to1),
            list(TRT=TRT), mean)
> # print the chanhe
> print(MCh)
```

```
  TRT diff2to1 diff3to1 diff4to1 diff5to1
1   A    -3.05    -5.85    -10.3    -15.2
2   B    -1.55    -2.70     -4.3     -4.8
```

It can be seen that the changes from baseline from time 2 to 5 for treatment "A" are -3.05, -5.85, -10.3, and -15.2; and for Placebo "B" are -1.55, -2.70, -4.3, and -4.8, respectively.

To test the treatment differences considering all the 4-changes together, we can make use of the MANOVA for a multivariate analysis of variance as follow:

```
> # call "manova" to fit a manova
> maov1=manova(cbind(diff2to1,diff3to1,diff4to1,diff5to1)~TRT,dat)
> # then F-test with Pillai (default in R)
> summary(maov1)
```

```
            Df Pillai approx F num Df den Df  Pr(>F)
TRT          1  0.821      40.1       4      35 1.3e-12
Residuals 38
```

```
> # F-test with Hotelling-Lawley
> summary(maov1, test="Hotelling-Lawley")
```

```
            Df Hotelling-Lawley approx F num Df den Df  Pr(>F)
TRT          1             4.59      40.1       4      35  1.3e-12 ***
Residuals 38
```

```
> # F-test with Wilks
> summary(maov1, test="Wilks")
```

```
            Df Wilks approx F num Df den Df  Pr(>F)
TRT          1 0.179      40.1       4      35 1.3e-12
Residuals 38
```

```
> # F-test with Roy
> summary(maov1, test="Roy")
```

```
            Df  Roy approx F num Df den Df  Pr(>F)
TRT          1 4.59      40.1       4      35 1.3e-12 ***
Residuals 38
```

It can be seen from all these four tests in MANOVA that there is a highly statistically significant treatment effect in lowering the DBP.

3.3.2   Analysis of Duodenal Ulcer Healing Trial

3.3.2.1   Using Pearson's χ^2-test

A total of 168, 182, 165 and 188 patients were entered in the 0 mg C, 400 mg C, 800 mg C, and 1600 mg C groups, respectively. The corresponding cumulative number of patients whose ulcers healed by the end (Week 4) of the trial were 69, 113, 120, and 145, respectively. These data are loaded into R as:

```
> n  = c(168, 182, 165,188)
> p4 = c(.41, .62, .73, .77)
> x4 = c(69, 113, 120, 145)
```

We can employ Pearson's χ^2-test discussed in Section 3.2.2 to test the null hypothesis of equal probabilities of healing for the four treatment groups using the R function prop.test as:

```
> prop.test(x4, n)

        4-sample test for equality of proportions
        without continuity correction

data:  x4 out of n
X-squared = 60, df = 3, p-value = 2e-12
alternative hypothesis: two.sided
sample estimates:
prop 1 prop 2 prop 3 prop 4
 0.411  0.621  0.727  0.771
```

We note that the χ^2 statistic has a value 57.799 with 3 degrees of freedom, which gives a p-value of 1.735e-12. This means that there is strong evidence to reject the null hypothesis. This is not surprising since the observed proportions healed are 41%, 62%, 73% and 77%, in the 0 mg C, 400 mg C, 800 mg C, and 1600 mg C groups, respectively.

We again use **prop.test** for comparisons among two treatment groups. For example, to compare 800 mg C to 0 mg C, we use:

```
> prop.test(x4[c(1,3)], n[c(1,3)])

        2-sample test for equality of proportions
        with continuity correction

data:  x4[c(1, 3)] out of n[c(1, 3)]
X-squared = 30, df = 1, p-value = 1e-08
alternative hypothesis: two.sided
95 percent confidence interval:
 -0.423 -0.210
sample estimates:
prop 1 prop 2
 0.411  0.727
```

which gives a p-value $< 10^{-8}$ indicating 800 mg C is statistically more effective than the 0 mg C. We compare 800 mg C to 400 mg C using:

```
> prop.test(x4[c(2,3)], n[c(2,3)])

        2-sample test for equality of proportions
        with continuity correction

data:  x4[c(2, 3)] out of n[c(2, 3)]
X-squared = 4, df = 1, p-value = 0.05
alternative hypothesis: two.sided
95 percent confidence interval:
 -0.21008 -0.00271
```

```
sample estimates:
prop 1 prop 2
 0.621  0.727
```

which gives a p-value < 0.05 indicating 800 mg C is superior to 400 mg C. We compare 1600 mg C to 800 mg C using:

```
> prop.test(x4[c(3,4)], n[c(3,4)])

        2-sample test for equality of proportions
        with continuity correction

data:  x4[c(3, 4)] out of n[c(3, 4)]
X-squared = 0.7, df = 1, p-value = 0.4
alternative hypothesis: two.sided
95 percent confidence interval:
 -0.1404  0.0524
sample estimates:
prop 1 prop 2
 0.727  0.771
```

which produces a p-value $= 0.406$ and a 95% CI of (-0.140, 0.052), indicating that 1600 mg C and 800 mg C are not statistically significantly different. Therefore, the study demonstrated that 800 mg C was clinically optimal (is effective as compared to 0 mg C; is more effective than 400 mg C; and is not statistically nor clinically inferior to 1600 mg C).

3.3.2.2   Using Contingency Table

We create a dataframe named "Ulcer" to hold all these values as:

```
> # create a dataframe for the Ulcer trial
> Ulcer = data.frame(
 # use ``factor" to create the treatment factor
 trt = factor(rep(c("0 mg C","400 mg C","800 mg C","1600 mg C"),
 each=2),levels=c("0 mg C","400 mg C","800 mg C","1600 mg C") ),
 Heal = c("Yes","No","Yes","No","Yes","No","Yes","No"),
 y    = c(x4[1],n[1]-x4[1],x4[2],n[2]-x4[2],x4[3],
          n[3]-x4[3],x4[4],n[4]-x4[4]))
> Ulcer

        trt Heal   y
1    0 mg C  Yes  69
2    0 mg C   No  99
3  400 mg C  Yes 113
4  400 mg C   No  69
5  800 mg C  Yes 120
```

```
6  800 mg C    No   45
7 1600 mg C   Yes  145
8 1600 mg C    No   43
```

Then call **xtabs** to transform the dataframe into a contingency table as:

```
> tab.Ulcer = xtabs(y~trt+Heal,Ulcer)
> tab.Ulcer

          Heal
trt         No Yes
  0 mg C    99  69
  400 mg C  69 113
  800 mg C  45 120
  1600 mg C 43 145
```

We can plot the information in the contingency table using **dotchart** and **mosaicplot** as shown in Figure 3.4, and view the ulcer healing status by treatment group using the R code chunk:

```
> # layout for the plot
> par(mfrow=c(1,2), mar=c(4,2,1,1))
> # call ``dotchart"
> dotchart(tab.Ulcer)
> # call ``mosaicplot"
> mosaicplot(tab.Ulcer,color=T,las=1, main=" ",
        xlab="Treatment",ylab="Heal Status" )
```

In this figure, the left side is a dot chart showing the number of patients healed or not healed in each treatment group. The right side of the figure is a mosaic plot that shows the percentages healed or not healed in each treatment group. With the contingency table, we can verify the total number of patients in each treatment using:

```
> margin.table(tab.Ulcer,1)

trt
  0 mg C  400 mg C  800 mg C 1600 mg C
    168       182       165       188
```

We can also utilize Pearson's χ^2-test for contingency table to test the null hypothesis of equal proportions healed as:

```
> summary(tab.Ulcer)

Call: xtabs(formula = y ~ trt + Heal, data = Ulcer)
Number of cases in table: 703
Number of factors: 2
Test for independence of all factors:
        Chisq = 58, df = 3, p-value = 2e-12
```

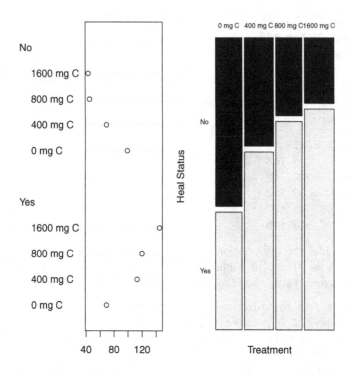

FIGURE 3.4: Ulcer Healing Distribution

This reproduces the results from Section 3.3.2.1. In Chapter 4, we re-analyze the ulcer healing data using logistic regression.

3.4   Summary and Conclusions

In this chapter, we illustrated how to perform analyses of treatment comparisons using continuous and dichotomous data arising in clinical trials using the R system. For continuous data, the simplest test is the t-test for a two treatment comparison which is then extended to the one-way analysis of variance if there are multiple treatments to be compared. When there is more than one factor (i.e., other than the treatment effect only), the two-way or three-way ANOVA should be used to investigate the interactions among these multiple factors. For clinical trials with multiple outcomes which could be correlated, the multivariate analysis of variance can be used. For clinical trials with categorical outcome, the classical ANOVA and MANOVA cannot be directly applied and the χ^2-test should be employed. Readers may adapt the R code presented to analyze their own trial results.

3.5　Appendix: SAS Programs

The SAS program below corresponds to the R program in Section 3.3.

```
/*Section 3.3.1.1*/
Data dat;
/*read data from the path of dataset*/
infile "Your file path/DBP.csv" delimiter="," firstobs=2;
input Subject TRT$ DBP1 DBP2 DBP3 DBP4 DBP5 Age Sex$;
/*create a column "diff"*/
diff= DBP5-DBP1;
RUN;

/*show the first 6 observations using proc print*/
PROC PRINT data=dat(obs=6); RUN;

/*Section 3.3.1.2*/
/*call two-side t-test with equal variance*/
PROC TTEST data=dat sides=2 alpha=0.05 h0=0;
/*specifies the title line of result*/
title "Two sample two side t-test";
/*defines the grouping variable*/
class TRT;
/*variable whose means will be compared*/
var diff;
RUN;

/*welch t-test with unequal variance*/
/*check the lines labeled "Satterthwaite" from above results*/
/*test the null hypothesis for equal variance*/
/*check the table named "Equality of Variance" from above
    results*/

/*nonparametric t-test(Wilcoxon rank-sum test)*/
PROC NPAR1WAY wilcoxon data=dat;
title "Wilcoxon rank-sum test";
class TRT;
var diff;
exact wilcoxon;                    /*request for exact p-value*/
```

```
RUN;

/*call one-side t-test */
/*alternative hypothesis: means(A)<means(B)*/
PROC TTEST data=dat sides=L alpha=0.05 h0=0;
title "Two sample one-side t-test";
class TRT;
var diff;
RUN;

/*Section 3.3.1.3*/
/*bootstrap method*/
/*call bootstrap with 1000 replication*/
PROC SURVEYSELECT data=dat out=boot_samples seed=123
/* specify the type of random sampling */
method=urs
/* get a sample of the same size as original dataset */
samprate=1
/*give the times a record chosen*/
outhits              /
* specify the number of bootstrap samples */
rep=1000;
/*bootstrapping by TRT without overlap*/
strata TRT / alloc = proportional;
RUN;

/*calculate the means of each replication*/
PROC MEANS data=boot_samples mean;
var diff;
class Replicate TRT;
/*output the results*/
output out=temp1(where=(_type_=3) drop= _freq_) Mean=mean;
RUN;

/*transform the data to contingency table*/
PROC TRANSPOSE data=temp1(drop=_type_) out=temp2(drop=_:);
id Trt;
var Mean;
by Replicate; RUN;

/*calculate the mean difference*/
Data boot_diff;
set temp2;
mean_diff=A-B;
drop A B; RUN;
```

```
/*calculate and show the bootstraps quantiles*/
PROC UNIVARIATE data= boot_diff;
var mean_diff;
output out= result PCTLPTS= 2.5 50 97.5 PCTLPRE = q; RUN;

/*Section 3.3.1.4*/
/*extract the means by treatment group*/
PROC MEANS data= dat;
/*defines the grouping variable*/
class TRT;
/*variable whose means will be extracted*/
var DBP1 DBP2 DBP3 DBP4 DBP5; RUN;

/*rearrange the dataframe of dat into a "long" format*/
DATA Dat_L;
set dat;
/*create an array*/
array ADBP(1:5) DBP1-DBP5;
/*set new variable (DBP) equal to the value of
                the array for the given time*/
do time= 1 to 5;
DBP= ADBP(time);
/*output the results*/
output;
end;
/*drop unused variables*/
drop DBP1-DBP5 diff; RUN;

/* sort data in ascending order by time*/
PROC SORT data= Dat_L out= Dat_L;
by time; RUN;

/*show the first 6 observations*/
PROC PRINT data= Dat_L(obs=6); RUN;

/*test treatment "A"*/
DATA datA(where=(TRT='A'));
set Dat_L; RUN;

PROC ANOVA data= datA;
title "one-way ANOVA to test treatment 'A'";
class time;
model DBP= time;
/*determines the times at which DBP
```

```
      means are significantly different*/
means time/ tukey cldiff; RUN;

/*test treatment "B"*/
DATA datB(where=(TRT='B'));
set Dat_L; RUN;

PROC ANOVA data= datB;
title "one-way ANOVA to test treatment 'B'";
class time;
model DBP= time;
means time / tukey cldiff; RUN;

/*determines the times at which DBP means are significantly
   different*/
/*check the result from table named
"Tukey's Studentized Range (HSD) Test for DBP"*/

/*Section 3.3.1.5*/
/*two-way anova test the significance of interaction using glm*/
PROC GLM data= Dat_L;
title "two-way ANOVA test using glm";
class TRT time;
model DBP= TRT time TRT*time;
lsmeans TRT time TRT*time/ pdiff adjust= tukey;
RUN;

/*Section 3.3.2.1*/
DATA Ulcer;                      /*load data*/
input Trt$ x_4 n @@;
Heal="Yes"; Count=x_4; output;
Heal="No"; Count=n-x_4; output;
datalines;
d1 69 168 d2 113 182 d3 120 165 d4 145 188
RUN;

/*test equal probabilities of healing for the four treatment
   groups
using Pearson's chi square test*/
PROC FREQ data= Ulcer order=data;
weight Count;
tables Trt*Heal/ chisq; RUN;

/*comparison between two treatment groups*/
/*load data of group1(0 mg)and group3(800 mg)*/
```

```
DATA dat_1_1(where=(Trt="d1"|Trt="d3"));
Set Ulcer;
RUN;
PROC FREQ data= dat_1_1 order=data;
weight Count;
tables Trt*Heal/ chisq; RUN;

/*load data of group2(400 mg)and group3(800 mg)*/
DATA dat_1_2(where=(Trt="d2"|Trt="d3"));
Set Ulcer;
RUN;
PROC FREQ data= dat_1_2 order=data;
weight Count;
tables Trt*Heal/ chisq; RUN;

/*load data of group3(800 mg)and group4(1600 mg)*/
DATA dat_1_3(where=(Trt="d3"|Trt="d4"));
Set Ulcer;
RUN;
PROC FREQ data= dat_1_3 order=data;
weight Count;
tables Trt*Heal/ chisq; RUN;


/*transform dataframe to contingency table*/
/*sort data in ascending order by Trt*/
PROC SORT data= Ulcer out=tab_Ulcer;
by Trt; RUN;

PROC TRANSPOSE data=tab_Ulcer out=tab_Ulcer(drop=_:);
   id  Heal;
   var Count;
   by  Trt; RUN;
```

Chapter 4

Treatment Comparisons in Clinical Trials with Covariates

In this chapter, we present data analyses methods for treatment comparisons in clinical trials adjusting for covariates using the R system. Analysis of Covariance (ANCOVA) for univariate outcome and multivariate analysis of covariance (MANCOVA) for multiple correlated outcomes are the natural extension of the ANOVA methods illustrated in Chapter 3. Three actual clinical trial datasets are considered and appear in Section 4.1. These datasets reflect response variables or endpoints arising from continuous, binomial, and count data.

The associated statistical models for analyzing these types of data include the well-known ANCOVA/MANCOVA for continuous data, logistic regression for binomial data and Poisson regression for count data. These models are presented in Section 4.2. For both logistic and Poisson regression, we emphasize diagnostics for detecting over/underdispersion for correct modeling and present several remedies whenever over/underdispersion is pinpointed. In Section 4.3, we demonstrate how to use R and the R functionalities to analyze the data. The chapter concludes with a brief discussion and recommendations 4.4.

4.1 Data from Clinical Trials

4.1.1 Diastolic Blood Pressure

The diastolic blood pressure (DBP) dataset presented in Table 3.1 for which analyses of variance (ANOVA) were presented in Chapter 3 is an example of continuous response data and also includes patients' age and sex at baseline as potential covariates. In this chapter, we further analyze the DBP data taking into account the effects of the covariates: "Age" and "Sex". This analysis is referred to as an "analysis of covariance (ANCOVA)". Statistical inference on comparisons of treatment groups are based on adjusted treatment group means (i.e., observed treatment group response means are adjusted for the linear relationship response has with the covariates).

4.1.2 Clinical Trials for Betablockers

The data for this example is from Yusuf et al. (1985) who present an overview of mortality data from a 22-center clinical trial in which betablockers were used to reduce mortality after myocardial infarction. Further, McLachlan and Peel (2000) used these data for mixture models. The data are reproduced in Table 4.1.

TABLE 4.1: Data for Betablocker Clinical Trial

Center	Control Deaths	Control Total	Treated Deaths	Treated Total	Center	Control Deaths	Control Total	Treated Deaths	Treated Total
1	3	39	3	38	12	47	266	45	263
2	14	116	7	114	13	16	293	9	291
3	11	93	5	69	14	45	883	57	858
4	127	1520	102	1533	15	31	147	25	154
5	27	365	28	355	16	38	213	33	207
6	6	52	4	59	18	6	154	8	151
7	152	939	98	945	17	12	122	28	251
8	48	471	60	632	19	3	134	6	174
9	37	282	25	278	20	40	218	32	209
10	188	1921	138	1916	21	43	364	27	391
11	52	583	64	873	22	39	674	22	680

In this table, "Deaths" is the number of deaths and "Total" is the total number of patients enrolled at each clinical "Center". "Treatment" represents whether patients at each center were randomized to "Control" or "Treated" (betablocker). The objective of the analysis is to demonstrate that betablocker treatment is effective in reducing mortality after myocardial infarction, as compared to control. The data (death or non-death) are binomial and are used to demonstrate the application of logistic regression as well as remedies for overdispersion using a quasi-likelihood approach.

4.1.3 Clinical Trial on Familial Adenomatous Polyposis

A placebo-controlled clinical trial of a non-steroidal anti-inflammatory drug (NSAID) in treating familial adenomatous polyposis (FAP) is reported by Giardiello et al. (1993) and by Piantadosi (1997). A planned interim analysis of the number of colonic polyps revealed significant evidence favoring NSAID treatment to warrant termination of the trial. Table 4.2 lists the numbers of colonic polyps after 12 months of treatment and the age at baseline for patients in the NSAID and placebo treated groups. The primary objective of the trial was to assess the effectiveness of NSAID treatment as compared to placebo in reducing polyps at one year, taking into account age as a covariate. Everitt and Hothorn (2006) analyzed these data using Poisson regression which revealed overdispersion. Using quasi-likelihood techniques, we re-analyze data from this trial assuming a negative-binomial regression model and illustrate how to deal with overdispersion.

TABLE 4.2: Number of Polyps in FAP Clinical Trial

NSAID		Placebo	
number	age	number	age
2	16	63	20
17	22	28	18
1	23	61	13
25	17	7	34
3	23	15	50
33	23	44	19
3	23	28	22
1	722	10	30
4	42	40	27
		46	22
		50	34

4.2 Statistical Models Incorporating Covariates

4.2.1 ANCOVA Models for Continuous Endpoints

When covariates are available, such as "Age" and "Sex" in the DBP trial, the analysis of variance of DBP in Chapter 3 can be extended to incorporate them into the statistical analysis of DBP, which is known as analysis of covariance (ANCOVA). In statistics, ANCOVA represents a combination of analysis of variance and regression. Accordingly, ANCOVA refers to regression to deal with the mixture of qualitative and quantitative predictors where the qualitative 'predictors' may include the treatments in the clinical trial as well as other factors.

Therefore, ANCOVA can be cast into regression theory model framework as $y = X\beta + \epsilon$ where y is the measured clinical endpoint (e.g., DBP) and X is the so-called design matrix with one column for treatment. β is the vector of regression parameters and ϵ is the error term which is commonly assumed to follow a normal distribution with mean 0 and variance σ^2 (Note that this assumption requires the treatment groups to have homogeneous variances).

Then regression theory can be drawn on for estimation, inference and model diagnostics.

The basic strategy for incorporating covariates into regression is to introduce *dummy variables* for the qualitative covariates within the $y = X\beta + \epsilon$ framework and keep the continuous (quantitative) covariates as they are in the design matrix X. We illustrate this strategy using DBP at month 4 as the clinical endpoint (i.e., $y = DBP5$; alternatively, if of clinical interest, we could consider the DBP change from baseline as the clinical endpoint, etc.). Treatment is a qualitative covariate which can be incorporated into the regression using a *dummy variable*, X_1 as:

$$X_1 = \begin{cases} 0 & \text{TRT} = \text{A} \\ 1 & \text{TRT} = \text{B} \end{cases} \tag{4.1}$$

The same approach can be taken for other qualitative covariates, such as "Sex" in this trial. Continuous covariates, such as "Age" and baseline DBP, can be incorporated into the regression as quantitative covariates or regression predictors, such as, $X_2 = Age$ and $X_3 = DBP1$. This strategy has been implemented in many statistical analysis software packages, such as R and SAS.

With this strategy, the ANOVA in Chapter 3 and ANCOVA can be merged into the regression framework as:

$$y = X\beta + \epsilon \tag{4.2}$$

where y is a vector of the observed clinical endpoint, X is the design matrix, β is the vector of regression parameters, $X\beta$ is called the structural or systematic component of the model, and ϵ is the error term (or random component).

We briefly present the theory of estimation and inference in this chapter. Readers may refer to regression books, such as Draper and Smith (1998) and Kutner et al. (2004), for more comprehensive discussions.

The regression Equation (4.2) expresses the clinical response measurement as the sum of a systematic component, denoted by $X\beta$, and a random non-observable component, ϵ. The fundamental idea in estimating the parameter β is to find values (estimates) such that the systematic component explains as much of the response variation as possible. This is equivalent to finding values of the parameters that make the deviations between the clinical response measurement and systematic component as small as possible. This is called least squares estimation; i.e., find β so that the error sum of squares (or residual sum of squares) is as small as possible. Therefore, the least squares estimate (LSE) of β, denoted by $\hat{\beta}$, may be obtained by minimizing:

$$\begin{aligned} \sum_i \epsilon_i^2 &= \epsilon'\epsilon = (y - X\beta)'(y - X\beta) \\ &= y'y - 2\beta X'y + \beta'X'X\beta \end{aligned} \tag{4.3}$$

Taking the derivative of the error sum of squares with respect to β and setting to zero leads to the so-called "normal equations":

$$X'X\hat{\beta} = X'y \tag{4.4}$$

when $X'X$ is **invertible**, we have

$$\hat{\beta} = (X'X)^{-1}X'y \tag{4.5}$$

We list below some results associated with least squares estimation:

1. **The predicted values:** $\hat{y} = X\hat{\beta} = X(X'X)^{-1}X'y = Hy$. We denote $H = X(X'X)^{-1}X'$ which is called the "hat-matrix" to turn observed y into "hat" y.

2. **The residuals for diagnostics:** $\hat{\epsilon} = y - \hat{y} = y - X\hat{\beta} = (I - H)y$.

3. **Residual sum of squares:** $RSS = \hat{\epsilon}'\hat{\epsilon} = y'(I - H)'(I - H)y = y'(I - H)y$.

4. **Unbiasedness:** $\hat{\beta}$ is unbiased with variance $var(\hat{\beta}) = (X'X)^{-1}\sigma^2$ if $var(\epsilon) = \sigma^2 I$.

5. **Variance estimate:** It is easy to show $E(\hat{\epsilon}'\hat{\epsilon}) = \sigma^2(n - p)$ (where p is the number of columns of the design matrix X, i.e., the number of parameters in the linear model).

   We then **estimate σ^2** using:

$$\hat{\sigma}^2 = \frac{\hat{\epsilon}'\hat{\epsilon}}{n - p} = \frac{RSS}{n - p} \tag{4.6}$$

   where $n - p$ is the *degrees of freedom* of the model.

6. R^2, is called the **coefficient of determination** or percentage of response variation explained by the systematic component (which is usually used as a goodness-of-fit measure):

$$R^2 = \frac{\sum(\hat{y}_i - \bar{y})^2}{\sum(y_i - \bar{y})^2} = 1 - \frac{\sum(y_i - \hat{y}_i)^2}{\sum(y_i - \bar{y})^2}. \tag{4.7}$$

R^2 ranges from 0 to 1 with values closer to 1 indicating a better fit of the model.

We note that no distributional assumption needs to be made in order to find the least squares estimates of the model parameters. However, if ϵ or the error term of the model is assumed to be a random variable with distribution $N(0, 1)$, parameter estimates of the model via maximum likelihood estimation would be the same as the least squares estimates.

4.2.2   Logistic Regression for Binary/Binomial Endpoints

When the observed clinical response is Bernoulli (or binary such as, death/alive or cured/uncured) or binomial (such as the number of deaths among a fixed total number of patients as described in Table 4.1) and there are covariates that may be correlated with response, regressing the response data (1, 0) on the covariates using the (normal-based) regression method in Section 4.2.1 may yield biased estimates of the covariate parameters. Logistic regression provides a preferred alternative for this type of data.

In this situation, the response variable Y_i for $i = 1, \cdots, n_i$ is binomially distributed with n_i fixed, independent trials ($n_i = 1$ for binary data where $Y_i = 1$ or 0) and probability p_i which is denoted by $Y_i \sim B(n_i, p_i)$. The probability distribution can then be written as:

$$P(Y_i = y_i) = \binom{n_i}{y_i} p_i^{y_i} (1 - p_i)^{n_i - y_i} \tag{4.8}$$

The binomial clinical response variable Y_i may be related to q clinical covariates such as treatment received, sex, age, etc., which are denoted by $(x_{i1}, \cdots, x_{iq})$. The fundamental difference between logistic regression and the multiple linear regression in Section 4.2.1 is that the response variable is binomially distributed. We then model the probability p_i as a linear function of the q covariates. This is the basic idea behind logistic regression which is described as part of the *generalized linear model* developed for the exponential family of distributions. In the generalized linear model framework, we use *a linear predictor* to model the linear relationship and a *link function* to link the *linear predictor* to the binomial probability p_i.

Specifically, the *linear predictor* is denoted by:

$$\eta_i = \beta_0 + \beta_1 x_{i1} + \cdots + \beta_q x_{iq} = X_i \beta \tag{4.9}$$

where $X_i = (1, x_{i1}, \cdots, x_{iq})$ is the matrix of observed covariates and $\beta = (\beta_0, \beta_1, \cdots, \beta_q)$ is the associated parameter vector. Various *link functions* are possible for linking the *linear predictor* η to the probabilities p_i we want to model. It is easy to see that the identity link of $p_i = \eta_i$ is not appropriate since the binomial probability p_i has to be constrained to the [0; 1] interval. For binomial response, the most commonly used link function is the so-called *logit* (and therefore giving rise to the term logistic regression) given by:

$$\eta = log\left(\frac{p}{1-p}\right) \tag{4.10}$$

Other link functions used in the logistic regression of binomial response data are *probit link function*: $\eta = \Phi^{-1}(p)$, where Φ^{-1} is the inverse normal cumulative distribution function, and the *complementary log-log link function*: $\eta = log[-log(1 - p)]$.

Maximum likelihood methods may be used for parameter estimation and statistical inference. We briefly describe maximum likelihood estimation (MLE) as follows:

To perform MLE, we first specify the likelihood function to be maximized. The general likelihood function is defined as:

$$P(Y = y) = \prod_{i=1}^{n} f(y_i|\theta) = L(\theta|y) \tag{4.11}$$

For binomial data, the likelihood becomes:

$$L(\beta|y) = \prod_{i=1}^{n} \binom{n_i}{y_i} p_i^{y_i}(1 - p_i)^{n_i - y_i} \tag{4.12}$$

The likelihood is a function of the unknown parameters and the observed response data and covariates. MLE of the unknown parameters requires finding values of the parameters that maximize the likelihood function.

Maximizing the likelihood function is equivalent to maximizing the log-likelihood function (or minimizing negative log-likelihood function, which is convenient when using likelihood ratio tests:

$$l(\theta|y) = log L(\theta|y) \tag{4.13}$$

For binomial data:

$$l(\beta|y) = \sum_{i=1}^{n} \left[log\binom{n_i}{y_i} + y_i log(p_i) + (n_i - y_i)log(1 - p_i) \right] \tag{4.14}$$

If we use the **logit link function** of $\eta = log\left(\frac{p}{1-p}\right)$, then $p = \frac{e^\eta}{1+e^\eta}$. The log-likelihood function becomes:

$$
\begin{aligned}
l(\beta|y) &= \sum_{i=1}^{n} \left[log\binom{n_i}{y_i} + y_i log(p_i) + (n_i - y_i)log(1 - p_i) \right] \\
&= \sum_{i=1}^{n} \left[y_i\eta_i - n_i log(1 + e^{\eta_i}) + log\binom{n_i}{y_i} \right]
\end{aligned} \tag{4.15}
$$

This function is then maximized to obtain the parameter estimates. There is no analytical closed form solution for the parameter estimates as there was in normal based multiple linear regression. Numerical search methods are required and maximum likelihood estimation theory is drawn upon for parameter estimates and their standard errors, confidence intervals, p-values as well as model selection. Readers are referred to McCullagh and Nelder (1995). This logistic regression is implemented in R system as R function `glm`.

4.2.3   Poisson Regression for Clinical Endpoint with Counts

When the observed clinical response data are counts, such as the number of polyps as described in Table 4.2, further extension of the methods proposed is needed. If Y is Poisson distributed with mean $\mu \geq 0$, then:

$$P(Y = y) = \frac{e^{\mu} \mu^y}{y!} \tag{4.16}$$

for $y = 0, 1, 2 \cdots$. It is important to note that for a Poisson random variable Y, $E(Y) = Var(Y) = \mu$.

Suppose Y_i represents count data and that we want to model Y_i as a function of a set of clinical covariates of $(x_1, \cdots, x_q)$. If $Y_i \sim Pois(\mu_i)$, we need a link function to link the μ_i to $(x_1, \cdots, x_q)$ with the linear predictor $\eta_i = X_i\beta$ as described in Equation (4.9). We require that $\mu_i \geq 0$, which can be ensured by the canonical log-link function as:

$$log(\mu_i) = \eta_i = X_i\beta \tag{4.17}$$

Now we can construct the likelihood function using (4.11), or the log likelihood function using (4.13). The log-likelihood function is:

$$
\begin{aligned}
l(\beta) &= \sum_{i=1}^{n} log P(Y = y) = \sum_{i=1}^{n} log \left[\frac{e^{\mu_i} \mu_i^{y_i}}{y_i!} \right] \\
&= \sum_{i=1}^{n} \left[y_i x_i^T \beta - exp(x_i^T \beta) - log(y_i!) \right]
\end{aligned}
\tag{4.18}
$$

Differentiating with respect to β gives the MLE for $\hat{\beta}$ as the solution to:

$$\sum_{i=1}^{n} \left[y_i - exp(x_i^T \hat{\beta}) \right] x_j = 0 \tag{4.19}$$

Again there is no closed form analytic solution for $\hat{\beta}$ from this equation and some numerical search algorithms are needed to find the solution. This Poisson regression is implemented in R system as R function glm.

4.2.4   Overdispersion

Overdispersion is a common phenomenon in generalized linear regression including logistic and Poisson regression. Overdispersion is evident if the deviance from the fitted model is too large. In the theory of maximum likelihood estimation, residual deviance is asymptotically distributed as χ^2 with appropriate degrees of freedom. For χ^2 distributed deviance, its value should be close to its degrees of freedom. If this is not the case, overdispersion occurs when the deviance is greater than the degrees of freedom. Conversely, we have underdispersion if the deviance is smaller than the degrees of freedom.

There may be several explanations for over/underdispersion; e.g., dependence between the n_i trials, heterogeneity arising from clusters, etc., which led to specifying the wrong model structure for the observed clinical data. For example, in the application of Poisson regression, we embed an underlying assumption unconsciously; i.e., the variance of the clinical response is the same as its mean and therefore there is only one parameter μ to model the data. Therefore, Poisson regression is not very flexible for model fitting. This is also true for binomial data.

There are several remedies to deal with under/overdispersion as outlined below:

1. *Estimate and Adjust the Dispersion Parameter: A Two-Stage Approach.*
   To overcome this stringent mean-variance assumption, we can generalize the binomial/Poisson regression by introducing a dispersion parameter ϕ for over/underdispersion such that $var(Y) = \phi E(Y) = \phi\mu$. If $\phi=1$, then we have regular Poisson regression. If $\phi \geq 1$, then we have overdispersion and if $\phi \leq 1$ we have underdispersion. The first step in this two-stage approach is to estimate the dispersion parameter using Pearson's χ^2 as:

$$\hat{\phi} = \frac{\chi^2}{n - p} \tag{4.20}$$

   After the dispersion parameter is estimated, the second stage is to use the estimated dispersion parameter to adjust the model fit for further statistical inference. We illustrate this in the R system.

2. *Using Quasi-Likelihood: A Combined Approach.* Instead of estimating the dispersion parameter from Equation (4.20) after model fitting and then adjusting the statistical inference, the quasi-likelihood approach permits estimating the dispersion parameter along with the model parameters simultaneously – without assuming an error distribution. This approach requires only the mean and variance functions to be specified. This approach is implemented in R glm and we illustrate its application in data analyses.

3. *Fit Negative Binomial Regression.* Another remedy is to use a more general distribution to relax the dependence of the mean and variance function, such as the negative binomial (NB) or gamma distribution to model the overdispersion. We now describe negative binomial regression.

   The original definition of negative binomial (NB) distribution is: for a series of independent trials with probability of success p for each trial (repetitions, not to be confused with clinical trials), the random variable N for the number of trials until the kth success is observed has a NB distribution with distribution function given by:

$$P(N = n) = \binom{n - 1}{k - 1} p^k (1 - p)^{n-k} \qquad n = k, k + 1, \cdots \tag{4.21}$$

The NB distribution as described above would be the same were we interested in failures instead of successes. As such the NB may be thought of as the distribution of the waiting time to the kth failure. This means that k-1 failures would have occurred among N-1 trials, and the kth failure occurred on the Nth trial.

The NB is an extension of the Poisson distribution from a Bayesian perspective where the Poisson parameter λ is assumed to vary according to a gamma distribution. The resulting distribution is commonly known as the "Gamma-Poisson mixture". It can be shown that the negative binomial distribution is a continuous mixture of Poisson distributions where the mixing distribution of the Poisson rate parameter is a gamma distribution. That is, we can view the negative binomial as a Poisson(λ) distribution, where λ is itself a random variable with a distribution $\Gamma\left(k, \frac{p}{1-p}\right)$.

Mathematically, the NB distribution in Equation (4.21) is re-parameterized for convenience in model fitting by defining $Y = N - k$ and $p = \frac{1}{1+\alpha}$ as:

$$P(Y = y) = \binom{y + k - 1}{k - 1} \frac{\alpha^y}{(1 + \alpha)^{y+k}}, \quad y = 0, 1, 2, \cdots \quad (4.22)$$

With this re-parameterization, $E(Y) = \mu = k\alpha$ and $var(Y) = k\alpha + k\alpha^2 = \mu + \mu^2/k$. Therefore, we have an extra term $k\alpha^2$ in the variance to model overdispersion. The log-likelihood function may be written as:

$$l(\alpha, k) = \sum_{i=1}^{n} \left(y_i log \frac{\alpha}{1 + \alpha} - klog(1 + \alpha) + \sum_{j=0}^{y_j - 1} log(j + k) - log(y!) \right) \quad (4.23)$$

The *link function* to link mean response μ to a linear combination of the clinical covariates X is:

$$\eta = X\beta = log\frac{\alpha}{1 + \alpha} = log\frac{\mu}{\mu + k} \quad (4.24)$$

The NB regression is discussed in Venables and Ripley (2002) and is implemented in the MASS (Modern Applied Statistics with S) library as glm.nb.

4.3 Data Analysis in **R**

4.3.1 Analysis of DBP Trial

4.3.1.1 Analysis of Baseline Data

Similar to Chapter 3, we read the data into R using R function `read.csv` and create a new dataframe named `dat`. We first investigate whether the treatment groups are balanced at baseline in terms of diastolic blood pressure (DBP1), Age, and Sex. We can easily plot baseline `DBP1` for the two treatment groups using a boxplot to see the distributions as well as the difference in treatment group means. This can be generated by `boxplot` with the following R code chunk which produces Figure 4.1:

```
> boxplot(DBP1~TRT,dat,xlab="Treatment",ylab="DBP at Baseline")
```

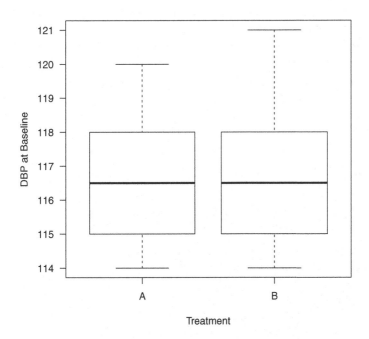

FIGURE 4.1: Boxplot for Baseline DBP

It can be seen from this plot that the treatment group distributions of DBP at baseline are similar, and we conclude that the treatment groups are balanced at baseline in terms of DBP. Similarly, a plot for age at baseline `Age` may be generated and we leave that as an exercise for readers.

We can also statistically test whether the treatment group baseline DBP means are different by using `t.test` as:

```
> t.test(DBP1~TRT, dat)

        Welch Two Sample t-test

data:  DBP1 by TRT
t = -0.3, df = 40, p-value = 0.8
alternative hypothesis: true difference in means is not equal to 0
95 percent confidence interval:
 -1.52  1.12
sample estimates:
mean in group A mean in group B
            117             117
```

This shows that mean DBP at baseline is 116.55 mmHg for treatment group A and 116.75 mmHg for treatment group B. The (p-value) for the difference (-0.20 mmHg) is 0.76, which is not statistically significant. The same test can be performed for `Age` to conclude that the treatment groups are balanced at baseline.

The `Sex` in the dataset is a categorical variable. We can perform a test on the difference in treatment group proportions as:

```
> # call function table to make the 2 by 2 table
> SexbyTRT = table(dat$TRT,dat$Sex)
> # print it
> SexbyTRT

     F  M
  A  8 12
  B 10 10

> # call prop.test to test the difference
> prop.test(SexbyTRT)

        2-sample test for equality of proportions
        with continuity correction

data:  SexbyTRT
X-squared = 0.1, df = 1, p-value = 0.8
alternative hypothesis: two.sided
95 percent confidence interval:
 -0.457  0.257
sample estimates:
prop 1 prop 2
   0.4    0.5
```

We see that there are 8 females and 12 males in treatment "A" and 10 each in treatment "B", which corresponds to 40% and 50% females in the respective treatment groups. The test yielded a *p*-value of 0.75 which again indicates the treatment groups are not statistically significantly different. In summary, the treatment groups are balanced at baseline in terms of the three covariates, indicating that randomization was successful in balancing the treatment groups in terms of baseline covariates.

It is of further interest to investigate the relationship of baseline DBP to "Age" and "Sex" using linear regression as:

```
> # Fit the main effect model on "Sex" and "Age"
> bm1=lm(DBP1~Sex+Age, dat)
> # Show the result
> summary(bm1)

Call:
lm(formula = DBP1 ~ Sex + Age, data = dat)

Residuals:
   Min     1Q Median    3Q    Max
-2.199 -0.560  0.169  0.524  1.951

Coefficients:
            Estimate Std. Error t value Pr(>|t|)
(Intercept) 104.3834    1.1288   92.48  < 2e-16 ***
SexM         -0.6422    0.3016   -2.13    0.04 *
Age           0.2639    0.0228   11.55  7.8e-14 ***

Residual standard error: 0.945 on 37 degrees of freedom
Multiple R-squared:  0.795,      Adjusted R-squared:  0.784
F-statistic: 71.6 on 2 and 37 DF,  p-value: 1.9e-13
```

We observe that both "Age" and "Sex" are statistically significant at the 5% level. These results are graphically shown in Figure 4.2 below using the following R code chunk. In this figure, "F" and "M" denote the two levels of "Sex". The solid line is the regression line for "F" and the dashed line is the regression line for "M". From these data, the DBP increases with "Age" for both "F" and "M" at the rate of 0.264 mmHg per year.

```
> # plot the ``Age" to ``DBP1"
> plot(DBP1~Age,las=1,pch=as.character(Sex), dat,
        xlab="Age", ylab="Baseline DBP")
> # add the regression lines using ``abline"
> abline(bm1$coef[1], bm1$coef[3],lwd=2, lty=1)
> abline(bm1$coef[1]+bm1$coef[2], bm1$coef[3],lwd=2, lty=4)
```

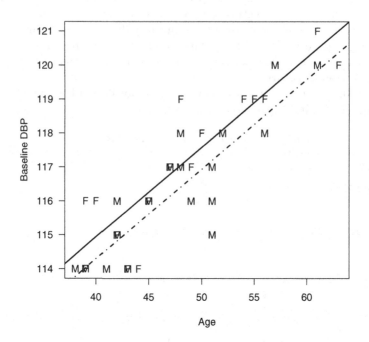

FIGURE 4.2: Baseline DBP as Function of "Age" and "Sex"

4.3.1.2   ANCOVA of DBP Change from Baseline

We now use analysis of covariance (ANCOVA) to analyze change from baseline in DBP at the end of trial which is defined as "diff". We start with the full model that contains all "covariates": "TRT", "Age" and "Sex" and their interactions, and then perform stepwise model selection to simplify the model as follows:

```
> # start with full model
> m0 = lm(diff~TRT*Age*Sex, dat)
> # stepwise model selection
> m1 = step(m0)

Start:  AIC=79.5
diff ~ TRT * Age * Sex

              Df Sum of Sq RSS  AIC
- TRT:Age:Sex  1      2.71 198 78.1
<none>                    196 79.5
```

```
Step:   AIC=78.1
diff ~ TRT + Age + Sex + TRT:Age + TRT:Sex + Age:Sex

            Df Sum of Sq RSS  AIC
- TRT:Sex  1       1.33 200 76.3
- TRT:Age  1       9.56 208 78.0
<none>                  198 78.1
- Age:Sex  1      17.07 216 79.4

Step:   AIC=76.3
diff ~ TRT + Age + Sex + TRT:Age + Age:Sex

            Df Sum of Sq RSS  AIC
<none>                  200 76.3
- TRT:Age  1       10.3 210 76.3
- Age:Sex  1       16.2 216 77.4

> # output the ANOVA
> anova(m1)

Analysis of Variance Table

Response: diff
            Df Sum Sq Mean Sq F value  Pr(>F)
TRT          1   1082    1082 184.06 2.8e-15 ***
Age          1     51      51   8.69  0.0057 **
Sex          1      1       1   0.18  0.6744
TRT:Age      1     10      10   1.76  0.1939
Age:Sex      1     16      16   2.75  0.1064
Residuals   34    200       6
```

After the stepwise model selection, we are left with the main effects with two two-way interaction terms of *TRT:Age* and *Age:Sex*. However, these two two-way interactions are not statistically significant as well as the main effect for "Sex". We drop them and further fit a model with the rest of the terms as follows:

```
> # fit the reduced model
> m2 = lm(diff~TRT+Age, dat)
> # output the anova
> anova(m2)

Analysis of Variance Table

Response: diff
            Df Sum Sq Mean Sq F value  Pr(>F)
```

```
TRT           1    1082    1082  176.04 1.2e-15 ***
Age           1      51      51    8.31  0.0065 **
Residuals 37         227       6
```

```
> # output the model fit
> summary(m2)
```

```
Call:
lm(formula = diff ~ TRT + Age, data = dat)
```

```
Residuals:
   Min     1Q  Median     3Q     Max
-5.904 -1.652 -0.009  1.156   5.230
```

```
Coefficients:
             Estimate Std. Error t value Pr(>|t|)
(Intercept)  -6.7809     2.9724   -2.28   0.0284 *
TRTB         10.1315     0.7894   12.84 3.4e-15 ***
Age          -0.1732     0.0601   -2.88   0.0065 **
```

```
Residual standard error: 2.48 on 37 degrees of freedom
Multiple R-squared:  0.833,       Adjusted R-squared:  0.824
F-statistic: 92.2 on 2 and 37 DF,  p-value: 4.24e-15
```

Now we see that "TRT" and "Age" are statistically significant. The model p-value is 4.24e-15 with $R^2 = 0.833$ indicating satisfactory model fit. We now perform model diagnostics for the normality and homogeneity of variance assumptions based upon model residuals.

We summarize the results of this analysis graphically using Figure 4.3 with the following R code chunk:

```
> plot(diff~Age,las=1,pch=as.character(TRT), dat,
          xlab="Age", ylab="DBP Change")
> abline(m2$coef[1], m2$coef[3],lwd=2, lty=1)
> abline(m2$coef[1]+m2$coef[2], m2$coef[3],lwd=2, lty=4)
```

The final model is

$$\text{DBP Change} = -6.78 - 0.173 \times Age + 10.132 \times TRT \qquad (4.25)$$

Therefore, the new treatment (B) dropped DBP by 10 mmHg compared to placebo (A). "Age" is a significant covariate reflecting decreasing trend. For every 10 years of aging, the change in DBP would be about 1.7 (0.17×10) mmHg.

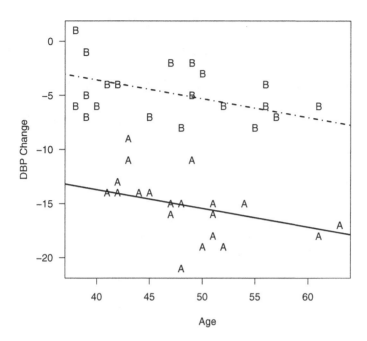

FIGURE 4.3: DBP Change as Function of "Age" for each "TRT"

4.3.1.3 MANCOVA for DBP Change from Baseline

Continuing the MANOVA in Section 3.2.1.4 for treatment difference, we now use multivariate Analysis of Covariance (MACOVA) to incorporate covariates in correlated multivariate outcomes to test treatment difference for the changes from baseline.

Taking the same data structure from Section 3.2.1.4 with changes from baseline at the four time points, the test of treatment differences considering all the four-changes together adjusting for covariate `Age` can be implemented using the MACOVA for a multivariate analysis of covariance as follows:

```
> # call "manova" to fit a manova adjusting for "Age"
> macov1=manova(cbind(diff2to1,diff3to1,diff4to1,
                      diff5to1)~TRT+Age,dat)
> # then F-test with Pillai (default in R)
> summary(macov1)

        Df Pillai approx F num Df den Df Pr(>F)
TRT      1  0.836    43.3      4     34  7e-13 ***
```

```
Age          1  0.287      3.4      4      34  0.019 *
Residuals 37
```

```
> # F-test with Hotelling-Lawley
> summary(macov1, test="Hotelling-Lawley")

          Df Hotelling-Lawley approx F num Df den Df  Pr(>F)
TRT        1             5.09     43.3      4     34  7e-13 ***
Age        1             0.40      3.4      4     34  0.019 *
Residuals 37
```

```
> # F-test with Wilks
> summary(macov1, test="Wilks")

          Df Wilks approx F num Df den Df Pr(>F)
TRT        1 0.164    43.3      4     34 7e-13 ***
Age        1 0.713     3.4      4     34 0.019 *
Residuals 37
```

```
> # F-test with Roy
> summary(macov1, test="Roy")

          Df  Roy approx F num Df den Df Pr(>F)
TRT        1 5.09    43.3      4     34 7e-13 ***
Age        1 0.40     3.4      4     34 0.019 *
Residuals 37
```

It can be seen from all these four tests in MACOVA that there is a highly statistically significant treatment effect in lowering the DBP and the `Age` is also a significant covariate which is consistent with the conclusion in Section 4.3.1.2.

4.3.2   Analysis of Betablocker Trial

We read the data into R and create a new dataframe named as "betablocker". We print this "betablocker" dataframe as follows:

```
> betablocker

  Deaths Total Center    TRT
1      3    39      1 Control
2     14   116      2 Control
3     11    93      3 Control
```

4	127	1520	4	Control
5	27	365	5	Control
6	6	52	6	Control
7	152	939	7	Control
8	48	471	8	Control
9	37	282	9	Control
10	188	1921	10	Control
11	52	583	11	Control
12	47	266	12	Control
13	16	293	13	Control
14	45	883	14	Control
15	31	147	15	Control
16	38	213	16	Control
17	12	122	17	Control
18	6	154	18	Control
19	3	134	19	Control
20	40	218	20	Control
21	43	364	21	Control
22	39	674	22	Control
23	3	38	1	Treated
24	7	114	2	Treated
25	5	69	3	Treated
26	102	1533	4	Treated
27	28	355	5	Treated
28	4	59	6	Treated
29	98	945	7	Treated
30	60	632	8	Treated
31	25	278	9	Treated
32	138	1916	10	Treated
33	64	873	11	Treated
34	45	263	12	Treated
35	9	291	13	Treated
36	57	858	14	Treated
37	25	154	15	Treated
38	33	207	16	Treated
39	28	251	17	Treated
40	8	151	18	Treated
41	6	174	19	Treated
42	32	209	20	Treated
43	27	391	21	Treated
44	22	680	22	Treated

These data correspond to the data in Table 4.1. We first fit a **logistic regression model** using glm as:

```
> # fit a logistic regression using glm
> beta.glm = glm(cbind(Deaths,Total-Deaths)~TRT+Center,
                  family=binomial,data=betablocker)
> # print the model fitting
> anova(beta.glm)

Analysis of Deviance Table

Model: binomial, link: logit

Response: cbind(Deaths, Total - Deaths)

Terms added sequentially (first to last)


          Df Deviance Resid. Df Resid. Dev
NULL                      43          333
TRT        1    27.2      42          306
Center 21     282.1       21           24
```

From the model fitting, we can see both "Treatment" and "Center" are statistically significant with *p*-value associated with "Treatment" is 1.80e-07. The details of the model fit can be printed as:

```
> summary(beta.glm)

Call:
glm(formula = cbind(Deaths, Total - Deaths) ~ TRT + Center,
                 family = binomial, data = betablocker)

Deviance Residuals:
    Min      1Q   Median      3Q      Max
 -1.828  -0.618    0.004   0.535    1.921

Coefficients:
             Estimate Std. Error z value Pr(>|z|)
(Intercept)   -2.3493     0.4260   -5.52  3.5e-08 ***
TRTTreated    -0.2610     0.0499   -5.23  1.7e-07 ***
Center2        0.1739     0.4832    0.36    0.719
Center3        0.2428     0.5004    0.49    0.628
Center4       -0.0391     0.4309   -0.09    0.928
Center5       -0.0217     0.4480   -0.05    0.961
Center6        0.1685     0.5395    0.31    0.755
Center7        0.5966     0.4308    1.38    0.166
Center8        0.2715     0.4373    0.62    0.535
Center9        0.3888     0.4462    0.87    0.384
```

```
Center10     0.0958     0.4293    0.22    0.823
Center11     0.0520     0.4363    0.12    0.905
Center12     0.9153     0.4406    2.08    0.038 *
Center13    -0.6357     0.4720   -1.35    0.178
Center14    -0.3065     0.4375   -0.70    0.484
Center15     1.0016     0.4505    2.22    0.026 *
Center16     0.8799     0.4449    1.98    0.048 *
Center17     0.3997     0.4573    0.87    0.382
Center18    -0.5635     0.5059   -1.11    0.265
Center19    -1.0144     0.5436   -1.87    0.062 .
Center20     0.8759     0.4447    1.97    0.049 *
Center21     0.1966     0.4436    0.44    0.658
Center22    -0.5812     0.4451   -1.31    0.192
```

(Dispersion parameter for binomial family taken to be 1)

```
    Null deviance: 332.993  on 43  degrees of freedom
Residual deviance:  23.621  on 21  degrees of freedom
AIC: 287.1
```

Number of Fisher Scoring iterations: 4

The residual deviance is 23.621 with 21 degrees of freedom indicating a reasonable model fit and the overdispersion is not very serious. However, for illustration purposes, we still show the application of methods in dealing with overdispersion using this data. For this data, the dispersion parameter is estimated using the Pearson residual as:

```
> est.dp = sum(resid(beta.glm, type="pearson")^2)/beta.glm$df.res
> est.dp
```

```
[1] 1.12
```

i.e., the estimate of dispersion is 1.12 (again, small and not serious for this data). With this estimate, we can adjust the model fitting as follows:

```
> summary(beta.glm, dispersion=est.dp)
```

```
Call:
glm(formula = cbind(Deaths, Total - Deaths) ~ TRT + Center,
    family = binomial, data = betablocker)
```

```
Deviance Residuals:
   Min      1Q   Median      3Q     Max
-1.828  -0.618    0.004   0.535   1.921
```

Coefficients:

```
              Estimate Std. Error z value Pr(>|z|)
(Intercept)    -2.3493     0.4512   -5.21  1.9e-07 ***
TRTTreated     -0.2610     0.0529   -4.93  8.1e-07 ***
Center2         0.1739     0.5118    0.34  0.734
Center3         0.2428     0.5300    0.46  0.647
Center4        -0.0391     0.4564   -0.09  0.932
Center5        -0.0217     0.4745   -0.05  0.964
Center6         0.1685     0.5714    0.29  0.768
Center7         0.5966     0.4563    1.31  0.191
Center8         0.2715     0.4632    0.59  0.558
Center9         0.3888     0.4727    0.82  0.411
Center10        0.0958     0.4547    0.21  0.833
Center11        0.0520     0.4621    0.11  0.910
Center12        0.9153     0.4667    1.96  0.050 *
Center13       -0.6357     0.4999   -1.27  0.204
Center14       -0.3065     0.4634   -0.66  0.508
Center15        1.0016     0.4772    2.10  0.036 *
Center16        0.8799     0.4713    1.87  0.062 .
Center17        0.3997     0.4843    0.83  0.409
Center18       -0.5635     0.5358   -1.05  0.293
Center19       -1.0144     0.5758   -1.76  0.078 .
Center20        0.8759     0.4710    1.86  0.063 .
Center21        0.1966     0.4698    0.42  0.676
Center22       -0.5812     0.4715   -1.23  0.218

(Dispersion parameter for binomial family taken to be 1.12)

    Null deviance: 332.993  on 43  degrees of freedom
Residual deviance:  23.621  on 21  degrees of freedom
AIC: 287.1

Number of Fisher Scoring iterations: 4
```

We see that same conclusion is obtained. This two-stage approach may be combined into the quasi-likelihood approach as follows:

```
> # fit quasi-likelihood for binomial data
> beta.glm2 = glm(cbind(Deaths,Total- Deaths)~TRT+Center,
        family=quasibinomial,data=betablocker)
> # print the model fit
> summary(beta.glm2)

Call:
glm(formula = cbind(Deaths, Total - Deaths) ~ TRT + Center,
    family = quasibinomial,   data = betablocker)
```

```
Deviance Residuals:
    Min      1Q   Median      3Q      Max
 -1.828  -0.618    0.004   0.535    1.921
```

```
Coefficients:
             Estimate Std. Error t value Pr(>|t|)
(Intercept)   -2.3493     0.4512   -5.21 3.7e-05 ***
TRTTreated    -0.2610     0.0529   -4.93 7.0e-05 ***
Center2        0.1739     0.5118    0.34   0.737
Center3        0.2428     0.5300    0.46   0.652
Center4       -0.0391     0.4564   -0.09   0.933
Center5       -0.0217     0.4745   -0.05   0.964
Center6        0.1685     0.5714    0.29   0.771
Center7        0.5966     0.4563    1.31   0.205
Center8        0.2715     0.4632    0.59   0.564
Center9        0.3888     0.4727    0.82   0.420
Center10       0.0958     0.4547    0.21   0.835
Center11       0.0520     0.4621    0.11   0.911
Center12       0.9153     0.4667    1.96   0.063 .
Center13      -0.6357     0.4999   -1.27   0.217
Center14      -0.3065     0.4634   -0.66   0.516
Center15       1.0016     0.4772    2.10   0.048 *
Center16       0.8799     0.4713    1.87   0.076 .
Center17       0.3997     0.4843    0.83   0.419
Center18      -0.5635     0.5358   -1.05   0.305
Center19      -1.0144     0.5758   -1.76   0.093 .
Center20       0.8759     0.4710    1.86   0.077 .
Center21       0.1966     0.4698    0.42   0.680
Center22      -0.5812     0.4715   -1.23   0.231
```

```
(Dispersion parameter for quasibinomial family taken to be 1.12)

    Null deviance: 332.993  on 43  degrees of freedom
Residual deviance:  23.621  on 21  degrees of freedom
AIC: NA
```

```
Number of Fisher Scoring iterations: 4
```

We observe from the model fitting (i.e., **beta.glm2**) that the dispersion parameter is estimated as 1.1218, which equals to what we obtained from the two-stage approach. The p-value for "Treatment" is now 7.02e-5, slightly different from the two-stage result, but with the same conclusion of statistical significance of the betablocker.

This data will be re-analyzed in Chapter 8 as an example for meta-analysis.

4.3.3   Analysis of Data from Familial Adenomatous Polyposis Trial

The data from the placebo-controlled clinical trial of a non-steroidal anti-inflammatory drug in treating familial adenomatous polyposis (FAP) is shown in Table 4.2. We read this data into R and name it `polyps`. The data may be printed using:

```
> polyps
```

	number	treat	age
1	63	placebo	20
2	2	drug	16
3	28	placebo	18
4	17	drug	22
5	61	placebo	13
6	1	drug	23
7	7	placebo	34
8	15	placebo	50
9	44	placebo	19
10	25	drug	17
11	3	drug	23
12	28	placebo	22
13	10	placebo	30
14	40	placebo	27
15	33	drug	23
16	46	placebo	22
17	50	placebo	34
18	3	drug	23
19	1	drug	22
20	4	drug	42

We first fit a Poisson model to this count data using:

```
> # Poisson Regression
> m0.polyps = glm(number~treat*age, polyps, family=poisson())
> # print the model fit
> summary(m0.polyps)

Call:
glm(formula = number ~ treat * age, family = poisson(),
        data = polyps)

Deviance Residuals:
    Min      1Q   Median      3Q     Max
 -4.241  -3.040   -0.086   1.439   5.849
```

```
Coefficients:
                Estimate Std. Error z value Pr(>|z|)
(Intercept)      4.51912    0.15336   29.47  < 2e-16
treatdrug       -1.25726    0.47163   -2.67   0.0077
age             -0.03840    0.00625   -6.15  7.8e-10
treatdrug:age   -0.00463    0.02082   -0.22   0.8240

(Dispersion parameter for poisson family taken to be 1)

    Null deviance: 378.66  on 19  degrees of freedom
Residual deviance: 179.49  on 16  degrees of freedom
AIC: 275.8

Number of Fisher Scoring iterations: 5
```

On the surface, both treatment and age appear statistically significant. However, there is overdispersion with residual deviance of 179.49 on 16 degrees of freedom. The dispersion parameter is estimated as:

```
> est.dp = sum(resid(m0.polyps, type="pearson")^2)/m0.polyps$df.res
> est.dp

[1] 11.4
```

which is 11.4. Using this estimate, we can adjust the model fitting as:

```
> summary(m0.polyps, dispersion=est.dp)

Call:
glm(formula = number ~ treat * age, family = poisson(),
        data = polyps)

Deviance Residuals:
   Min      1Q  Median      3Q     Max
-4.241  -3.040  -0.086   1.439   5.849

Coefficients:
                Estimate Std. Error z value Pr(>|z|)
(Intercept)      4.51912    0.51725    8.74   <2e-16
treatdrug       -1.25726    1.59067   -0.79    0.429
age             -0.03840    0.02106   -1.82    0.068
treatdrug:age   -0.00463    0.07023   -0.07    0.947

(Dispersion parameter for poisson family taken to be 11.4)

    Null deviance: 378.66  on 19  degrees of freedom
Residual deviance: 179.49  on 16  degrees of freedom
```

AIC: 275.8

Number of Fisher Scoring iterations: 5

We now observe that no term is statistically significant. Since the interaction is strongly not statistically significant, we re-fit the reduced model without the interaction term and adjust for dispersion:

```
> # refit the model without interaction
> m1.polyps = glm(number~treat+age, polyps, family=poisson())
> # estimate the dispersion parameter
> est.dp = sum(resid(m1.polyps, type="pearson")^2)/m1.polyps$df.res
> # print the estimated dispersion parameter
> est.dp
```

[1] 10.7

```
> # print the model fit adjusting the overdispersion
> summary(m1.polyps, dispersion=est.dp)
```

Call:
glm(formula = number ~ treat + age, family = poisson(),
        data = polyps)

Deviance Residuals:
    Min   1Q Median   3Q   Max
  -4.22   -3.05   -0.18   1.45   5.83

Coefficients:
              Estimate Std. Error z value Pr(>|z|)
(Intercept)   4.5290   0.4811   9.41 < 2e-16 ***
treatdrug   -1.3591   0.3853   -3.53 0.00042 ***
age   -0.0388   0.0195   -1.99 0.04651 *

(Dispersion parameter for poisson family taken to be 10.7)

    Null deviance: 378.66 on 19 degrees of freedom
Residual deviance: 179.54 on 17 degrees of freedom
AIC: 273.9

Number of Fisher Scoring iterations: 5

We now observe that the estimated dispersion parameter is 10.7, and both "Treatment" and the covariate "age" are statistically significant at 5% level. This two-step approach can be combined into the *quasi-likelihood* approach as:

```
> # fit the quasi Poisson
> m2.polyps = glm(number~treat+age, polyps, family=quasipoisson())
> # print the model fit
> summary(m2.polyps)

Call:
glm(formula = number ~ treat + age, family = quasipoisson(),
    data = polyps)

Deviance Residuals:
   Min      1Q   Median      3Q     Max
 -4.22   -3.05    -0.18    1.45    5.83

Coefficients:
            Estimate Std. Error t value Pr(>|t|)
(Intercept)   4.5290     0.4811    9.41  3.7e-08 ***
treatdrug    -1.3591     0.3853   -3.53   0.0026 **
age          -0.0388     0.0195   -1.99   0.0628 .

(Dispersion parameter for quasipoisson family taken to be 10.7)

    Null deviance: 378.66  on 19  degrees of freedom
Residual deviance: 179.54  on 17  degrees of freedom

Number of Fisher Scoring iterations: 5
```

From the quasi-likelihood approach, the estimated dispersion is 10.7. "Treatment" is still statistically significant with p-value $= 0.0026$. However, the covariate "age" is no longer statistically significant at the 5% level, but is marginally statistically significant with p-value$=0.0628$.

As further exploration, we fit the negative binomial model using the function `glm.nb` in MASS library using:

```
> # load the MASS library
> library(MASS)
> # fit the negative binomial model
> m3.polyps = glm.nb(number~treat+age, polyps)
> # print the model fit
> summary(m3.polyps)

Call:
glm.nb(formula = number ~ treat + age, data = polyps,
       init.theta = 1.719491,  link = log)

Deviance Residuals:
    Min       1Q   Median       3Q      Max
```

```
-1.8327  -1.1390  -0.0885   0.3364   1.8978
```

```
Coefficients:
            Estimate Std. Error z value Pr(>|z|)
(Intercept)   4.5260     0.5947    7.61 2.7e-14 ***
treatdrug    -1.3681     0.3690   -3.71 0.00021 ***
age          -0.0386     0.0210   -1.84 0.06575 .
```

```
(Dispersion parameter for Negative Binomial(1.72) family taken
   to be 1)
```

```
    Null deviance: 36.734  on 19  degrees of freedom
Residual deviance: 22.002  on 17  degrees of freedom
AIC: 164.9
```

```
Number of Fisher Scoring iterations: 1
```

```
            Theta:   1.719
        Std. Err.:   0.607
 2 x log-likelihood:  -156.880
```

We observe that the estimated parameter k in the negative binomial distribution is 1.719 with standard error equal to 0.607. Further "Treatment" is statistically significant with p-value $= 0.00021$, and the p-value for the covariate "age" is marginally significant with p-value 0.06575. These results are similar to those obtained from applying the quasi-likelihood approach to the Poisson regression model.

4.4   Summary and Conclusions

In this chapter, we illustrated analysis methodology for comparing treatments incorporating covariates in clinical trials using three real datasets. These datasets reflected clinical response variables for the continuous, binomial and count data cases. In conducting the analyses, we presented the associated statistical models as well as the R code for the analysis methods. Specifically, we cast the classical ANCOVA for continuous data into multiple linear regression, and illustrated logistic regression for binomial data and Poisson regression for count data. Further, we presented three remedies for dealing with over/underdispersion inherent in binomial and count data. Readers may use the models and the associated R code to analyze their own trials.

For further reading, we recommend McCullagh and Nelder (1995) for theoretical background and Venables and Ripley (2002) for application in R/S with its MASS (Modern Applied Statistics with S) library.

4.5   Appendix: SAS Programs

The SAS program below corresponds to the R program in Section 4.3.

```
/********************************
Chapter 4: SAS Programs
******************************/
/*read data from the path of dataset*/
Data dat;
infile "Your data path/DBP.csv" delimiter="," firstobs=2;
input Subject TRT$ DBP1 DBP2 DBP3 DBP4 DBP5 Age Sex$;
/*create a column diff*/
diff= DBP5-DBP1; RUN;


/***********************************************
Section 4.3.1.1
*********************************************/
/*test whether the DBP means are different*/
PROC TTEST data= dat;
title "Two sample two sided t-test";
class Trt;
var DBP1; RUN;

/*make 2 by 2 table using variable "Sex"*/
PROC FREQ data= dat;
tables Trt*Sex / out= freqs ; RUN;

PROC TRANSPOSE data= freqs out= SexbyTrt(drop=_:);
   id  Sex;
   var count;
   by  Trt;
RUN;

/*print the table*/
PROC PRINT data= SexbyTrt; RUN;

/*test equality of proportions of 2 treatment groups
using Pearson's Chi squares*/
PROC FREQ data= freqs;
weight count;
tables Trt*Sex/ chisq; RUN;

/*Fit the main effect model on "Sex" and "Age"*/
PROC GLM data= dat;
```

```
class Sex(ref="F");
model DBP1= Sex Age / solution;
RUN;


/***********************************************
Section 4.3.1.2
***********************************************/
/*stepwise model selection */
PROC GLMSELECT data= dat;
class Trt Sex;
model diff= Trt|Sex|Age
/ selection= stepwise(select= AIC) stats= all;
RUN;

/*fit the reduced model*/
PROC GLM data= dat;
class TRT(ref="A");
model diff= Age Trt / solution;
RUN;


/*****************************
Section 4.3.1.3: MACNOVA for Treatment Difference
***********************************/
/* create the data*/
data mdat;
set dat;
diff2to1 = DBP2-DBP1;
diff3to1 = DBP3-DBP1;
diff4to1 = DBP4-DBP1;
diff5to1 = DBP5-DBP1;
run;
/* manova using glm*/
PROC glm data= mdat;
class TRT;
model diff2to1 diff3to1 diff4to1 diff5to1= TRT Age/ss3;
contrast '1 vs 2' TRT 1 -1;
manova h=_all_;
RUN;


/***********************************************
Section 4.3.2
***********************************************/
/*read data from the path of dataset*/
Data dat1;
infile "your path/betablocker.csv" delimiter="," firstobs=2;
```

```
input Deaths Total Center Treatment$;
RUN;


/*fit the logistic regression model*/
PROC GENMOD data= dat1;
class Center(ref="1") Treatment(ref="Control");
model Deaths/Total= Center Treatment/dist= binomial link= logit;
RUN;


/*disperson of parameter*/
/*check table "Criteria For Assessing Goodness Of Fit"
line "pearson chi sqaure*/


/*adjust model fitting with estimate of dispersion*/
PROC GENMOD data= dat1;
class Center(ref="1") Treatment(ref="Control");
model Deaths/Total= Center Treatment
/dist= binomial link= logit scale= pearson;
RUN;


/*fit quasi-likelihood for binomial data*/
PROC GLIMMIX data= dat1;
class Center(ref="1") Treatment(ref="Control");
model Deaths/Total= Center Treatment
/ link=logit dist=binomial solution;
/*specify the overdispersion parameter*/
random _residual_;
RUN;


/*Section 4.3.3*/
/*read data from the path of dataset*/
Data dat2;
infile "your path/polyps.csv" delimiter="," firstobs=2;
input number treat$ age;
RUN;


/*fit poisson regression model*/
PROC GENMOD data= dat2;
class treat(ref="placebo");
model number= age|treat / dist= poisson link= log;
RUN;


/*disperson of parameter*/
/*check table "Criteria For Assessing Goodness Of Fit"
line "pearson chi sqaure*/
```

```
/*adjust model fitting with estimate of dispersion*/
PROC GENMOD data= dat2;
class treat(ref="placebo");
model number= age|treat / dist= poisson link= log
scale= PEARSON;
RUN;

/*refit the model without interaction*/
PROC GENMOD data= dat2;
class treat(ref="placebo");
model number= age treat / dist= poisson link= log
scale= PEARSON;
RUN;

/*disperson of parameter*/
/*check table "Criteria For Assessing Goodness Of Fit"
line "pearson chi sqaure*/

/*fit the quasi poisson*/
PROC GLIMMIX data= dat2;
class treat(ref="placebo");
model number= age treat / dist= poisson link= log solution;
random _residual_;
RUN;

/*fit the negative-binomial model*/
PROC GENMOD data= dat2;
class treat(ref="placebo");
model number= age treat / dist= negbin;
RUN;

/*parameter estimate: k=1/dispersion: 1/0.5816= 1.7194*/
```

Chapter 5

Analysis of Clinical Trials with Time-to-Event Endpoints

In this chapter, we analyze time-to-event data arising from clinical trials using the R system. Time-to-event data are produced in a variety of clinical trials where the primary endpoint is some critical event. For example, in analgesic studies such as post-dental extraction pain or post-partum pain, the event is relief of pain. In an anti-infective study of chronic urinary tract infection, the event is microbiological cure or the abatement of clinical signs and symptoms of the infection. In the study of bladder tumors, for example, important events in patient followup are remission or progression. In transplantation studies involving renal allografts, although death is ultimately primary, rejection may be the primary event reflecting the experimental objective. If the event is recurrence, then time-to-event is progression free interval. If the event is death, then time-to-event is survival time.

Data on the times to the event and the times of censoring (as well as any information about the censoring mechanisms) from such populations may be analyzed to provide meaningful information about parameters of the underlying population distributions. However, the data structure is different from that of complete (no censored observations) data or data reflecting only the occurrence or non-occurrence of the event (e.g., binomially distributed data), and therefore require special statistical analysis methods. The primary difference is that times-to-event are positive and are generally skewed to the right. Another key difference is that times-to-event are censored for some patients. For these patients, we know that they had not experienced the event at their last time of observation (e.g., clinic visit). Thus we only know that times-to-event are greater than those recorded, but the exact survival times (if the event is death) cannot be directly observed. We again need special methods to model this type of censoring, which in general gave rise to the statistical field called *survival data analysis.*

In this chapter, we start with the analysis of a typical clinical trial that produces right-censored data. Then, we consider more recent analysis methods for data from clinical trials that produce interval-censored data, such as cancer clinical trials. Therefore, datasets from two clinical trials are introduced in Section 5.1. We outline the associated statistical models in Section 5.2. Models for analyzing right-censored data appear in Section 5.3, and models for analyzing interval-censored data appear in Section 5.4. The use of R for analyzing survival data is presented in Section 5.5 followed by a summary and discussion in Section 5.6.

5.1   Clinical Trials with Time-to-Event Data

5.1.1   Phase II Trial of Patients with Stage-2 Breast Carcinoma

The objective of a Phase II trial was to assess the relative efficacy of chemotherapy (CT) and immunotherapy (IT) alone and in combination, as adjuvant to surgery in the treatment of patients with stage-2 carcinoma of the breast. The design of the trial was parallel with random assignment to the three treatment groups:

1. S+CT: Surgery plus one year of chemotherapy

2. S+IT: Surgery plus one year of immunotherapy

3. S+CT+IT: Surgery plus one year of chemotherapy and immunotherapy

The measures of efficacy were "time-to-death" and "time-to-evidence of disease" recorded in weeks. We analyze "time-to-death" in this chapter. Baseline information were collected and we use the patient's age as a covariate in the analyses presented. The data are shown in Table 5.1.

TABLE 5.1: Breast Carcinoma Data

S+CT			S+IT			S+CT+IT		
Time	Status	Age	Time	Status	Age	Time	Status	Age
48	1	26	102	0	52	36	0	60
55	0	65	105	0	72	73	0	72
58	1	48	144	0	52	139	1	48
63	0	53	151	0	54	158	0	60
102	0	55	182	1	52	185	1	47
133	0	63	191	1	62	198	1	51
144	0	62	192	0	62	239	1	55
177	1	49	196	1	50	239	1	56
182	1	50	222	1	43	240	1	61
216	1	63	251	1	31	242	1	35
217	0	58						

Note in this table, "Time" is "time-to-death" in weeks, "Status" is the censoring status with 0=died and 1=censored (i.e., alive at the last follow-up).

The primary objective for this analysis is to assess whether immunotherapy when added to surgery plus chemotherapy improves survival; i.e., is S+CT+IT better than S + CT? We also assess whether chemotherapy adds to the efficacy of surgery plus immunotherapy; i.e., is S+CT+IT better than S + IT? In addition, we assess the effect of age on survival in the analyses.

5.1.2 Breast Cancer Trial with Interval-Censored Data

In oncology clinical trials, time-to-event data are usually generated from diagnostic assessments performed when patients return to the clinic at protocol specified visits (such as at 8 weeks or 2 months, etc.) after baseline, resulting in interval-censored data. In this section, we use breast cosmesis data described in Finkelstein (1986) which is reproduced in Table 5.2.

TABLE 5.2: Breast Cancer Data

Radiation Only						Radiation+Chemotherapy					
t_L	t_U	Status	t_L	t_U	Status	t_L	t_U	Status	t_L	t_U	Status
0	7	1	32	NA	0	0	22	1	16	24	1
0	8	1	33	NA	0	0	5	1	16	60	1
0	5	1	34	NA	0	4	9	1	17	27	1
4	11	1	36	44	1	4	8	1	17	23	1
5	12	1	36	48	1	5	8	1	17	26	1
5	11	1	36	NA	0	8	12	1	18	25	1
6	10	1	36	NA	0	8	21	1	18	24	1
7	16	1	37	44	1	10	35	1	19	32	1
7	14	1	37	NA	0	10	17	1	21	NA	0
11	15	1	37	NA	0	11	13	1	22	32	1
11	18	1	37	NA	0	11	NA	0	23	NA	0
15	NA	0	38	NA	0	11	17	1	24	31	1
17	NA	0	40	NA	0	11	NA	0	24	30	1
17	25	1	45	NA	0	11	20	1	30	34	1
17	25	1	46	NA	0	12	20	1	30	36	1
18	NA	0	46	NA	0	13	NA	0	31	NA	0
19	35	1	46	NA	0	13	39	1	32	NA	0
18	26	1	46	NA	0	13	NA	0	32	40	1
22	NA	0	46	NA	0	13	NA	0	34	NA	0
24	NA	0	46	NA	0	14	17	1	34	NA	0
24	NA	0	46	NA	0	14	19	1	35	NA	0
25	37	1	46	NA	0	15	22	1	35	39	1
26	40	1				16	24	1	44	48	1
27	34	1				16	20	1	48	NA	0

This dataset has been used by many authors to illustrate different models. The event of interest is cosmetic deterioration - moderate or severe breast retraction. The data on time-to-event derive from a retrospective study comparing two treatments: radiotherapy alone ($TRT=1$) versus radiotherapy plus adjuvant chemotherapy ($TRT=0$) in 94 women with early breast cancer.

For these 94 patients, 46 were treated with radiation alone and 48 were treated with radiation plus chemotherapy. Patients were monitored initially every 4-6 months and the interval between visits lengthened as their recovery progressed. The data of interest in this analysis is time to first appearance of moderate or severe breast retraction. Since patients could be only observed during their clinic visits, the exact time of breast retraction was known only to be within the interval between visits and therefore the data are interval-censored. For the 94 patients, 56 were interval-censored ($Status = 1$) and 38 were right-censored ($Status = 0$) observations as seen in Table 5.2 [reproduced from Finkelstein (1986) for easy reference].

In this table, the interval-censored data are denoted by $Status = 1$ and have specific values for t_L and t_U. The right-censored data are denoted by $Status = 0$ for patients who had not achieved moderate or severe breast retraction by the last visit and $t_U = NA$.

The objective of this clinical trial was to test whether the time-to-breast retraction increased by adding chemotherapy to radiation treatment. We also use these data to compare various statistical analysis methods for interval-censored data.

5.2   Statistical Models

5.2.1   Primary Functions and Definitions

Prior to proceeding with analyses of these two datasets, the reader may find the following review of definitions of key functions in survival analysis helpful.

The primary functions in depicting survival are the *hazard function* or *force of mortality*, the *survival function*, the *death density function* and the *cumulative death distribution function*. These functions are symbolized in this chapter as $h(t)$, $S(t)$, $f(t)$ and $F(t)$, respectively, where t denotes survival time. We will briefly define and explain these functions; greater detail may be found in Peace (2009) in general, Sun (2006), and Chen et al. (2012) for interval-censored data.

5.2.1.1   The Hazard Function

The mathematical definition of the *hazard function* $h(t)$ is:

$$h(t) = \lim_{\Delta t \to 0} \frac{Pr\,(t \le T \le t + \Delta t | T \ge t)}{\Delta t} \tag{5.1}$$

where T denotes the random variable survival time. Ignoring limit considerations, $h(t)$ is the proportion of a population expiring in the interval $[t; t + \Delta t]$ among those at risk of expiring at the beginning of the interval, averaged over the length of the interval. So $h(t)$ may be thought of as the conditional probability of dying at time $= t$, given that death did not occur prior to t; or $h(t)$ is the conditional instantaneous risk of death at time t given that death did not occur prior to t.

A hazard function may remain constant with respect to time (corresponding to an exponential density), may increase as a function of time according to some power function (corresponding to a Weibull density), may increase linearly with time (corresponding to a Rayleigh density), or may increase exponentially with time (corresponding to a Gompertz density). In addition, there may be intervals of time where the hazard may alternatingly decrease or increase according to some power, linear, or exponential function of time.

Associated with this *hazard function*, $h(t)$, is the *integrated or cumulative hazard function* $H(t)$ which is widely used in survival modeling and is defined as:

$$H(t) = \int_{u=0}^{t} h(u)du \tag{5.2}$$

5.2.1.2   The Survival Function

Besides the *hazard function*, the *survival function* is another fundamental function of interest in the analysis of survival data. The mathematical definition of the *survival function* $S(t)$ is:

$$S(t) = Pr\left(T \geq t\right) \tag{5.3}$$

where T denotes the random variable survival time. The survival function $S(t)$ may be interpreted as the probability of surviving to at least time t, the t-year survival rate, the cumulative proportion surviving to at least time t, or the proportion of a population surviving to at least time t.

5.2.1.3   The Death Density Function

For modeling survival data using a likelihood approach, the *death density function* is usually employed. The mathematical definition of the *death density function* $f(t)$ is:

$$f(t) = \lim_{\Delta t \to 0} \frac{Pr\left(t \leq T \leq t + \Delta t\right)}{\Delta t} \tag{5.4}$$

where T denotes the random variable survival time. Ignoring limit considerations, $f(t)$ is the proportion of all individuals in a population expiring in the interval $[t; t + \Delta t]$ divided by the length of the interval. So $f(t)$ may be thought of as the unconditional probability of dying at time $= t$; or $f(t)$ is the instantaneous unconditional risk of death at time t.

Associated with this *death density function*, $f(t)$, the *cumulative death distribution function* $F(t)$, which is the complement of the survival function; i.e.,

$$F(t) = 1 - S(t) \tag{5.5}$$

5.2.1.4   Relationships between These Functions

The *hazard, density, survival,* and *cumulative death distribution functions* are interrelated. If one knows the survival function, its complement is the cumulative death distribution function, and the death density may be obtained by differentiating the negative of the survival function with respect to t; i.e.,

$$f(t) = -\frac{d[S(t)]}{dt} \tag{5.6}$$

The hazard function may then be obtained by dividing the death density by the survival function; i.e.,

$$h(t) = \frac{f(t)}{S(t)} = -\frac{d[lnS(t)]}{dt} \tag{5.7}$$

Also, if the hazard function is specified, the survival function may be obtained by exponentiating the negative integral of the hazard; i.e.,

$$S(t) = exp\left[-\int_0^t h(u)du\right] = exp\left[-H(t)\right] \tag{5.8}$$

Thus knowledge of any one of the four enables one to determine the other three.

5.2.2   Parametric Models

For a particular set of survival data, the functions defined in Section 5.2.1, may be parametrically estimated by assuming survival follows some parametric distribution or model, "fitting" the data to the model and estimating model parameters by some valid estimation method (such as maximum likelihood). Five commonly used parametric models are the exponential, Weibull, Rayleigh, Gompertz, and log-normal. We describe different settings to which the models may apply.

5.2.2.1   The Exponential Model

The exponential model is used to model a constant hazard function: $h(t) = \lambda_0 > 0$. The exponential death density function is $f(t) = \lambda_0 exp(-\lambda_0 t)$. The exponential survival function is $S(t) = exp(-\lambda_0 t)$. The cumulative death distribution function is $F(t) = 1 - exp(-\lambda_0 t)$.

5.2.2.2   The Weibull Model

The Weibull model derives from a power law hazard function: $h(t) = \lambda_0 \lambda_1 t^{\lambda_1 - 1}$, where $\lambda_0 > 0$ and $\lambda_1 > 0$. It may be noted that $\lambda_1 > 1$ guarantees that $h(t)$ is monotone increasing.

The Weibull death density function is $f(t) = \lambda_0 \lambda_1 t^{\lambda_1 - 1} exp[-\lambda_0 t^{\lambda_1}]$, the Weibull survival function is $S(t) = exp[-\lambda_0 t^{\lambda_1}]$, and the Weibull cumulative death distribution function is $F(t) = 1 - exp[-\lambda_0 t^{\lambda_1}]$.

5.2.2.3   The Rayleigh Model

The Rayleigh model is used to model a linear hazard function: $h(t) = \lambda_0 + 2\lambda_1 t$, where $\lambda_0 > 0$ and $\lambda_1 \geq 0$. It may be noted that if $\lambda_1 > 0$ then $h(t)$ is monotone increasing. The Rayleigh death density function is $f(t) = (\lambda_0 + 2\lambda_1 t)exp[-(\lambda_0 t + \lambda_1 t^2)]$; the Rayleigh survival function is $S(t) = exp[-(\lambda_0 t + \lambda_1 t^2)]$; and the Rayleigh cumulative death distribution function is $F(t) = 1 - exp[-(\lambda_0 t + \lambda_1 t^2)]$.

5.2.2.4   The Gompertz Model

The Gompertz model derives from an exponential hazard function; i.e., $h(t) = exp(\lambda_0 + \lambda_1 t)$. Note that if $\lambda_1 > 0$, then $h(t)$ is monotone increasing. The Gompertz death density function is $f(t) = exp(\lambda_0 + \lambda_1 t) \times exp\left\{\frac{1}{\lambda_1}\left[exp(\lambda_0) - exp(\lambda_0 + \lambda_1 t)\right]\right\}$; the Gompertz survival function is $S(t) = exp\left\{\frac{1}{\lambda_1}\left[exp(\lambda_0) - exp(\lambda_0 + \lambda_1 t)\right]\right\}$; and the cumulative death distribution function is $F(t) = 1 - exp\left\{\frac{1}{\lambda_1}\left[exp(\lambda_0) - exp(\lambda_0 + \lambda_1 t)\right]\right\}$.

5.2.2.5   The Lognormal Model

The lognormal death density function is given by:

$$f(t) = \frac{1}{\sqrt{2\pi}\sigma t}exp\left[-\frac{(log(t) - \mu)^2}{2\sigma^2}\right] \tag{5.9}$$

The lognormal survival function is $S(t) = 1 - \Phi\left[\frac{log(t) - \mu}{\sigma}\right]$, where Φ is the standard cumulative normal distribution. The hazard function is $h(t) = \frac{f(t)}{S(t)}$. The cumulative death distribution function is $F(t) = \Phi\left[\frac{log(t) - \mu}{\sigma}\right]$.

5.3   Statistical Methods for Right-Censored Data

5.3.1   Nonparametric Models: Kaplan-Meier Estimator

Nonparametric approaches to estimate the functions in Section 5.2.1 make no distributional or specific model assumptions about the observed survival times. Therefore, these *nonparametric* methods are sometimes called *distribution-free* methods. The *Kaplan-Meier* estimator is the most commonly used non-parametric method to estimate the survival function.

Based on the definition of survival function, $S(t)$, we can estimate $S(t)$ from a sample of n observations as

$$\hat{S}(t) = \frac{\text{number of patients with observed times} \geq t}{n} \tag{5.10}$$

when there are no censored survival times in the sample. In this case, this estimate in Equation (5.10) is simply the proportion (binomial) of deaths in the total n sample. If one wanted to display uncertainty about the estimates at the times of death, confidence intervals can be constructed at each time of death t using the variance estimate:

$$Var\left[\hat{S}(t)\right] = \frac{\hat{S}(t)[1 - \hat{S}(t)]}{n} \tag{5.11}$$

When there are censored observations, the survival function is estimated by the *Kaplan-Meier* estimator, which extends the simple binomial estimate in Equation (5.10) to incorporate censored observations.

The estimator is presented in detail in Kaplan and Meier (1958) and is based on conditioning on the exact times at which deaths occur. We briefly describe its computation here. First, the observed survival times are ordered from smallest to the largest as $t_{(1)} \leq t_{(2)} \leq \cdots \leq t_{(n)}$, where $t_{(j)}$ is the jth ordered survival time. The Kaplan-Meier estimator of the survival function can be constructed as:

$$\hat{S}(t) = \prod_{R(j)} \left(1 - \frac{e_j}{r_j}\right) \tag{5.12}$$

where r_j is the dimension of the risk set of $R(j) = \{j : t_{(j)} \leq t\}$ and e_j is the number of patients who die at time t_j. The estimated variance of $\hat{S}(t)$ can be obtained as:

$$Var\left[\hat{S}(t)\right] = \left[\hat{S}(t)\right]^2 \prod_{R(j)} \frac{e_j}{r_j(r_j - e_j)} \tag{5.13}$$

5.3.2   Cox Proportion Hazards Regression

The methods presented above do not account for covariate information that might be correlated with survival. In many clinical trials, there exists concomitant, covariate or regressor information on patients in addition to their observed survival times. In such settings, there is interest in assessing the statistical significance of the concomitant information as it relates to the distribution of times-to-death.

Generally this is accomplished using the proportional hazards model proposed by Sir David Cox (1972) (Cox (1972)). The model is specified in terms of the hazard function instead of the survival function, and assumes that additive changes in the concomitant variables correspond to multiplicative changes in the hazard function or, equivalently, to additive changes in the log of the hazard.

In other words, the hazard function reflecting the proportional hazards model is defined as:

$$h(t|X) = exp(X\beta)h_0(t) \tag{5.14}$$

where X is a vector of concomitant, covariate or regressor information $X =$

$(x_1, x_2, \cdots, x_p)$, β is the column vector of parameters $(\beta_1, \beta_2, \cdots, \beta_p)$ corresponding to X, and $h_0(t)$ is the time-specific baseline hazard function defined in Section 5.2.1, sometimes referred to as a homogeneous or baseline hazard function.

Based on this structure in Equation (5.14), the hazard ratio for any two patients with different covariants X_1 and X_2 is constant over time since

$$\frac{h(t|X_1)}{h(t|X_2)} = \frac{exp(X_1\beta)}{exp(X_2\beta)} \tag{5.15}$$

$h_0(t)$ cancels from numerator and denominator of the ratio, and therefore the hazard for one subject is proportional to the hazard of another subject.

From the formulation in Equation (5.14), it is noted that the concomitant information acts in a multiplicative fashion on the time dependent only hazard function. Further, the term proportional hazards also arises by observing that if a x_i is an indicator of treatment group membership ($x_i = 1$ if treatment group 1; $x_i = 0$ if treatment group 0), then the ratio of the hazard for treatment group 1 to the hazard of treatment group 0 is $exp(\beta_i)$; or the hazard for treatment group 1 is proportional to the hazard of treatment group 0. Therefore, $exp(\beta)$ sometimes is referred to as *relative risk*.

As noted by Cox (1972), coefficients of the covariates in the Cox Proportional Hazards model may be estimated and used to provide inferences by maximizing the conditional likelihood arising from the Cox model. In doing so, the actual survival times are not explicitly used in the estimation process, rather they serve as bookkeepers of the covariate information; thus knowledge of the survival time ranks would equally suffice.

In the discussion of Cox's paper, several authors note that the likelihood is not strictly a conditional likelihood. Kalbfleisch and Prentice (2002) use the method of marginal likelihood. Cox (1975) later presents the notion of partial likelihood. Regardless of nomenclature, estimating the covariate coefficients in the Cox model enables one to test the significance of the covariates as well as provide estimates of the relative hazard of one group to another or of one patient to another (using the covariate information of those patients in addition to the estimates of the coefficients).

The survival function arising from the Cox specification of the hazard function in Equation (5.14) may be estimated. If we define $S(t|X)$ as the survival function (i.e., survival probability) at time t for patients with concomittant variable X, then

$$
\begin{aligned}
S(t|X) &= exp\left[-\int_0^t h(u|X)du\right] \\
&= exp\left[-\int_0^t exp(X\beta)h_0(t)du\right] \\
&= exp\left[-exp(X\beta) \times \int_0^t h_0(t)du\right] \\
&= \{exp\left[-H_0(t)\right]\}^{exp(X\beta)} \qquad\qquad (5.16)
\end{aligned}
$$

where $H_0(t)$ is the baseline cumulative hazard. Therefore, when the estimates of $\hat{\beta}$ are obtained, survival probabilities can be estimated for any covariates from clinical trials if we can also estimate the baseline cumulative hazard.

The estimation is based on the principal of maximum partial likelihood. We refer the reader to Cox (1975) or the excellent texts of Lawless (1982), Kalbfleisch and Prentice (2002), and Collett (2003). We demonstrate the implementation in the R system.

5.4   Statistical Methods for Interval-Censored Data

In oncology clinical trials, but also in many other clinical trials, time-to-event data are generated by subjecting the patient to questioning, physical examination or other diagnostic methods at scheduled clinic followup visits. In such trials, the exact times of the event (e.g., cancer, remission, etc.) are not known, rather if the event is present at a particular clinic visit, what one knows is that the event occurred between the last visit and the current visit. Hence, such times-to-event reflect **interval-censored data**. Interval-censored data are commonly produced in clinical trials where there is a non-lethal endpoint, such as the progression-free survival (PFS), time-to-no evidence of disease or time-to-remission in oncology trials.

Due to lack of knowledge of more appropriate statistical methods or inaccessibility of the appropriate statistical software, the common *ad hoc* practice is to approximate the interval-censored data using the left or right endpoint or the midpoint of the interval. Under this convention, well-known statistical methods developed for exact failure time data for right censored data may be utilized. The inference from force fitting exact times-to-event methods to interval censored data may introduce bias and may render inferences therefrom invalid.

Since the seminal Cox proportional hazards regression is not applicable to interval censored data, we introduce the so-called proportional hazards model using an iterative convex minorant (ICM) algorithm for interval censored data as proposed by Pan (1999). This approach is implemented as a *intcox* in the R system. In addition, we introduce Turnbull's nonparametric estimator for interval-censored data as well as some parametric models to fit interval-censored data. A comprehensive discussion can be found in Sun (2006) and Chen et al. (2012). Most of these developed methods are implemented in R package `interval` which is documented in Fay and Shaw (2010) and we will use this package to analyze the interval-censored data in this chapter.

5.4.1 Turnbull's Nonparametric Estimator

For interval censored data, Turnbull (1976) proposed an analog to the Kaplan-Meier product-limit estimator. This is based on an iterative procedure to estimate the survival function $S(t)$ corresponding to the interval-censored data such as those presented in Table 5.2.

To construct Turnbull's estimator, the observed times-to-event are ordered in the same manner as in Kaplan and Meier estimator. Let $0 = \tau_0 < \tau_1 < \tau_2 < \cdots < \tau_m$ be the ordered time points including all left t_{Li} and right t_{Ui} time points in all intervals of $(t_{Li}, t_{Ui}), i = 1, 2, \cdots, n$, from n patients. Notice that m is usually larger than n because of the interval data.

Then, for the ith patient, define an indicator I_{ij} to keep track of whether the interval (τ_{j-1}, τ_j) is completely within the interval $(t_{Li}, t_{Ui}]$ as:

$$I_{ij} = \begin{cases} 1 & \text{if } (\tau_{j-1}, \tau_j) \in (t_{Li}, t_{Ui}] \\ 0 & \text{otherwise} \end{cases} \tag{5.17}$$

where I_{ij} also indicates whether the event that occurred in $(t_{Li}, t_{Ui}]$ could have occurred at τ_j. Based on this indicator, Turnbull's estimator is obtained from the following iterative steps:

1. Make an initial guess at $S(\tau_j)$ and compute

$$p_j = S(\tau_{j-1}) - S(\tau_j) \quad j = 1, 2, \cdots, m$$

2. Compute the number of events occurred at τ_j using

$$e_j = \sum_{i=1}^{n} \frac{p_j I_{ij}}{\sum_{k=1}^{m} p_k I_{ik}} \quad j = 1, 2, \cdots, m$$

3. Compute the estimated number at risk at time τ_j using

$$r_j = \sum_{k=j}^{m} e_k$$

4. Compute the updated product-limit estimator $S(\tau_j)$ using the constructed pseudo-data from Steps 2 to 3.

5. Iterate Steps 1 to 4 and update $S_{new}(\tau_j)$ from the previous step. If $S(\tau_j)$ is close to its value in the previous step for all τ's, stop the iterative process. The convergence of the iterative approach depends on the initial guess of $S(\tau_j)$, which are typically estimated using the Kaplan-Meier estimator.

5.4.2   Parametric Likelihood Estimation with Covariates

The usual likelihood approach starts with the proportional hazards assumption as in Equation (5.14) to combine the covariates $\mathbf{X}$ and the vector of regression coefficients $\boldsymbol{\beta}$ via a linear predictor with the baseline hazard $h_0(t)$.

We are interested in the effect the covariates have on the probability of the occurrence of events as formulated by the survival function

$$S(t|X) = 1 - F(t|X) \tag{5.18}$$

where F is the cumulative distribution function. Similar mathematical manipulation as in Equation (5.16), we have:

$$S(t|X) = S_0(t)^{\exp\{\beta'X\}}. \tag{5.19}$$

where $S_0(t)$ is the baseline survival function which is independent of the covariates. Therefore,

$$
\begin{aligned}
1 - F(t|\mathbf{X}) &= S(t|\mathbf{X}) \\
&= S_0(t)^{\exp(\beta'\mathbf{X})} \\
&= [1 - F_0(t)]^{\exp(\beta'\mathbf{X})}
\end{aligned}
\tag{5.20}
$$

Therefore, for n patients with observed interval censored data of (t_{Li}, t_{Ui}), $i = 1, \cdots, n$, the log-likelihood function with regression parameter vector β and the parameters θ from the baseline distribution can be constructed as follows:

$$LL(F_0, \boldsymbol{\beta}, \theta) = \sum_{i=1}^{n} log\left\{ [1 - F_0(t_{Li}, \theta)]^{\exp(\beta'\mathbf{X}_i)} - [1 - F_0(t_{Ui}, \theta)]^{\exp(\beta'\mathbf{X}_i)} \right\}. \tag{5.21}$$

Commonly used baseline distribution functions F_0 are defined in Section 5.2.2. Statistical estimation and inference is then based on maximum likelihood methods from the Equation (5.21), which has been implemented in R *survival*.

The advantage of this likelihood approach is that we can estimate the regression parameter vector β and the baseline parameters θ simultaneously (see Peace and Flora (1978)). The disadvantage is that we need to specify the baseline F_0 which is contrary to the essence of Cox regression if interest is only in estimates and inferences on the regression parameters.

5.4.3 Semiparametric Estimation: the IntCox

From Section 5.4.2, Pan's semiparametric method is used to estimate the regression parameters β as the parametric part (Pan (1999)). This requires utilizing a nonparametric piecewise constant function to represent the baseline cumulative density function $F_0(t)$ in the likelihood function of Equation (5.21) using the iterative convex minorant (ICM) algorithm. Since the parameter vector θ associated with $F_0(t)$ is eliminated, the log-likelihood function in Equation (5.21) now becomes:

$$L(F_0, \beta) = \sum_{i=1}^{n} log\left\{ [1 - F_0(t_{Li})]^{\exp(\beta' \mathbf{X}_i)} - [1 - F_0(t_{Ui})]^{\exp(\beta' \mathbf{X}_i)} \right\}. \quad (5.22)$$

Henschel, Heiss, and Mansmann implemented Pan's ICM in the R package *intcox*, which can be obtained from following link:

http://cran.r-project.org/web/packages/intcox/

This package has not been further updated and has been removed from the CRAN repository. However, formerly available versions can still be obtained from this weblink. In this section, we briefly describe this implementation. The reader may use the above link to access more information for further development. The implementation requires maximizing the log-likelihood in Equation (5.22) by a modified Newton-Raphson algorithm assuming that the baseline function $F_0(t)$ is a piecewise constant represented by a finite dimensional vector – which is estimated together with the regression parameter β.

With the log-likelihood function in Equation (5.22), the gradients are $\nabla_1 L(F_0, \beta) = \frac{\partial L(F_0, \beta)}{\partial F_0}$ and $\nabla_2 L(F_0, \beta) = \frac{\partial L(F_0, \beta)}{\partial \beta}$. The full Hessian matrix in the original Newton-Raphson algorithm is replaced by the diagonal matrices of the negative second partial derivatives $G_1(F_0, \beta)$ and $G_2(F_0, \beta)$.

The Newton-Raphson algorithm updates $F^{(m+1)}$ from $F^{(m)}$ iteratively by utilizing the stepsize α with initial starting value $\alpha = 1$ as follows:

$$F_0^{(m+1)} = \text{Proj}\left[F_0^{(m)} + \alpha G_1(m)^{-1} \nabla_1 L(m), G_1(m), \mathcal{R} \right]$$
$$\beta^{(m+1)} = \beta^{(m)} + \alpha G_2(m)^{-1} \nabla_2 L(m).$$

To ensure $F_0^{(m+1)}$ is a distribution function, the authors used a projection into the restricted range $\mathcal{R}$ weighted by G as

$$\text{Proj}[y, G, \mathcal{R}] = \arg\min_x \left\{ \sum_{i=1}^{k} (y_i - x_i)^2 G_{ii} : 0 \leq x_1 \leq \cdots \leq x_k \leq 1 \right\}.$$

If $L(F^{(m+1)}) < L(F^{(m)})$, α is halved and the step is reiterated. To expedite convergence, starting values are computed by treating the data as right-censored and using the classical proportional hazards model.

5.5   Step-by-Step Implementations in **R**

We now proceed with data analyses using the R system with a step-by-step approach. We start with the phase-II clinical trial for patients with Stage-2 breast carcinoma given in Table 5.1. This is a typical right-censored survival dataset with interest in the comparative analyses of three treatments. The second dataset is publicly available and represents data from a breast cancer cosmesis trial with interval-censored data where interest is to compare radiotherapy alone versus radiotherapy and adjuvant chemotherapy in the delay of breast retraction. The data is given in Table 5.2.

We read data from Table 5.1 into R with R function `read.csv` and name it as *dat*:

```
> dat          = read.csv("CTCarcinoma.csv", header=T)
> # show first 6 observations using R function "head"
> head(dat)

  TRT Time Status Age
1 S+CT   48      1  26
2 S+CT   55      0  65
3 S+CT   58      1  48
4 S+CT   63      0  53
5 S+CT  102      0  55
6 S+CT  133      0  63
```

5.5.1   Stage-2 Breast Carcinoma

5.5.1.1   Fit Kaplan-Meier

We now load the R package *survival* (maintained by Terry Therneau at the Mayo Clinic) to fit the Kaplan-Meier estimator as described in Section 5.3.1:

```
> # load the R library
> library(survival)
> # fit Kaplan-Meier
> fit.km = survfit(Surv(Time,Status==0)~TRT,
                   type=c("kaplan-meier"),dat)

> # print the model fitting
> fit.km

Call: survfit(formula = Surv(Time, Status == 0) ~ TRT, data = dat,
    type = c("kaplan-meier"))

              n events median 0.95LCL 0.95UCL
```

```
TRT=S+CT     11      6    144    102    NA
TRT=S+CT+IT  10      3    NA     158    NA
TRT=S+IT     10      5    192    144    NA
```

Note that in *fit.km*, *Surv(Time, Status==0)* we create a survival object to be used as the response variable in the survival model fitting of *survfit*. The default for *Status* as event is 1. Since we use 0=dead as the event, we need to tell *Surv* to set *Status = 0* as the event. The model fit object *fit.km* above shows the summary of the model fitting as well as the estimated median survival and the 95% confidence interval.

The estimated survival function by Kaplan-Meier method in Section 5.3.1 may be printed from the fitting object *fit.km* as shown in Table 5.3, and is graphically illustrated in Figure 5.1 with following R code chunk:

```
> plot(fit.km, lty=c(1,4,8),lwd=2,xlab="Time in Weeks",ylab="S(t)")
        legend("bottomleft",title="Line Types",
        c("S+CT","S+CT+IT","S+IT"),lty=c(1,4,8), lwd=2)
```

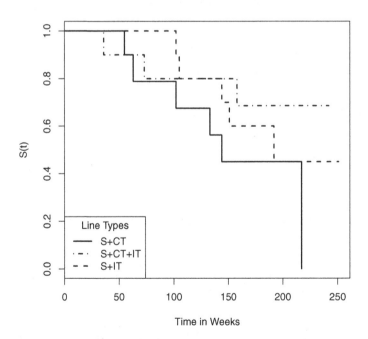

FIGURE 5.1: Kaplan-Meier Estimator for Survival Function

TABLE 5.3: Kaplan-Meier Estimator for Survival Function

time	n.risk	n.event	survival	std.err	lower 95% CI	upper 95% CI
			TRT=S+CT			
48	11	0	1.000	0.0000	1.000	1.000
55	10	1	0.900	0.0949	0.732	1.000
58	9	0	0.900	0.0949	0.732	1.000
63	8	1	0.787	0.1340	0.564	1.000
102	7	1	0.675	0.1551	7 0.430	1.000
133	6	1	0.562	0.1651	0.316	1.000
144	5	1	0.450	0.1660	0.218	0.927
177	4	0	0.450	0.1660	0.218	0.927
182	3	0	0.450	0.1660	0.218	0.927
216	2	0	0.450	0.1660	0.218	0.927
			TRT=S+IT			
102	10	1	0.90	0.0949	0.732	1.000
105	9	1	0.80	0.1265	0.587	1.000
144	8	1	0.70	0.1449	0.467	1.000
151	7	1	0.60	0.1549	0.362	0.995
182	6	0	0.60	0.1549	0.362	0.995
191	5	0	0.60	0.1549	0.362	0.995
192	4	1	0.45	0.1743	0.211	0.961
196	3	0	0.45	0.1743	0.211	0.961
222	2	0	0.45	0.1743	0.211	0.961
251	1	0	0.45	0.1743	0.211	0.961
			TRT=S+CT+IT			
36	10	1	0.900	0.0949	0.732	1
73	9	1	0.800	0.1265	0.587	1
139	8	0	0.800	0.1265	0.587	1
158	7	1	0.686	0.1515	0.445	1
185	6	0	0.686	0.1515	0.445	1
198	5	0	0.686	0.1515	0.445	1
239	4	0	0.686	0.1515	0.445	1
240	2	0	0.686	0.1515	0.445	1
242	1	0	0.686	0.1515	0.445	1

From the table as well as the figure, we note descriptively that survival for chemotherapy and immunotherapy as combined adjuvant treatment to surgery (i.e., "S+CT+IT") is better than immunotherapy as a single adjuvant to surgery (i.e., "S+IT") and that immunotherapy as a single adjuvant (i.e., "S+IT") is better than chemotherapy as a single adjuvant to surgery (i.e., "S+CT"). This outcome is consistent with a priori belief that survival would be ordered as: "S+IT+CT" > "S+IT" > "S+CT".

Estimated median survival for "S+CT" is 144 (weeks) and is 192 (weeks) for "S+IT". For the combined treatment of "S+CT+IT", the estimated survival probability is always above 50%. This conclusion can be supported additionally by estimating the cumulative hazard function using the following R code and displaying the results in Figure 5.2.

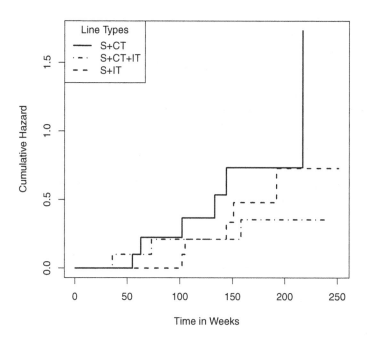

FIGURE 5.2: Nonparametric Estimation for Cumulative Hazard Function

We can test whether these differences are statistically significant as follows:

```
> # use "survdiff" to test difference
> fit.diff = survdiff(Surv(Time, Status==0)~TRT,data=dat)
> fit.diff

Call:
survdiff(formula = Surv(Time, Status == 0) ~ TRT, data = dat)
```

	N	Observed	Expected	(O-E)^2/E	(O-E)^2/V
TRT=S+CT	11	6	3.64	1.52842	2.12654
TRT=S+CT+IT	10	3	5.19	0.92444	1.51837
TRT=S+IT	10	5	5.17	0.00549	0.00887

```
Chisq= 2.5  on 2 degrees of freedom, p= 0.28
```

Since the p-value associated with the χ^2-test is 0.28, we may conclude there is no statistically significantly difference among the three treatments.

This is expected since this trial was a relatively small phase-II clinical trial not designed to have large power to detect specified treatment differences a priori.

5.5.1.2   Fit Weibull Parametric Model

To illustrate the parametric model approach for the baseline hazard described in Section 5.2.2, we use both the exponential and Weibull models. The reader can be guided by the R code to fit other models.

To fit the exponential and Weibull models, we use `survreg` as follows:

```
> # fit exponential model
> fit.exp =survreg(Surv(Time, Status==0)~TRT,dat,
                dist="exponential")
> summary(fit.exp)

Call:
survreg(formula = Surv(Time, Status == 0) ~ TRT, data = dat,
    dist = "exponential")
              Value Std. Error      z        p
(Intercept) 5.449      0.408  13.347  1.23e-40
TRTS+CT+IT  0.919      0.707   1.300  1.94e-01
TRTS+IT     0.401      0.606   0.662  5.08e-01

Scale fixed at 1

Exponential distribution
Loglik(model)= -95   Loglik(intercept only)= -96
        Chisq= 1.81 on 2 degrees of freedom, p= 0.4
Number of Newton-Raphson Iterations: 4
n= 31

> # fit Weibull model
> fit.Weibull =survreg(Surv(Time, Status==0)~TRT,dat)
> summary(fit.Weibull)

Call:
survreg(formula = Surv(Time, Status == 0) ~ TRT, data = dat)
              Value Std. Error      z        p
(Intercept) 5.263      0.221  23.842  1.23e-125
TRTS+CT+IT  0.611      0.388   1.574  1.16e-01
TRTS+IT     0.293      0.326   0.901  3.68e-01
Log(scale) -0.627      0.234  -2.679  7.39e-03

Scale= 0.534

Weibull distribution
```

```
Loglik(model)= -92.2   Loglik(intercept only)= -93.6
        Chisq= 2.77 on 2 degrees of freedom, p= 0.25
Number of Newton-Raphson Iterations: 5
n= 31
```

We note that treatment effects are not statistically significant from either parametric model. The p-values $> 10\%$, consistent with the conclusions from the nonparametric methods in the previous section. Between these two parametric models, the Weibull is statistically a better fit than the exponential since the negative log-likelihood function dropped from 95 to 92.2, resulting in a statistically significantly likelihood ratio test - since $2 \times (95 - 92.2) = 5.6 > \chi^2(0.95, 1) = 3.841$.

Note for the interpretations of the parameters in the `survreg`:

1. *Extreme distribution.* The estimated coefficients (when specifying the *exponential* or the *Weibull* model) are actually those for the extreme value distribution, i.e., the log transform of a random variable following a Weibull distribution.

2. *Exponential distribution.* The MLE of the usual exponential distribution, $\hat{\lambda}_0$ in Section 5.2.2.1 and the R output estimator is related by $\hat{\mu} = log(1/\hat{\lambda}_0) = -log(\hat{\lambda}_0)$, where $\hat{\mu} = (Intercept)$ in the Summary output. That is, $\hat{\lambda}_0 = exp[-(Intercept)]$. For this data, the estimated $\hat{\mu} = (Intercept) = 5.449$. Therefore, the estimated $\hat{\lambda}_0 = 0.0043$, which is statistically significant.

3. *Weibull distribution.* From the R output for the Weibull distribution $(Intercept) = \hat{\mu} = -\frac{ln\hat{\lambda}_0}{\hat{\lambda}_1}$ and $Scale = \hat{\sigma} = 1/\hat{\lambda}_1$. Therefore $\hat{\lambda}_0 = exp(-\hat{\mu} \times \hat{\lambda}_1) = exp\left(-\frac{\hat{\mu}}{\hat{\sigma}}\right) = exp\left(-\frac{(Intercept)}{Scale}\right)$ and $\hat{\lambda}_1 = 1/\hat{\sigma} = 1/Scale$. For this data, $(Intercept) = 5.263$ and $Scale = 0.566$, which are both statistically significant. The estimated parameters for Weibull distribution are then $\hat{\lambda}_0 = 9.1e - 05$ and $\hat{\lambda}_1 = 1.768$. In addition, the regression parameter vector $\hat{\beta}$ is estimated by the negative of the corresponding estimated `Value` from the R output divided by the estimated `Scale` value, i.e., $\hat{\beta} = -\frac{Value}{Scale}$.

Testing for the covariate (i.e., Age) effect can be easily incorporated into `survreg` as

```
> # fit exponential model +Age
> fit.exp.age = survreg(Surv(Time, Status==0)~TRT+Age,
                dat,dist="exponential")
> summary(fit.exp.age)

Call:
```

```
survreg(formula = Surv(Time, Status == 0)~ TRT + Age, data = dat,
    dist = "exponential")
                Value Std. Error      z        p
(Intercept) 11.0560      2.2253  4.968 6.76e-07
TRTS+CT+IT   0.7334      0.7072  1.037 3.00e-01
TRTS+IT      0.2329      0.6068  0.384 7.01e-01
Age         -0.0966      0.0366 -2.636 8.38e-03

Scale fixed at 1

Exponential distribution
Loglik(model)= -91   Loglik(intercept only)= -96
        Chisq= 9.91 on 3 degrees of freedom, p= 0.019
Number of Newton-Raphson Iterations: 5
n= 31

> # fit Weibull model+Age
> fit.Weibull.age = survreg(Surv(Time,Status==0)~TRT+Age,dat)
> summary(fit.Weibull.age)

Call:
survreg(formula = Surv(Time, Status == 0)~ TRT + Age, data = dat)
                Value Std. Error      z        p
(Intercept)  8.5885      1.3214  6.500 8.04e-11
TRTS+CT+IT   0.3899      0.3505  1.112 2.66e-01
TRTS+IT      0.1038      0.2947  0.352 7.25e-01
Age         -0.0569      0.0217 -2.620 8.78e-03
Log(scale)  -0.7294      0.2291 -3.184 1.45e-03

Scale= 0.482

Weibull distribution
Loglik(model)= -87.2   Loglik(intercept only)= -93.6
        Chisq= 12.8 on 3 degrees of freedom, p= 0.0051
Number of Newton-Raphson Iterations: 7
n= 31
```

From both models we note that the "Age" effect is a statistically significant factor for breast carcinoma although the treatment effect remains non-significant.

5.5.1.3   Fit Cox Regression Model

Cox regression eliminates the need to select baseline parametric models as was done in Section 5.5.1.2. Fitting of the Cox model is easily accomplished in the R system using R package *survival*. To do so, the R function coxph is called from the package as follows:

```
> # fit Cox
> fit.Cox = coxph(Surv(Time, Status==0)~TRT,dat)
> summary(fit.Cox)
```

Call:
coxph(formula = Surv(Time, Status == 0) ~ TRT, data = dat)

  n= 31, number of events= 14

	coef	exp(coef)	se(coef)	z	Pr(>|z|)
TRTS+CT+IT	-1.085	0.338	0.716	-1.52	0.13
TRTS+IT	-0.548	0.578	0.608	-0.90	0.37

	exp(coef)	exp(-coef)	lower .95	upper .95
TRTS+CT+IT	0.338	2.96	0.0831	1.37
TRTS+IT	0.578	1.73	0.1755	1.90

Concordance= 0.599 (se = 0.08)
Rsquare= 0.077   (max possible= 0.933)
Likelihood ratio test= 2.49 on 2 df,   p=0.289
Wald test   = 2.41 on 2 df,   p=0.3
Score (logrank) test = 2.57 on 2 df,   p=0.276

```
> # fit Cox +Age
> fit.Cox.age = coxph(Surv(Time, Status==0)~TRT+Age,dat)
> summary(fit.Cox.age)
```

Call:
coxph(formula = Surv(Time, Status == 0) ~ TRT + Age, data = dat)

  n= 31, number of events= 14

	coef	exp(coef)	se(coef)	z	Pr(>|z|)	
TRTS+CT+IT	-0.8621	0.4223	0.7185	-1.20	0.2301	
TRTS+IT	-0.2942	0.7451	0.6120	-0.48	0.6307	
Age	0.1125	1.1191	0.0412	2.73	0.0064	**

	exp(coef)	exp(-coef)	lower .95	upper .95
TRTS+CT+IT	0.422	2.368	0.103	1.73
TRTS+IT	0.745	1.342	0.225	2.47
Age	1.119	0.894	1.032	1.21

Concordance= 0.769 (se = 0.086)
Rsquare= 0.314   (max possible= 0.933)
Likelihood ratio test= 11.7 on 3 df,   p=0.00855
Wald test   = 9.13 on 3 df,   p=0.0276
Score (logrank) test = 9.72 on 3 df,   p=0.0211

Again, the associated p-values for treatment effects are high (all $> 10\%$) indicating non-significance from both fitting treatment alone ($fit.Cox$) as well as fitting treatment with Age as a covariate ($fit.Cox.age$). However, the "Age" effect is significant. This Cox model fitting again confirms the conclusions reached from both nonparametric and parametric model fittings.

5.5.2   Breast Cancer with Interval-Censored Data

Table 5.2 presented a cosmesis dataset for breast cancer patients who were treated with radiotherapy alone versus radiotherapy and adjuvant chemotherapy. The objective was to assess the efficacy of chemotherapy as adjuvant to radiotherapy in delaying the time to first appearance of moderate or severe breast retraction. We load the data into R as:

```
> dat           = read.csv("BreastCancer.csv", header=T)
> head(dat)

  tL tU TRT Status
1  0  7   1      1
2  0  8   1      1
3  0  5   1      1
4  4 11   1      1
5  5 12   1      1
6  5 11   1      1
```

5.5.2.1   Fit Turnbull's Nonparametric Estimator

We implement the Turnbull nonparametric estimator described in Section 5.4.1 in R to estimate the survival function. This implementation is based on Giolo's online paper available at:

http://www.est.ufpr.br/rt/suely04a.htm

Readers may refer to this paper for more detail. We make use of this R program so we can see how easy to implement this estimator in R. We made modifications in order to match the data structure in this chapter.

Based on the description in Section 5.4.1, we first order all time points from left to right for the τ's by creating a R function:

```
> cria.tau = function(data){
  l   = data$tL;r = data$tU
# sort all the time points
  tau = sort(unique(c(l,r[is.finite(r)])))
  return(tau)
  }
```

We obtain an initial estimate for the survival function for Turnbull's non-parametric estimator using Kaplan-Meier estimator by creating the R function:

```
> S.ini = function(tau){
 # take the ordered time
 m     = length(tau)
 # fit the Kaplan-Meier
 ekm   = survfit(Surv(tau[1:m-1],rep(1,m-1))~1)
 # Output the estimated Survival
 So    = c(1,ekm$surv)
 # estimate the step
 p     = -diff(So)
 return(p)
 }
```

Based on these two functions, Turnbull's nonparametric estimator is implemented in R as in the following R code chunk:

```
> cria.A = function(data,tau){
 tau12 = cbind(tau[-length(tau)],tau[-1])
 interv = function(x,inf,sup)
                 ifelse(x[1]>=inf & x[2]<=sup,1,0)
 A     = apply(tau12,1,interv,inf=data$tL,sup=data$tU)
 id.lin.zero = which(apply(A==0, 1, all))
 if(length(id.lin.zero)>0) A = A[-id.lin.zero, ]
 return(A)
 }
> # Turnbull function
> Turnbull = function(p, A, data, eps=1e-3,
          iter.max=200, verbose=FALSE){
 n =nrow(A);m=ncol(A);Q=matrix(1,m)
 iter     = 0
 repeat {
 iter = iter + 1; diff = (Q-p)
 maxdiff = max(abs(as.vector(diff)))
 if (verbose) print(maxdiff)
 if (maxdiff<eps | iter>=iter.max) break
 Q  = p; C  = A%*%p; p=p*((t(A)%*%(1/C))/n)
 }
 cat("Iterations = ", iter,"\n")
 cat("Max difference = ", maxdiff,"\n")
 cat("Convergence criteria: Max difference < 1e-3","\n")
 dimnames(p) = list(NULL,c("P Estimate"))
 surv        = round(c(1,1-cumsum(p)),digits=5)
 right       = data$tU
 if(any(!(is.finite(right)))){
 t = max(right[is.finite(right)])
 return(list(time=tau[tau<t],surv=surv[tau<t]))
 }
```

```
else return(list(time=tau,surv=surv))
}
```

With these functions, we can fit Turnbull's estimator for the breast cosmesis data. We first fit this estimator for $TRT=1$ (i.e., the treatment of "Radiation Only") as:

```
> # get the data for TRT=1
> dat1 = dat[dat$TRT==1,]
> dat1$tU[is.na(dat1$tU)] = Inf
> # sort the time points
> tau  = cria.tau(dat1)
> # Estimate the initial Survival
> p    = S.ini(tau=tau)
> # run Turnbull and name it as "mb1"
> A    = cria.A(data=dat1,tau=tau)
> mb1  = Turnbull(p,A,dat1)

Iterations =   40
Max difference =  0.000982
Convergence criteria: Max difference < 1e-3

> # print the estimates
> mb1

$time
 [1]  0  4  5  6  7  8 10 11 12 14 15 16 17 18 19 22
[17] 24 25 26 27 32 33 34 35 36 37 38 40 44 45 46

$surv
 [1] 1.000 1.000 0.954 0.954 0.920 0.832 0.832 0.832
 [9] 0.761 0.761 0.761 0.761 0.761 0.761 0.761 0.759
[17] 0.751 0.669 0.669 0.669 0.665 0.650 0.588 0.588
[25] 0.588 0.587 0.568 0.474 0.468 0.468 0.468
```

Then we call these functions again to fit Turnbull's estimator for $TRT = 0$ (i.e., the treatment of "Radiation+Chemotherapy") as:

```
> dat0  = dat[dat$TRT==0,]
> dat0$tU[is.na(dat0$tU)] = Inf
> tau   = cria.tau(dat0)
> p     = S.ini(tau=tau)
> A     = cria.A(data=dat0,tau=tau)
> mb0   = Turnbull(p,A,dat0)

Iterations =   30
Max difference =  0.000972
Convergence criteria: Max difference < 1e-3
```

```
> mb0

$time
 [1]  0  4  5  8  9 10 11 12 13 14 15 16 17 18 19 20
[17] 21 22 23 24 25 26 27 30 31 32 34 35 36 39 40 44
[33] 48

$surv
 [1] 1.0000 1.0000 0.9567 0.9134 0.9134 0.9134 0.9134
 [8] 0.8442 0.8442 0.8442 0.8442 0.8438 0.6988 0.6973
[15] 0.5587 0.4437 0.4430 0.4423 0.4408 0.4403 0.3532
[22] 0.3411 0.3392 0.3389 0.2812 0.2751 0.2665 0.2663
[29] 0.1170 0.1106 0.1106 0.1106 0.0553
```

The estimated survival functions for both treatments are shown graphically in Figure 5.3 using the following R code chunk:

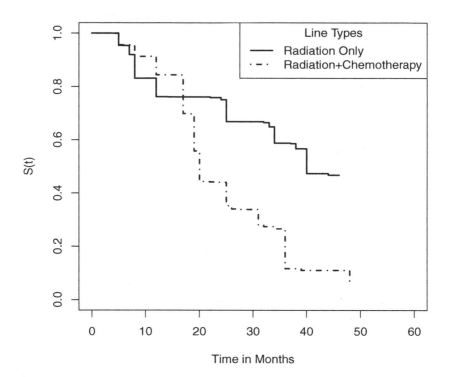

FIGURE 5.3: Turnbull's Nonparametric Estimator for Both Treatments

```
> # plot the TRT=1
> plot(mb1$time,mb1$surv,lty=1,lwd=2,type="s", ylim=c(0,1),
      xlim=range(c(0,60)),xlab="Time in Months",ylab="S(t)")
> # add a line for TRT=0
> lines(mb0$time,mb0$surv,lty=4,lwd=2,type="s")
> # put a legend
> legend("topright",title="Line Types",lty=c(1,4),lwd=2,
  c("Radiation Only","Radiation+Chemotherapy"))
```

From Figure 5.3, we note that the estimated survival (without breast retraction) functions do not differ noticeably in the early stage, say before 20 months. But after 20 months, there is a sharp decline in the curves; particularly for patients in the "Radiation+Chemotherapy" treatment group. For example, at $time = 44$ months, 11.06% of patients are estimated to be free of breast retraction in the "Radiation+Chemotherapy" group, as compared to 46.78% of patients in the "Radiation Only" treatment.

As previously pointed out, many analyses of interval-censored data were performed using non-interval censored data methods, after approximating the interval-censored observations with the midpoint or left or right endpoint of the interval in which they occurred. We noted in addition that this approach could lead to estimation bias. We briefly illustrate the bias using the midpoint approximation here:

```
> # get the midpoint
> time     = dat$tL+((dat$tU-dat$tL)/2)
> # get the censorship
> Status = ifelse(is.finite(time),1,0)
> # replace the NA with left-time
> time     = ifelse(is.finite(time),time,dat$tL)
> # fit Kaplan-Meier model
> ekm      = survfit(Surv(time, Status)~TRT,
                  type=c("kaplan-meier"),dat)
> # print the output
> ekm

Call: survfit(formula = Surv(time, Status) ~ TRT, data = dat,
        type = c("kaplan-meier"))

        n events median 0.95LCL 0.95UCL
TRT=0 48      35   21.5      20    27.5
TRT=1 46      21   40.5      31      NA
```

We overlay the Kaplan-Meier estimates based on midpoints with Turnbull's estimates in Figure 5.4 using following R the code chunk:

```
> plot(mb1$time,mb1$surv,lty=1,lwd=3,type="s",ylim=c(0,1),
    xlim=range(c(0,50)), xlab="Time in Months",ylab="S(t)")
```

```
> legend("bottomleft",title="Line Types",lty=c(1,4),lwd=3,
    c("Radiotherapy Only","Radiotherapy+Chemotherapy"))
> lines(mb0$time,mb0$surv,lty=4,lwd=3,type="s")
> lines(ekm[1]$time,ekm[1]$surv,type="s",lty=4,lwd=1)
> lines(ekm[2]$time,ekm[2]$surv,type="s",lty=1,lwd=1)
```

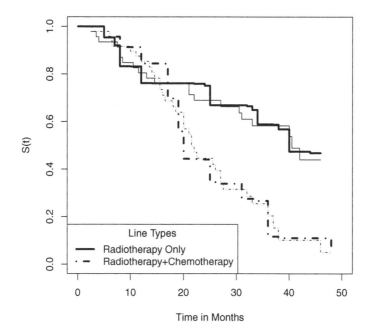

FIGURE 5.4: Turnbull's Estimator Overlaid with Midpoint Kaplan-Meier Estimator

In this figure, the solid lines reflect the "Radiation Only" treatment, and the dashed lines reflect the "Radiation+Chemotherapy" treatment. In addition, the thick lines reflect Turnbull's estimator and the thin lines reflect Kaplan-Meier estimator from the midpoint data. We note from this figure that although both methods have similar trends in estimating the survival curve, the midpoint Kaplan-Meier estimator tends to bias the estimation upward or downward. Readers may wish to reproduce this comparison using the left or right endpoints of the intervals.

5.5.2.2   Fit Turnbull's Nonparametric Estimator Using R Package interval

The analysis in the above section can be performed using the R package interval which can be summarized as follows:

```
> # load the library
> library(interval)
> # fit the NPMLE by calling "icfit" and name it as "fit
> fit.Int = icfit(Surv(tL,tU,type="interval2")~TRT,data=dat)
> # print the summary
> summary(fit.Int)
```

```
TRT=0:
   Interval Probability
1      (4,5]        0.0433
2      (5,8]        0.0433
3    (11,12]        0.0692
4    (16,17]        0.1454
5    (18,19]        0.1411
6    (19,20]        0.1157
7    (24,25]        0.0999
8    (30,31]        0.0709
9    (35,36]        0.1608
10   (44,48]        0.0552
11   (48,60]        0.0552
```

```
TRT=1:
   Interval Probability
1      (4,5]        0.0463
2      (6,7]        0.0334
3      (7,8]        0.0887
4    (11,12]        0.0708
5    (24,25]        0.0926
6    (33,34]        0.0818
7    (38,40]        0.1209
8    (46,48]        0.4656
```

This fit can be illustrated in Figure 5.5 with following R code chunk:

```
> # Call "plot" to plot the survival
> plot(fit.Int, XLAB="Time in Months",
      YLAB="Survival Probability", col=c("lightblue","pink"),
      LEGEND=F,estpar=list(col=c("blue","red"),lwd=3,lty=1))
> # add a legend
legend("bottomleft", col=c("red","blue"),lwd=2,
    legend=c("Radiotherapy Only","Radiotherapy+Chemotherapy"))
```

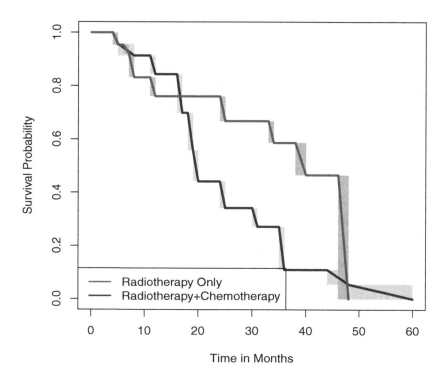

FIGURE 5.5: Turnbull's NPMLE from R Package `interval`

In this figure, the shaded rectangles represent gaps in the interval-censored data, where there is no information on the shape of the survival function. The solid slanted lines, which connect the right ends of each such interval with the left ends of the next, represent only one possible shape for the survival curve and any monotonic non-increasing connecting line would also be a valid estimate for the survival function. This ambiguity is a feature for the interval-censored data.

5.5.2.3 Fitting Parametric Models

The parametric likelihood estimation in Section 5.4.2 is implemented in the R package *survival* using the `survreg` function to call `Surv` with format *Surv(left,right,type = "interval2")*. At the time of writing this chapter, `survreg` cannot handle 0's on the left side of interval (i.e., ther t_L). Therefore, another dataset has to be created to treat the 0's as left-censored data as:

```
> # create a new dataset "breast" and keep "dat" for future use
> breast = dat
> # replace 0's with NA as left-censored
> breast$tL[breast$tL==0]= NA
> # print the first six observations
> head(breast)

  tL tU TRT Status
1 NA  7   1      1
2 NA  8   1      1
3 NA  5   1      1
4  4 11   1      1
5  5 12   1      1
6  5 11   1      1
```

As a check, note that the t_L in the first three observations changed from 0 to NA. Model fitting for the exponential and Weibull is as follows:

```
> # fit exponential
> fit.exp=survreg(Surv(tL,tU,type="interval2")~TRT,
                  breast,dist="exponential")
> summary(fit.exp)

Call:
survreg(formula = Surv(tL, tU, type = "interval2") ~ TRT,
    data = breast, dist = "exponential")
            Value Std. Error     z        p
(Intercept) 3.376      0.170 19.84 1.44e-87
TRT         0.742      0.277  2.68 7.39e-03

Scale fixed at 1

Exponential distribution
Loglik(model)= -150   Loglik(intercept only)= -153
        Chisq= 7.46 on 1 degrees of freedom, p= 0.0063
Number of Newton-Raphson Iterations: 4
n= 94

> # fit Weibull
> fit.Weibull=survreg(Surv(tL,tU,type="interval2")~TRT,data=breast)
> summary(fit.Weibull)

Call:
survreg(formula =Surv(tL,tU,type="interval2")~TRT,data=breast)
            Value Std. Error     z         p
(Intercept) 3.331      0.106 31.29 5.74e-215
TRT         0.568      0.176  3.23  1.23e-03
```

```
Log(scale)  -0.479      0.120 -3.99  6.49e-05
```

```
Scale= 0.619
```

```
Weibull distribution
Loglik(model)= -143   Loglik(intercept only)= -148
        Chisq= 10.9 on 1 degrees of freedom, p= 0.00093
Number of Newton-Raphson Iterations: 5
n= 94
```

We note that the treatment effect is statistically significant (p-value < 5%) from both models which corroborates the conclusion from the Turnbull method.

Between the two parametric models, the Weibull is statistically a better fit than the exponential since the value of the negative log-likelihood function dropped from 149.6 to 142 with one additional "scale" parameter in the Weibull, which resulted in a statistically significantly likelihood ratio test $[2 \times (150 - 143) = 14 > \chi^2(0.95, 1) = 3.841]$.

It is worth noting that the R function `survreg` can accomodate a user defined distribution using the R function `survreg.distributions`.

5.5.2.4 Testing Treatment Effect Using Semiparametric Estimation: IntCox

The method of "IntCox" described in Section 5.4.3 is implemented in the R package *intcox*. We load the package as:

```
> library(intcox)
```

and fit the breast cancer data by calling the `intcox` function as:

```
> fit.IntCox = intcox(Surv(tL,tU,type="interval2")~TRT,data=dat)
```

```
> # print the model fit
> fit.IntCox
```

```
intcox(formula=Surv(tL,tU,type="interval2")~TRT,data=dat)
```

```
      coef exp(coef) se(coef)  z  p
TRT -0.776      0.46       NA NA NA
```

It may be seen from the output of `fit.IntCox` that the estimated treatment coefficient is -0.776. With this fitting, we can extract the estimated piecewise baseline cumulative hazard function to calculate the estimated baseline survival functions for both treatments. We can then display them graphically as in Figure 5.6.

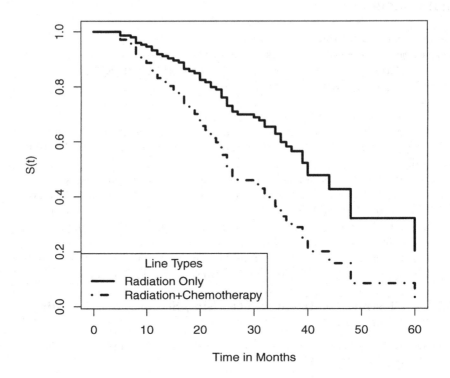

FIGURE 5.6: Estimated Survival Functions from IntCox

The reader may compare this figure with figures from Kaplan-Meier and other methods. Furthermore, we note that the output from intcox (i.e., *fit.IntCox*) is like that from the Cox regression coxph except that no standard errors of the regression parameters are available at the time of writing this chapter. Standard errors for the regression parameters may be estimated using standard bootstrap methods. We obtain random samples of the observed data with replacement for a large number of times and fit the intcox for the resultant bootstrap sample which can be implemented in R easily as:

```
> set.seed(12345678)
> # number of bootstrapping=1000
> num.boot    = 1000
> boot.intcox = numeric(num.boot)
> # the for-loop
> for(b in 1:num.boot){
        #sample with replacement
```

```
        boot.ID=sample(1:dim(dat)[1],replace=T)
        # fit intcox for the bootstrap sample
        boot.fit = intcox(Surv(tL,tU,type="interval2")~TRT,
                    dat[boot.ID,],no.warnings = TRUE)
        # keep track the coefficient
        boot.intcox[b] = coef(boot.fit)
  } # end of b-loop
```

The 95% confidence interval for the treatment effect can be obtained using the R function `quantile` as

```
> Boot.CI = quantile(boot.intcox, c(0.025,0.975))
> Boot.CI

  2.5%  97.5%
-1.412 -0.237
```

Therefore, from this bootstrapping sample, we see that the 95% confidence interval for treatment effect is $(-1.412, -0.237)$ with estimated regression parameter $\hat{\beta} = -0.776$, which again confirms the statistical significance of treatment effect.

In addition, we can use this bootstrapping sample to evaluate the bias between Pan's ICM estimate and the mean/median of the bootstrapping samples as:

```
> bias.IntCox =c(mean.bias=coef(fit.IntCox)-mean(boot.intcox),
          median.bias=coef(fit.IntCox)-median(boot.intcox))
> bias.IntCox

  mean.bias.TRT median.bias.TRT
          0.0248          0.0202
```

This shows that the bias is negligible. The bootstrapping distribution, the confidence interval, and the biases are depicted in Figure 5.7. Overlaying this bootstrapping distribution are the lower (left-most dashed vertical lines) and upper limits (right-most dashed vertical lines) for the 95% confidence interval. The three vertical lines in the middle depict the estimated treatment effect from "intcox", the mean and the median from the bootstrapping sample. Since they are so close, it is difficult to note any differences.

```
> # Histogram from bootstrap sample
> hist(boot.intcox,prob=T,las=1,
 xlab="Treatment Difference",ylab="Prob", main="")
> # put vertical lines for
> abline(v=c(Boot.CI[1],fit.IntCox$coef,mean(boot.intcox),
 median(boot.intcox),Boot.CI[2]), lwd=c(2,3,3,3,2),
 lty=c(4,1,2,3,4))
```

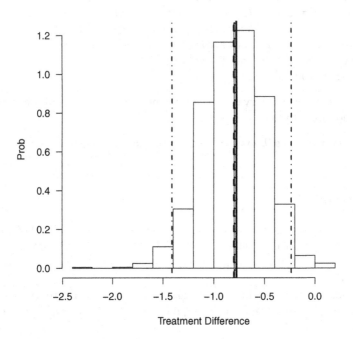

FIGURE 5.7: Bootstrapping Distribution for Treatment Difference

5.5.2.5 Testing Treatment Effect Using Semiparametric Estimation: `ictest`

By using R package `interval`, we can make use of the R function `ictest` to simplify the bootstrapping procedure in the previous section which can be implemented as follows:

```
> # call "ictest" to test "TRT" difference
> test.Int = ictest(Surv(tL,tU,type="interval2")~TRT,data=dat)
> # print the summary
> test.Int

        Asymptotic Logrank two-sample test
        (permutation form), Sun's scores

data:  Surv(tL, tU, type = "interval2") by TRT
Z = -2.68, p-value = 0.007339
alternative hypothesis: survival distributions not equal
```

```
  n Score Statistic*
1 46           -9.25
0 48            9.25
* like Obs-Exp, positive implies earlier failures than expected
```

This gives a $Z = -2.6811$ with p-value $= 0.007339$ indicating statistically significantly different survival functions for these two treatments of "Radiation Only" and "Radiation + Chemotherapy".

5.6 Summary and Discussions

In this chapter, we presented a variety of methods and models for analyzing time-to-event data in clinical trials with step-by-step implementation in the R system. Readers may use the R code and explanations provided in this chapter to analyze their own clinical trial data.

For further reading, we recommend the book by Peace (2009) specifically on design and analysis of variety of clinical trials with time-to-event endpoints. Other general texts on survival analysis can be referred to Lawless (1982), Kalbfleisch and Prentice (2002) and Collett (2003).

For interval-censored data, Lindsey and Ryan (1998) is an excellent article with which to begin to obtain a broad review of the statistical methods for interval-censored data. In this paper, the same breast cancer data in Table 5.2 was used for illustration and the reader may compare the results from this article to those in this chapter (they are exactly the same!). For a comprehensive understanding of theory and analysis of interval-censored data, we recommend the book by Sun (2006) which collects and unifies statistical models and methods in analyzing interval-censored data. Chen et al. (2012) further upgraded the recent development in interval-censored data. As a further extension of interval-censoring, progressive type-I interval-censoring is commonly seen. Readers may refer to Chen and Lio (2010) and the references cited therein.

5.7 Appendix: SAS Programs

The SAS program below corresponds to the R program in Sections 5.3, 5.4, and 5.5.

```
/*read data from the path of dataset*/
Data dat3;
```

```
infile "your path/CTCarcinoma.csv" delimiter="," firstobs=2;
input TRT$ Time Status Age; RUN;

/*print the first 3 observations*/
PROC PRINT data= dat3(obs=3); RUN;

PROC SORT data= dat3 out= dat3;
by descending TRT; RUN;

/***** Section 5.5.1.1 ****************************/
/*fit Kaplan-Meier and
estimate suvival and cumulative harzard function and plot*/
PROC LIFETEST data= dat3;
time Time*Status(1);        /*0 is event, 1 is censored*/
strata TRT; RUN;

/***** Section 5.5.1.2 *********************/
/*fit exponential model*/
PROC LIFEREG data= dat3 order= data;
class TRT;
model Time*Status(1)= TRT / dist= exponential; RUN;

/*fit Weibull model*/
PROC LIFEREG data= dat3 order= data;
class TRT;
model Time*Status(1)= TRT / dist=weibull; RUN;

/*fit exponential model+Age*/
PROC LIFEREG data= dat3 order= data;
class TRT;
model Time*Status(1)= TRT Age / dist= exponential;
RUN;

/*fit Weibull model+Age*/
PROC LIFEREG data= dat3 order= data;
class TRT;
model Time*Status(1)= TRT Age / dist= weibull; RUN;

/**** Section 5.5.1.3   ****************/
/*fit Cox regression model*/
PROC PHREG data= dat3;
class TRT(ref= "S+CT");
model Time*Status(1)= TRT/ ties=efron; RUN;

/*fit Cox regression model+Age*/
```

```
PROC PHREG data= dat3;
class TRT(ref= "S+CT");
model Time*Status(1)= TRT Age/ ties=efron; RUN;

/***     Section 5.5.2  ******************/
/*read data from the path of dataset*/
Data dat4;
infile "your path/BreastCancer.csv" delimiter="," firstobs=2;
input tL tU$ TRT Status;
if tU= "NA" then tU= .;
ntU= tU+0;       /* transform the type of variable "tU"
                       from char to int*/
if ntU= . then time= tL;
else time= (tL+ntU)/2;
if tL= 0 then ntL= .;
else ntL= tL; RUN;

PROC SORT data= dat4 out= dat4;
by descending TRT; RUN;

/****** Section 5.5.2.1  ******************/
/*fit Turnbull's estimator*/
PROC ICLIFETEST data= dat4 impute(seed= 123) method= turnbull;
strata TRT;
time (tL,ntU);
RUN;

/*fit Kaplan-Meier estimator with midpoint or left point*/
PROC LIFETEST data= dat4;
time time*Status(0);         /*0 is censored, 1 is event*/
strata TRT; RUN;

/*** Section 5.5.2.2 ********************/
/*fit exponential model*/
PROC LIFEREG data= dat4 order= data;
class TRT;
model (ntL, ntU)= TRT / dist= exponential;RUN;

/*fit Weibull model*/
PROC LIFEREG data= dat4 order= data;
class TRT;
model (ntL, ntU)= TRT / dist= weibull; RUN;
```

Chapter 6

Longitudinal Data Analysis for Clinical Trials

In this chapter, we analyze response data from longitudinal clinical trials using the R system. The primary feature of response data from longitudinal clinical trials is that it is measured over time on each clinical trial participant in addition to the baseline covariates. Therefore, an objective in the analysis of such data is to model its change over time along with the effects of treatment and covariates incorporating the correlations from time to time.

Two clinical trial datasets are used in this chapter to illustrate the analysis of longitudinal data as outlined in Section 6.1. Specifically, we continue the analyses in Chapters 3 and 4 and use the same diastolic blood pressure data which are observed longitudinally with four post-randomization measurements to illustrate the longitudinal modeling for continuous data. In addition, we use a clinical trial on duodenal ulcer healing to illustrate the longitudinal modeling for categorical data. The statistical models used to analyze these data appear in Section 6.2. Step-by-step implementation of the models in R is illustrated in Section 6.3. A summary and discussion session follow in Section 6.4.

6.1 Clinical Trials

6.1.1 Diastolic Blood Pressure Data

We re-analyze the diastolic blood pressure data in Table 3.1 from Chapter 3. In this table, diastolic blood pressure (DBP) was measured (mmHg) in the supine position at baseline (i.e., "DBP1") before randomization and monthly thereafter up to 4 months as indicated by "DBP2", "DBP3", "DBP4", and "DBP5". Patients' age and sex were recorded at baseline and represent potential covariates. The primary objective for this analysis is to test whether treatment A (new drug) may be effective in lowering DBP as compared to B (placebo). Secondary objectives are to test for longitudinal effects and assess the effect of the two covariates.

6.1.2 Clinical Trial on Duodenal Ulcer Healing

A duodenal ulcer healing trial was considered in Chapter 3. Specifically, we analyzed the cumulative 4-week healing data from that trial. We will revisit that trial in this chapter by providing a longitudinal analysis of the data available at the interim analysis in that trial.

Patients were followed by endoscopic evaluation at week 1 (Days 7-8), week 2 (Days 13-15), and week 4 (Days 26-30). Patients whose ulcers were healed at any followup endoscopy were considered trial completers and received no further treatment or endoscopic assessment. The primary efficacy data was ulcer healing at week 1, 2, or 4. Ulcer healing was defined as complete reepitheliation of the ulcer crater (normal or hyperemic mucosa), documented by endoscopy. The primary efficacy endpoint was cumulative ulcer healing at week 4. Baseline data from patients were collected for age, height, weight, sex, race, day or night pain, ulcer size, and smoking status. Since ulcer healing was expected to be negatively correlated with smoking and baseline ulcer size, and many centers were recruited with relatively few patients per treatment group per strata per center, 12 analysis blocks reflecting smoking status (2 levels)-by-baseline ulcer size (6 levels) were defined a priori (see Table 12.2 in Peace and Chen (2010)).

An interim analysis was performed when approximately half the planned number of patients had completed (N = 337 patients). There were 76, 83, 85, and 93 patients in the Placebo, 400 mg C, 800 mg C, and 1600 mg C, respectively. The cumulative duodenal ulcer healing rates were: 19%, 18%, 16%, and 21% at week 1; 29%, 37%, 38%, and 49% at week 2; and 41%, 62%, 72%, and 74% at week 4; for the Placebo, 400 mg C, 800 mg C, and 1600 mg C groups, respectively. At week 4: 800 mg C was effective (p-value < 0.00001) as compared to Placebo; 800 mg C was marginally superior to 400 mg C; and 1600 mg C provided no clinically significant greater benefit than did 800 mg C. Even though 800 mg C healed 10% more ulcers than did 400 mg C, the p-value for this comparison did not achieve statistical significance. Therefore, the interim analysis did not confirm the trial objective; i.e., that 800 mg C was clinically optimal.

In this chapter, the interim data were generated (simulated) using summary information from Chapter 12 in Peace and Chen (2010) to demonstrate the application of statistical methods in the analysis of non-normal endpoints from longitudinal clinical trials. Table 6.1 summarizes this generation. The detailed patient data appear in Section 6.3.

TABLE 6.1: Ulcer Trial Data

	Placebo	400 mg C	800 mg C	1600 mg C
Total	76	83	85	93
Week 1 (n_1)	14	15	14	19
Week 2 (n_2)	22	31	33	45
Week 4 (n_4)	31	51	62	68
Week 1 (p_1)	18.42%	18.07%	16.47%	20.43%
Week 2 (p_2)	28.95%	37.35%	38.82%	48.39%
Week 4 (p_4)	40.79%	61.45%	72.94%	73.12%

6.2 Statistical Models

6.2.1 Linear Mixed Models

We begin with the basic regression model. When modeling a response variable y in terms of a vector of explanatory variables X (such as treatment effect and the covariates: age, weight, etc.) in clinical trials, the typical model is the linear regression model that includes factors from the usual ANOVA and ANCOVA models. The regression model may be written in matrix form as:

$$y = X\beta + \epsilon \tag{6.1}$$

This model is also called the "fixed-effects model" with common assumption of normal errors and may be written as:

$$y \sim N(X\beta, \sigma^2 I) \tag{6.2}$$

where X is an $n \times p$ model matrix and β is a vector of length p. The parameter vector β is estimated using least squares or maximum likelihood methods, which are the same under the assumption of normally distributed errors.

In clinical trials to investigate the effectiveness of a new treatment on a sample of patients, treatment effect is usually assumed to be fixed in the modeling process, whereas patient effects are considered to be random. We are interested in the average trend/effect of the patient population instead of the effect for a particular patient. The regression model above indicates that the response (y) on a particular patient is explained by an effect $X\beta$ common to all patients plus a component ϵ reflecting random error in measuring y in each patient.

Fundamental to random-effects modeling is to estimate the distribution characteristics (such as the mean and variance) for the random-effects. The fixed-effects model in Equation (6.1) may be generalized to a mixed-effects model with an additional term for random-effects γ of dimension q with associated $n \times q$ model matrix Z. Therefore, this mixed-effects model may be written to model the response y, given the value of the random-effects as:

$$y = X\beta + Z\gamma + \epsilon \quad \text{i.e.,} \quad y|\gamma \sim N(X\beta + Z\gamma, \sigma^2 I) \tag{6.3}$$

Since γ is the random effect, it is usually assumed that $\gamma \sim N(0, \sigma^2 D)$ then we can show $var(y) = var(Z\gamma) + var(\epsilon) = \sigma^2 ZDZ' + \sigma^2 I = \sigma^2(ZDZ' + I)$. Therefore, the random-effects model in Equation (6.3) may be re-written as:

$$y \sim N\left(X\beta, \sigma^2(I + ZDZ')\right) \tag{6.4}$$

The random-effects model in Equation (6.4) may be further generalized (repeated measures) to clinical trials where several measurements are taken repeatedly on each patient. So-called longitudinal clinical trials are those when repeated measurements are taken over time, which includes almost all clinical trials. It is expected that measurements taken repeatedly over time would be correlated. The random-effects model in Equation (6.3) may be further generalized to incorporate the correlation structure as:

$$y|\gamma \sim N\left(X\beta + Z\gamma, \sigma^2\Lambda\right) \tag{6.5}$$

where Λ is a covariance matrix used to model the correlation structure. With this generalization, we can show $V = var(y) = var(Z\gamma) + var(\epsilon) = \sigma^2 ZDZ' + \sigma^2\Lambda = \sigma^2(\Lambda + ZDZ')$. Therefore, the general mixed-effects model which models the fixed-effects of treatment and covariates and the random-effects (such as patient effects, etc.) as well repeated/longitudinal measurements may be re-written as:

$$y \sim N\left(X\beta, \sigma^2(\Lambda + ZDZ')\right) = N(X\beta, V) \tag{6.6}$$

Several methods are employed for parameter estimation and statistical inference. One method is classical maximum likelihood estimation, which requires finding values of the unknown parameters that maximize the log-likelihood function as follows:

$$l(\beta, \sigma, D, \Lambda|y) \propto -log|\sigma^2 V| - \frac{1}{\sigma^2}(y - X\beta)'V^{-1}(y - X\beta) \tag{6.7}$$

A commonly used method for parameter estimation for the model in Equation (6.6) is the *restricted maximum likelihood (REML)* estimator. The basic idea is to search for a linear combination of k to make $k'X = 0$. With this k, we would have:

$$k'y \sim N(0, k'Vk) \tag{6.8}$$

This pivotal transformation eliminates the fixed-effects $X\beta$ from the estimation so that we can estimate the parameters associated with V only from maximizing the likelihood. This *REML* has been shown to produce less biased estimates than MLE.

Pinheiro and Bates (2000) describe the theory and implementation of

REML in the R system. Their book includes an R package *nlme* to fit these models. An updated version of this package called *lme4* is available in CRAN. However, this package does not list the p-values for their fixed-effects estimates as discussed by the creator, Professor Bates in (`https://stat.ethz.ch/pipermail/r-help/2006-May/094765.html`). More discussions can be found in `http://glmm.wikidot.com/faq`. Dr. Alexandra Kuznetsova (`alku@dtu.dk`) expanded *lme4* to *lmerTest* with different kinds of tests on `lmer` objects which include 1) F-tests of types I-III hypotheses for the fixed-effects, 2) likelihood-ratio tests for the random-effects, 3) least squares means (population means), and 4) differences of least squares means for the factors of the fixed-effects with corresponding plots. This package also provides a function step to perform backward elimination of non-significant effects starting from the random-effects and then going to fixed-effects. We use this package in this chapter to illustrate the longitudinal data analysis. We would like to note that we used *lme4* in the first edition of this book. Interested readers can compare the results from both packages and it can be seen that all parameter estimates are the same for both packages of *lme4* and *lmerTest* except the p-values are given in *lmerTest* in this revision.

6.2.2 Generalized Linear Mixed Models

Extending the linear mixed-effects models from Section 6.2.1 to generalized linear mixed-effects models (GLMM), we can analyze non-normal repeated endpoints from longitudinal clinical trials. In principle, the generalized linear mixed model synchronizes ideas from both the linear mixed-effects model described in Section 6.2.1 and the generalized linear model where the clinical response/endpoint is a random variable following a distribution from an exponential family; i.e.,

$$f(y|\theta,\phi) = exp\left[\frac{y\theta - b(\theta)}{a(\phi)} + c(y,\phi)\right] \qquad (6.9)$$

Similarly the link function $\eta = g(\mu)$ is used to link the mean function of $E(Y) = \mu = \theta$ (assume canonical link) to the linear predictor $\eta = X\beta + Z\gamma$. Then the likelihood function with n observations is written as:

$$L(\beta,\phi,V|y) = \prod_{i=1}^{n}\int f(y_i|\beta,\phi,\gamma)h(\gamma|V)d\gamma \qquad (6.10)$$

Where $h(\gamma|V)$ denotes the random-effects γ with parameter V. The integral in this likelihood for non-normal clinical endpoints makes the computations necessary to maximize this likelihood difficult. Therefore, approximation approaches are used. There are several ways to approximate the likelihood as well as numerous ways to implement the GLMM in R. A commonly used method is the so-called "Penalized Quasi-Likelihood method" in the *MASS* by Venables and Ripley (2002). The R packages *lme4* and *nlme* may also be used to fit this GLMM.

6.2.3   Generalized Estimating Equation

The generalized estimating equation (GEE) approach is the version of quasi-likelihood approach for repeated measures and/or longitudinal studies derived when no distributional assumptions are made. GEE was first proposed by Liang and Zeger (1986). The GEE is essentially the multivariate extension of the generalized linear model and the quasi-likelihood method. This quasi-likelihood approach requires only the link function and the variance. Suppose that y is a vector of random variables representing the responses or endpoints on patients from clinical trials and let $E(y) = \mu$. Again, a link function is used to link this mean function to the linear predictor with parameter β as $\eta = X\beta$. We specify the variance function as:

$$var(y) = var(y; \beta, \alpha) \tag{6.11}$$

where α is a vector of parameters to model the correlation structure within patients in clinical trials. Therefore, the GEE for regression parameters, β, is

$$\sum_i \left(\frac{\partial \mu_i}{\partial \beta} \right)' \frac{Y_i - \mu_i}{var(Y_i)} = 0 \tag{6.12}$$

Similar GEE for α may be derived. Note that we only need to specify the mean and variance functions. The mean function may be specified as a link function of the regression parameters. This makes fitting and specification simpler. As seen from Hardin and Hilbe (2003), the estimates of β are consistent even if the variance is misspecified. For a complete description, the reader is referred to this book and the implementation of GEE in the R package *gee*.

6.3   Longitudinal Data Analysis for Clinical Trials

6.3.1   Analysis of Diastolic Blood Pressure Data

We read in the data from Table 3.1 into R with the R function `read.csv` and name it as *dat*:

```
> dat  = read.csv("DBP.csv",header=T)
> # show first a few observations
> head(dat)

  Subject TRT DBP1 DBP2 DBP3 DBP4 DBP5 Age Sex
1       1   A  114  115  113  109  105  43   F
2       2   A  116  113  112  103  101  51   M
3       3   A  119  115  113  104   98  48   F
```

4	4	A	115	113	112	109	101	42	F
5	5	A	116	112	107	104	105	49	M
6	6	A	117	112	113	104	102	47	M

Readers may refer to Table 3.1 for all the data. Summary information for the data is produced as:

```
> summary(dat)
    Subject        TRT        DBP1            DBP2
 Min.   : 1.0   A:20   Min.   :114   Min.   :111
 1st Qu.:10.8   B:20   1st Qu.:115   1st Qu.:113
 Median :20.5          Median :116   Median :115
 Mean   :20.5          Mean   :117   Mean   :114
 3rd Qu.:30.2          3rd Qu.:118   3rd Qu.:115
 Max.   :40.0          Max.   :121   Max.   :119
      DBP3            DBP4            DBP5            Age        Sex
 Min.   :100   Min.   :102   Min.   : 97   Min.   :38.0   F:18
 1st Qu.:112   1st Qu.:107   1st Qu.:102   1st Qu.:42.0   M:22
 Median :113   Median :109   Median :106   Median :48.0
 Mean   :112   Mean   :109   Mean   :107   Mean   :47.8
 3rd Qu.:113   3rd Qu.:113   3rd Qu.:112   3rd Qu.:51.2
 Max.   :118   Max.   :117   Max.   :115   Max.   :63.0
```

6.3.1.1 Data Graphics and Response Feature Analysis

We start the data analysis with data graphics to illustrate the data and reveal the data trend longitudinally. The dataframe `dat` is in *wide* format and should be transformed into *long* format for further longitudinal data analysis. The R function **reshape reshapes** the data from "wide" to "long" as follows:

```
> # reshape the data into "long" direction
> Dat = reshape(dat, direction="long",
  varying=c("DBP1","DBP2","DBP3","DBP4","DBP5"),
  idvar = c("Subject","TRT","Age","Sex"),sep="")
> # rename the variables
> colnames(Dat) = c("Subject","TRT","Age","Sex","Time","DBP")
```

As a preliminary data analysis, we plot the DBP as a function of time points for each patient as seen in Figure 6.1. In this figure, the first 20 patients (from treatment A) are plotted using a solid line and the next 20 patients (from treatment B) are plotted using dashed lines. This figure is produced with the following R code chunk:

```
> # load the library
> library(lattice)
> # use "xyplot"
> print(xyplot(DBP~Time|as.factor(Subject),type="l",
    groups=TRT,lty=c(1,8),lwd=2,layout=c(10,4), Dat))
```

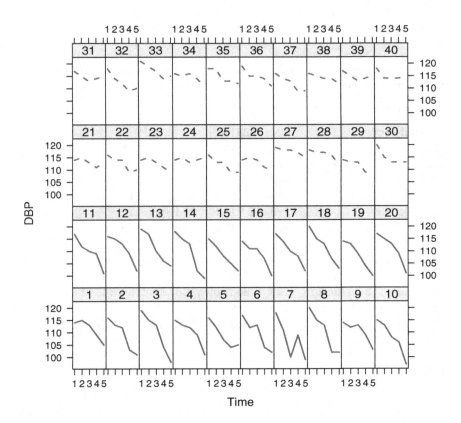

FIGURE 6.1: DBP as a Function of Time for Each Patient

For a better presentation of trend, this plot may be grouped for all patients as seen in Figure 6.2 with following R code chunk:

```
> print(xyplot(DBP~Time|TRT,type="l",Dat,
                groups=as.factor(Subject)))
```

From this figure, the obvious trend is revealed; i.e., that on average DBP declines at a faster rate in treatment A than in treatment B. We also note that the magnitude of the decline in treatment A is greater than that in treatment B. However, the rate and extent of decline varies across the 40 patients.

Further presentation of trend may be generated in a boxplot as seen in Figure 6.3 with boxplots.

```
> print(bwplot(DBP~as.factor(Time)|TRT,Dat, xlab="Time"))
```

Again, we note that the rate and extent of the decline in DBP is greater in treatment group A than in treatment group B. We further investigate the

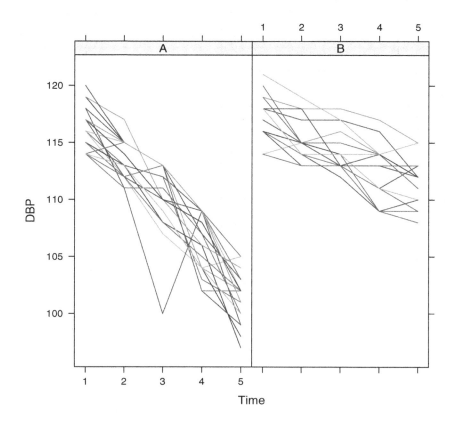

FIGURE 6.2: DBP as a Function of Time Grouped for All Patients

declining trend by estimating the slope and intercept for each patient as depicted in Figures 6.1 and 6.2. To do so, we first loop-over the 40 patients to fit linear regressions and then extract the intercepts and slopes to make a dataframe as follows:

```
> num.Subj = 40
> # initiate the intercept and slope
> intercept = slope = numeric(num.Subj)
> # loop-over
> for(i in 1:num.Subj){
 # fit regression model
 mod         = lm(DBP~Time, Dat[Dat$Subject==i,])
 # extract the intercept and slope
 intercept[i] = coef(mod)[1]
 slope[i]    = coef(mod)[2]
 }
```

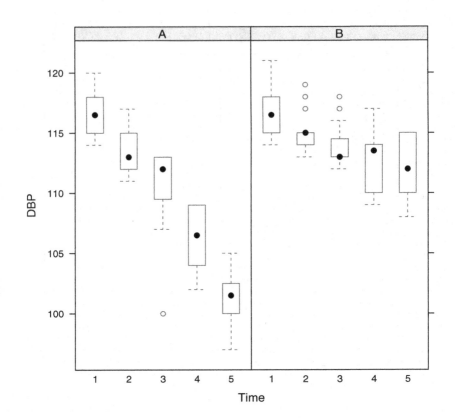

FIGURE 6.3: Boxplot by Treatments

```
> # make a dataframe "dat.coef"
> dat.coef = data.frame(Subject=dat$Subject,TRT=dat$TRT,
          Intercept = intercept, Slope=slope)
> # print it out
> dat.coef

  Subject TRT Intercept Slope
1       1   A       118  -2.4
2       2   A       121  -4.0
3       3   A       126  -5.3
4       4   A       120  -3.2
5       5   A       118  -3.0
6       6   A       121  -3.8
7       7   A       119  -4.0
8       8   A       125  -4.9
9       9   A       118  -2.5
```

10	10	A	121	-4.3
11	11	A	120	-3.5
12	12	A	121	-3.4
13	13	A	124	-4.1
14	14	A	125	-5.1
15	15	A	118	-3.3
16	16	A	118	-3.2
17	17	A	121	-3.6
18	18	A	124	-4.2
19	19	A	119	-3.7
20	20	A	122	-3.8
...Removed	......			
31	31	B	116	-0.5
32	32	B	119	-2.1
33	33	B	122	-1.7
34	34	B	118	-1.1
35	35	B	120	-1.7
36	36	B	120	-1.7
37	37	B	118	-1.9
38	38	B	117	-0.9
39	39	B	116	-0.5
40	40	B	117	-0.6

We note that the intercepts vary about 120 **mmHg** with a slope of about -2.5 mmHg/month. A bivariate plot of the intercept and slope from the 40 patients is shown in Figure 6.4 with following R code:

```
> # Make histogram for both intercept and slope
> int.hist   = hist(intercept,plot=F)
> slope.hist = hist(slope,plot=F)
> # make layout for plotting
> top=max(c(int.hist$counts, slope.hist$counts))
> nf =layout(matrix(c(2,0,1,3),2,2,byrow=T),c(3,1),c(1,3),T)
> par(mar=c(5,4,1,1))
> # plot the intercept and slope
> plot(Slope~Intercept,las=1,dat.coef,xlab="Intercept",
            ylab="Slope",pch=as.character(TRT))
> par(mar=c(0,4,1,1))
> # add the intercept and slope histograms
> barplot(int.hist$counts, axes=FALSE,ylim=c(0,top),space=0)
> par(mar=c(5,0,1,1))
> barplot(slope.hist$counts,axes=FALSE,xlim=c(0,top),
            space=0,horiz=TRUE)
```

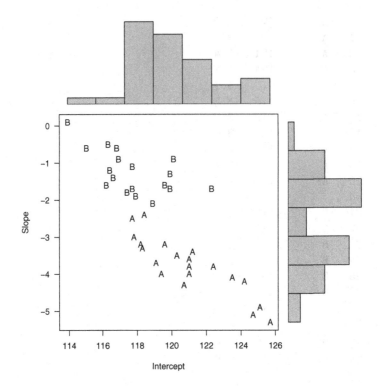

FIGURE 6.4: Bivariate Plot for Intercept and Slope

This figure clearly shows the declining trend by treatment group. The slope declines faster in treatment group A than in treatment group B. The average baseline DBP is about 120 mmHg as characterized by the intercept. The variations embedded in the intercepts and slopes illustrate the modeling of random-effects for both intercept and slope.

We now model the slope and intercept relationship by a linear regression as follows (in doing so, we fit two models: one with and one without interaction):

```
> # fit model 1 with interation
> mod1.coef = lm(Slope~Intercept*TRT, dat.coef)
> summary(mod1.coef)

Call:
lm(formula = Slope ~ Intercept * TRT, data = dat.coef)

Residuals:
    Min      1Q  Median      3Q     Max
-0.6636 -0.2947 -0.0314  0.3470  0.7532
```

```
Coefficients:
                Estimate Std. Error t value Pr(>|t|)
(Intercept)      28.3374     4.6874    6.05  6.0e-07
Intercept        -0.2654     0.0387   -6.85  5.2e-08
TRTB             -8.2964     7.3796   -1.12    0.27
Intercept:TRTB    0.0848     0.0620    1.37    0.18
```

```
Residual standard error: 0.429 on 36 degrees of freedom
Multiple R-squared:  0.919,       Adjusted R-squared:  0.912
F-statistic:  136 on 3 and 36 DF,  p-value: <2e-16
```

```
> # fit model 2 without interaction
> mod2.coef = lm(Slope~Intercept+TRT, dat.coef)
> summary(mod2.coef)
```

```
Call:
lm(formula = Slope ~ Intercept + TRT, data = dat.coef)
```

```
Residuals:
    Min     1Q  Median     3Q     Max
-0.7332 -0.3849  0.0281  0.3348  0.8727
```

```
Coefficients:
            Estimate Std. Error t value Pr(>|t|)
(Intercept) 24.3322     3.7022    6.57  1.1e-07 ***
Intercept   -0.2323     0.0306   -7.59  4.7e-09 ***
TRTB         1.7914     0.1683   10.64  8.2e-13 ***
```

```
Residual standard error: 0.434 on 37 degrees of freedom
Multiple R-squared:  0.915,       Adjusted R-squared:  0.91
F-statistic:  198 on 2 and 37 DF,  p-value: <2e-16
```

From Model 1, the interaction (Intercept: TRTB) is not statistically significant. From Model 2, there is a significant difference between the two treatments (TRT B). Further analysis of the difference between treatments may be performed using the t-test as:

```
> # test slope difference
> t.test(Slope~TRT, dat.coef)
```

```
        Welch Two Sample t-test
```

```
data:  Slope by TRT
t = -10, df = 40, p-value = 1e-13
alternative hypothesis: true difference in means is not equal to 0
95 percent confidence interval:
```

```
 -2.97 -2.09
sample estimates:
mean in group A mean in group B
          -3.76             -1.23

> # test intercept difference
> t.test(Intercept~TRT, dat.coef)

        Welch Two Sample t-test

data:  Intercept by TRT
t = 4, df = 40, p-value = 1e-04
alternative hypothesis: true difference in means is not equal to 0
95 percent confidence interval:
 1.70 4.66
sample estimates:
mean in group A mean in group B
          121             118
```

In the analysis of data from longitudinal clinical trials, the preliminary data analysis in this section is called *response feature* analysis. The analysis extracts fundamental features from each patient for simple and preliminary data exploration and summarization. This feature analysis provides basic summary information from the data for simple conclusions in addition to providing directions for further analysis. However, the analysis loses information since other features are included. A more efficient analysis is to use all the information from the data in a comprehensive manner; i.e., capture the longitudinal or repeated measures nature of the data.

6.3.1.2   Longitudinal Modeling

In this analysis, we fit a series models to help in determining the best model using the updated R package *lme4*. Interested readers can follow the analysis using R package *nlme* to reproduce the results. First we fit "Model 1" with TRT-by-Time interaction as random-effects on the intercept and slope on Time and compare it to the "Model 2" with random-intercept only:

```
> # load the library lmerTest
> library(lmerTest)
> # Fit Model 1
> mod1DBP =  lmer(DBP~TRT*Time+(Time|Subject), Dat)
> # Fit Model 2
> mod2DBP =  lmer(DBP~TRT*Time+(1|Subject), Dat)
> # model comparison
> anova(mod1DBP, mod2DBP)
```

```
Data: Dat
Models:
..1: DBP ~ TRT * Time + (1 | Subject)
object: DBP ~ TRT * Time + (Time | Subject)
       Df AIC BIC logLik deviance Chisq Chi Df  Pr(>Chisq)
..1     6 885 904   -436      873
object  8 886 913   -435      870  2.12      2  0.35
```

Model 1 includes an interaction effect between "TRT" and "Time" with both intercept and slope as random-effects; whereas Model 2 relaxes the random-effects on slope and includes intercept as the random effect. From the "anova" test for model comparison, we note that the *p*-value is 0.35 which means that these two models are not statistically significantly different. The simpler "Model 2" is thus recommended. The summary of this model fit can be printed as follows:

> *summary(mod2DBP)*

```
Linear mixed model fit by REML t-tests use
  Satterthwaite approximations to degrees of  freedom
  [lmerMod]
Formula: DBP ~ TRT * Time + (1 | Subject)
   Data: Dat

REML criterion at convergence: 878

Scaled residuals:
    Min     1Q Median     3Q    Max
 -4.203 -0.542 -0.051  0.554  2.333

Random effects:
 Groups    Name        Variance Std.Dev.
 Subject   (Intercept) 1.38     1.17
 Residual              3.81     1.95
Number of obs: 200, groups:  Subject, 40

Fixed effects:
             Estimate Std. Error      df t value  Pr(>|t|)
(Intercept)  120.965      0.528 159.200  229.14  < 2e-16 ***
TRTB          -3.180      0.747 159.200   -4.26  3.5e-05 ***
Time          -3.765      0.138 158.000  -27.26  < 2e-16 ***
TRTB:Time      2.530      0.195 158.000   12.95  < 2e-16 ***

Correlation of Fixed Effects:
          (Intr) TRTB    Time
TRTB      -0.707
```

```
Time        -0.785  0.555
TRTB:Time   0.555  -0.785 -0.707
```

We can further investigate the interaction effect between TRT and Time using two additional models ("Model 3" and "Model 4") as follows:

```
> # fit Model 3
> mod3DBP = lmer(DBP~TRT+Time+(Time|Subject), Dat)
> # fit Model 4
> mod4DBP = lmer(DBP~TRT+Time+(1|Subject), Dat)
> # model comparison
> anova(mod3DBP, mod4DBP)
```

```
Data: Dat
Models:
..1: DBP ~ TRT + Time + (1 | Subject)
object: DBP ~ TRT + Time + (Time | Subject)
        Df AIC  BIC  logLik deviance Chisq Chi Df  Pr(>Chisq)
..1      5 998  1015 -494            988
object   7 945  968  -466            931   57    2   4.2e-13 ***
```

In Model 3, we removed the interaction effect between TRT and Time, but transferred the interaction into the random-effects by keeping the random-effects for both intercept and slope to contrast with Model 2. Model 4 is a further simplified version of Model 3 that has intercept as the only random-effects. From the comparison of these two models, we note that Model 3 is statistically significantly different from Model 4 as indicated by the small p-value (< 0.0001). We therefore utilize Model 3 further to investigate the effects from the covariates. The summary for Model 3 fitting can be printed as follows:

```
> summary(mod3DBP)
```

```
Linear mixed model fit by REML t-tests use
  Satterthwaite approximations to degrees of  freedom
  [lmerMod]
Formula: DBP ~ TRT + Time + (Time | Subject)
   Data: Dat

REML criterion at convergence: 933

Scaled residuals:
   Min     1Q Median     3Q    Max
-4.331 -0.552 -0.005  0.520  2.523

Random effects:
 Groups   Name        Variance Std.Dev. Corr
 Subject  (Intercept) 12.62    3.55
```

```
            Time              1.75    1.32    -0.95
  Residual                    3.54    1.88
Number of obs: 200, groups:  Subject, 40


Fixed effects:
              Estimate Std. Error      df t value  Pr(>|t|)
(Intercept)   117.648      0.681  26.900  172.63  <2e-16 ***
TRTB            3.454      0.455  38.000    7.59  4e-09 ***
Time           -2.500      0.229  39.000  -10.91  2e-13 ***


Correlation of Fixed Effects:
     (Intr) TRTB
TRTB -0.334
Time -0.881  0.000
```

Based on this exercise, the final Model 3 corresponds to

$$DBP_{ijk} = (\beta_0 + \gamma_{0k}) + (\beta_1 + \gamma_{1k}) \times Time_j + TRT_i + \epsilon_{ijk} \qquad (6.13)$$

where i indexes treatment A or B, j indexes time from 1 to 5 and k indexes patient (from 1 to 40). The fixed-effects are estimated as $\hat{\beta}_0 = 117.6$ and $\hat{\beta} = -2.5$ which indicates that DBP declines at a rate of 2.5 mmHg per month. The estimated difference between the rates of decline of treatments B and A is 3.45 mmHg/month and all parameters are statistically significant. For random-effects, the estimated $\hat{\sigma} = 3.54$ and $\hat{D} = \begin{pmatrix} 12.62 & -4.44 \\ -4.44 & 1.75 \end{pmatrix}$.

Model diagnostics may be produced using the residuals from the model fitting. To check the normal assumption for the random-effects, we can use the QQ-plot to graph the quantiles from the residuals and the theoretical normal as follows:

```
> print(qqmath(~resid(mod3DBP)|TRT,Dat,
      xlab="Theoretical Normal", ylab="Residuals"))
```

It may be seen from Figure 6.5 that the QQ-plot exhibits a straight line for each treatment indicating no violation of the normality assumption.

We also plot the residuals as a function of time by treatment group as seen in Figure 6.6 using the following R code chunk, which indicates that Model 3 is reasonable.

```
> print(bwplot(resid(mod3DBP)~as.factor(Time)|TRT,Dat,
      xlab="Time",ylim=c(-5,5), ylab="Residuals"))
```

To investigate the effects of the covariates of "Age" and "Sex", we test these effects along with all other effects using the following Models 5 and 6. In Model 5, we fit the Model 3 incorporating the "Age" effect to test its significance as follows:

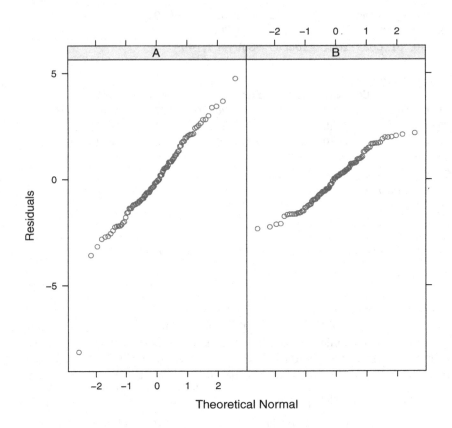

FIGURE 6.5: QQ-Plot for Model 3

```
> # fit Model 3 include ``Age" effect
> mod5DBP =  lmer(DBP~TRT+Time+Age+(Time|Subject), Dat)
> # call anova to test ``Age" effect
> anova(mod3DBP, mod5DBP)

Data: Dat
Models:
object: DBP ~ TRT + Time + (Time | Subject)
..1: DBP ~ TRT + Time + Age + (Time | Subject)
       Df AIC BIC logLik deviance Chisq Chi Df   Pr(>Chisq)
object  7 945 968   -466      931
..1     8 911 937   -448      895  36.3      1   1.7e-09 ***
```

We can see from the "anova" that the p-value associated with this test on "Age" effect is 1.6×10^{-9} which is statistically significant. We can further test "Sex" using Model 6 as follows:

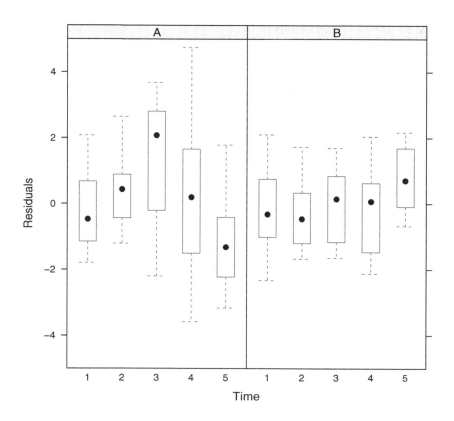

FIGURE 6.6: Boxplot for Residuals for all Subjects by Treatment

```
> # fit Model 6 including ``Age" and ``Sex"
> mod6DBP =  lmer(DBP~TRT+Time+Age+Sex+(Time|Subject), Dat)
> # test the ``Sex" effect
> anova(mod5DBP, mod6DBP)

Data: Dat
Models:
object: DBP ~ TRT + Time + Age + (Time | Subject)
..1: DBP ~ TRT + Time + Age + Sex + (Time | Subject)
       Df AIC BIC logLik deviance Chisq Chi Df  Pr(>Chisq)
object  8 911 937   -448      895
..1     9 912 942   -447      894  0.67      1   0.41
```

This gives a *p*-value of 0.41 indicating that "Sex" is not a statistically significant effect. This conclusion coincides with the conclusions in Section 4.3.1.2 of Chapter 4.

6.3.2   Analysis of Cimetidine Duodenal Ulcer Trial

6.3.2.1   Preliminary Analysis

We read the data into R as follows:

```
> dat  = read.csv("Ulcer.csv", header=T)
> # print the first 6 obs
> head(dat)

  Subject TRT WeekH Time0 Time1 Time2 Time4
1       1   3     0     0     0     0     0
2       2   4     2     0     0     1     1
3       3   2     2     0     0     1     1
4       4   3     2     0     0     1     1
5       5   4     1     0     1     1     1
6       6   1     0     0     0     0     0
```

The summary information in Table 6.1 for the four treatment groups and four time points is generated using the following R code chunk:

```
> # total n for each TRT
> n  = tapply(rep(1, dim(dat)[1]),dat$TRT,sum)
> # number for time 1
> n1 = tapply(dat$Time1,dat$TRT,sum)
> # number for time 2
> n2 = tapply(dat$Time2,dat$TRT,sum)
> # number for time 4
> n4 = tapply(dat$Time4,dat$TRT,sum)
> print(rbind(n,n1,n2,n4))

    1  2  3  4
n  76 83 85 93
n1 14 15 14 19
n2 22 31 33 45
n4 31 51 62 68

> # proportions
> print( round(rbind(n1/n,n2/n,n4/n),2))

        1    2    3    4
[1,] 0.18 0.18 0.16 0.20
[2,] 0.29 0.37 0.39 0.48
[3,] 0.41 0.61 0.73 0.73
```

6.3.2.2   Fit Logistic Regression to Binomial Data

For modeling, we reshape the data into "long" format using the following R code chunk:

```
> Dat      = reshape(dat, direction="long",
  varying = c("Time0","Time1","Time2","Time4"),
   idvar  = c("Subject","TRT","WeekH"),sep="")
> colnames(Dat) = c("Subject","TRT","WeekH","Time","Heal")
> # sort the data by Subject: very important for gee
> Dat      = Dat[order(Dat$Subject),]
> # Remove the baseline for model fitting
> Dat      = Dat[Dat$Time > 0,]
> # make the TRT and Time as factors
> Dat$TRT  = as.factor(Dat$TRT)
> Dat$Time = as.factor(Dat$Time)
> # show the first 6 observations
> head(Dat)
```

	Subject	TRT	WeekH	Time	Heal
1.3.0.1	1	3	0	1	0
1.3.0.2	1	3	0	2	0
1.3.0.4	1	3	0	4	0
2.4.2.1	2	4	2	1	0
2.4.2.2	2	4	2	2	1
2.4.2.4	2	4	2	4	1

As a preliminary analysis, we first fit logistic regression models with (Model 1) and without (Model 2) interaction to the data using R glm as follows:

```
> # fit Model 1: with interaction
> mod1glm = glm(Heal~TRT*Time, family=binomial, Dat)
> # fit Model 2: without interaction
> mod2glm = glm(Heal~TRT+Time, family=binomial, data=Dat)
> # test these two model using Chi-Square test
> anova(mod1glm,mod2glm, test="Chi")

Analysis of Deviance Table

Model 1: Heal ~ TRT * Time
Model 2: Heal ~ TRT + Time
  Resid. Df Resid. Dev Df Deviance Pr(>Chi)
1      999       1186
2     1005       1196 -6    -9.75     0.14
```

Model 1 models TRT-by-Time interaction. We note that the TRT-by-Time interaction effect is statistically significant. The TRT-by-Time interaction effect is removed from Model 2. We note that both treatment and time effects are significant. Since Models 1 and 2 are nested, we can employ the likelihood ratio test to test the model differences (using the χ^2-test). We note that these two models are not statistically significantly different, with p-value = 0.1355. We then select Model 2 for inference. The summary of the model fit is as follows:

```
> summary(mod2glm)

Call:
glm(formula = Heal ~ TRT + Time, family = binomial, data = Dat)

Deviance Residuals:
   Min      1Q  Median      3Q     Max
-1.573  -0.969  -0.616   0.976   2.088

Coefficients:
            Estimate Std. Error z value Pr(>|z|)
(Intercept)   -2.061      0.205  -10.06  < 2e-16 ***
TRT2           0.493      0.209    2.35   0.0186 *
TRT3           0.676      0.208    3.26   0.0011 **
TRT4           0.893      0.204    4.39  1.2e-05 ***
Time2          1.056      0.181    5.83  5.7e-09 ***
Time4          2.063      0.183   11.28  < 2e-16 ***

(Dispersion parameter for binomial family taken to be 1)

    Null deviance: 1361.3  on 1010  degrees of freedom
Residual deviance: 1195.5  on 1005  degrees of freedom
AIC: 1208

Number of Fisher Scoring iterations: 4
```

And we can see that both "Time" and "TRT" are statistically significant. A multiple comparison may be performed using "Tukey"-test. We first load the R package *multcomp* for general linear hypotheses and multiple comparisons using glht as follows:

```
> # load the ``multcomp" library
> library(multcomp)
> # multiple comparisons
> glht.mod2glm = glht(mod2glm, mcp(TRT="Tukey", Time="Tukey"))
> summary(glht.mod2glm)

        Simultaneous Tests for General Linear Hypotheses

Multiple Comparisons of Means: Tukey Contrasts

Fit: glm(formul=Heal~TRT+Time,family=binomial,data=Dat)

Linear Hypotheses:
                 Estimate Std. Error z value Pr(>|z|)
TRT: 2 - 1 == 0     0.493      0.209    2.35   0.1305
```

```
TRT: 3 - 1 == 0       0.676       0.208       3.26 0.0094 **
TRT: 4 - 1 == 0       0.893       0.204       4.39 <0.001 ***
TRT: 3 - 2 == 0       0.183       0.196       0.93 0.9178
TRT: 4 - 2 == 0       0.400       0.192       2.09 0.2337
TRT: 4 - 3 == 0       0.217       0.189       1.15 0.8242
Time: 2 - 1 == 0      1.056       0.181       5.83 <0.001 ***
Time: 4 - 1 == 0      2.063       0.183      11.28 <0.001 ***
Time: 4 - 2 == 0      1.006       0.161       6.25 <0.001 ***
(Adjusted p values reported -- single-step method)
```

In this multiple comparison, we note that ulcer healing rates differ across time points in a statistically significant manner. This means that ulcer healing is significant between weeks 2 and 1, weeks 4 and 1, and weeks 4 and 2. Further, there are statistically significant differences between treatments 3 and 1 and between treatments 4 to 1 only. This means that 800 mg C and 1600 mg C are statistically more effective than Placebo in ulcer healing. No statistically significant differences exist for other treatment comparisons, which is consistent with what is reported in Chapter 12 in Peace and Chen (2010).

6.3.2.3   Fit Generalized Linear Mixed Model

We know that there is variability among patients in terms of ulcer healing. We fit (Model 3) the generalized linear mixed effects model (GLMM). There are several ways to fit a GLMM. We illustrate the penalized quasi-likelihood methods in R using the library *MASS*. This may be implemented as follows:

```
> # load MASS library
> library(MASS)
> # fit the Model 3
> mod3glm = glmmPQL(Heal~TRT, random=~1|Subject,
          family=binomial, Dat)
> # print the summary
> summary(mod3glm)

Linear mixed-effects model fit by maximum likelihood
 Data: Dat
  AIC BIC logLik
   NA  NA     NA

Random effects:
 Formula: ~1 | Subject
        (Intercept) Residual
StdDev:        1.63    0.812

Variance function:
 Structure: fixed weights
 Formula: ~invwt
```

```
Fixed effects: Heal ~ TRT
              Value Std.Error  DF t-value p-value
(Intercept) -1.192    0.246 674   -4.85  0.0000
TRT2         0.603    0.332 333    1.82  0.0703
TRT3         0.827    0.327 333    2.53  0.0119
TRT4         1.047    0.321 333    3.26  0.0012
 Correlation:
     (Intr) TRT2   TRT3
TRT2 -0.741
TRT3 -0.751  0.556
TRT4 -0.765  0.567  0.575


Standardized Within-Group Residuals:
   Min     Q1    Med     Q3    Max
-1.559 -0.493 -0.390  0.631  1.865


Number of Observations: 1011
Number of Groups: 337
```

This model (*mod3glm*) fits treatment effect incorporating the longitudinal nature (i.e., Time) of the data with a generalized linear model. We note from the summary that there is a statistically significant treatment effect. The estimated standard deviations due to patients and residuals are 1.635 and 0.812, respectively.

We compare this GLMM to the binomial logistic regression (Model 4) as

```
> # fit Model 4
> mod4glm = glm(Heal~TRT, family=binomial, Dat)
> summary(mod4glm)

Call:
glm(formula = Heal ~ TRT, family = binomial, data = Dat)

Deviance Residuals:
   Min     1Q Median     3Q    Max
-1.132 -1.056 -0.834  1.304  1.565

Coefficients:
            Estimate Std. Error z value Pr(>|z|)
(Intercept)   -0.877      0.145   -6.03 1.6e-09 ***
TRT2           0.428      0.195    2.19  0.0283 *
TRT3           0.584      0.193    3.03  0.0024 **
TRT4           0.769      0.188    4.08 4.5e-05 ***

(Dispersion parameter for binomial family taken to be 1)
```

```
      Null deviance: 1361.3  on 1010   degrees of freedom
  Residual deviance: 1343.2  on 1007   degrees of freedom
  AIC: 1351
```

```
Number of Fisher Scoring iterations: 4
```

The same conclusion is drawn for treatment effect. However, for this Model 4, the residual deviation is 1343.2 with 1007 degrees of freedom. Therefore, the estimated standard deviation for residuals calculated as the square-root of $1343.2/1007$ is 1.155. This estimate is larger than the estimate of 0.812 from GLMM.

6.3.2.4   Fit GEE

The generalized estimation equation may be fitted using the R library **gee**. We first fit the *GEE* assuming independent patient effects to reproduce the binomial logistical regression as follows:

```
> # load the ``gee" library
> library(gee)
> # fit the gee model with independent patient effect
> fit.gee1 = gee(Heal~TRT,id=Subject,family=binomial,
  data=Dat,corstr="independence", scale.fix=T)
```

```
(Intercept)        TRT2         TRT3         TRT4
     -0.877       0.428        0.584        0.769
```

```
> # print the summary
> summary(fit.gee1)
```

```
  GEE:  GENERALIZED LINEAR MODELS FOR DEPENDENT DATA
  gee S-function, version 4.13 modified 98/01/27 (1998)
```

```
Model:
 Link:                     Logit
 Variance to Mean Relation: Binomial
 Correlation Structure:    Independent
```

```
Call:
gee(formula=Heal~TRT,id=Subject,data=Dat,family=binomial,
    corstr = "independence", scale.fix = T)
```

```
Summary of Residuals:
   Min    1Q Median    3Q    Max
-0.473 -0.427 -0.294  0.573  0.706
```

```
Coefficients:
```

	Estimate	Naive S.E.	Naive z	Robust S.E.	Robust z
(Intercept)	-0.877	0.145	-6.03	0.220	-3.99
TRT2	0.428	0.195	2.19	0.280	1.53
TRT3	0.584	0.193	3.03	0.268	2.18
TRT4	0.769	0.188	4.08	0.267	2.88

```
Estimated Scale Parameter:  1
Number of Iterations:  1

Working Correlation
      [,1] [,2] [,3]
[1,]    1    0    0
[2,]    0    1    0
[3,]    0    0    1
```

In this *independence* model fit, i.e., *fit.gee1*, we assume that responses are independent over time – which is essentially the binomial logistic regression in *mod4glm*. We compare this independence GEE model (i.e., *fit.gee1*) to the glm model in *mod4glm* and see that the model estimates and Naive SE are reproduced. In the output, the "Robust SE" and "Robust z" are adjusted using the *sandwich estimator*. The "Robust Standard Errors" are larger than those from the GLMs implying that the independence assumption is not reasonable.

We then fit an exchangeable correlation structure to estimate a single correlation parameter for each pair of repeated observations using the following R code chunk:

```
> fit.gee2 = gee(Heal~TRT,id=Subject,family=binomial,
 data=Dat,corstr="exchangeable", scale.fix=T)
```

(Intercept)	TRT2	TRT3	TRT4
-0.877	0.428	0.584	0.769

```
> summary(fit.gee2)

GEE:  GENERALIZED LINEAR MODELS FOR DEPENDENT DATA
gee S-function, version 4.13 modified 98/01/27 (1998)

Model:
 Link:                      Logit
 Variance to Mean Relation: Binomial
 Correlation Structure:     Exchangeable

Call:
gee(formula=Heal~TRT,id=Subject,data=Dat,family=binomial,
    corstr = "exchangeable", scale.fix = T)
```

Summary of Residuals:

Min	1Q	Median	3Q	Max
-0.473	-0.427	-0.294	0.573	0.706

Coefficients:

	Estimate	Naive S.E.	Naive z	Robust S.E.	Robust z
(Intercept)	-0.877	0.193	-4.54	0.220	-3.99
TRT2	0.428	0.259	1.65	0.280	1.53
TRT3	0.584	0.256	2.28	0.268	2.18
TRT4	0.769	0.250	3.07	0.267	2.88

Estimated Scale Parameter: 1
Number of Iterations: 1

Working Correlation

	[,1]	[,2]	[,3]
[1,]	1.000	0.381	0.381
[2,]	0.381	1.000	0.381
[3,]	0.381	0.381	1.000

This correlation structure is the so-called *compound symmetry* structure. With this correlation structure, the naive and robust standard errors are quite close indicating that the assumption of exchangeable structure is adequate for the repeated measurements in this dataset. The estimated correlation is 0.38. Both the Naive and Robust z-values for TRT2 (corresponding to 400 mg C) are 1.652 and 1.527, respectively, indicating non-significance between 400 mg C and Placebo. However, there are statistically significant differences between 800 mg C and Placebo and between 1600 mg C and Placebo from both Naive and Robust z-values. These conclusions are consistent with those in Chapter 12 from Peace and Chen (2010).

6.4   Summary and Discussion

In this chapter, we presented longitudinal analysis of data from two real clinical trials. Data from the DBP clinical trial reflected continuous measurements, whereas data from the Cimetidine duodenal ulcer trial reflected binary measurements. Data analyses were illustrated using R along with the statistical theory in Section 6.2.

For further reading, we recommend Fitzmaurice et al. (2004). As presented by the authors, this book provides "a rigorous and systematic description of modern methods for analyzing data from longitudinal studies" from health sciences. The book by Pinheiro and Bates (2000) is always a reference book for longitudinal data analysis with detailed account for *nlme*.

6.5   Appendix: SAS Programs

The SAS program below corresponds to the R program in Section 6.3.

```
/***** Section 6.3.1.1 ***********************/
/*read data from the path of dataset*/
Data dat;
infile "your path/DBP.csv" delimiter="," firstobs=2;
input Subject TRT$ DBP1 DBP2 DBP3 DBP4 DBP5 Age Sex$;
diff= DBP5-DBP1;        /*create a column "diff"*/
RUN;

/*rearrange the dataframe of dat into a "long" format*/
DATA Dat_L;
set dat;
array ADBP(1:5) DBP1-DBP5;  /*creat an array*/
/*set new variable (DBP) equal to the value of
             the array for the given time*/
do time= 1 to 5;
DBP= ADBP(time);
output;                 /*output the results*/
end;
drop DBP1-DBP5 diff;    /*drop unuseful variables*/
RUN;

PROC SORT data= Dat_L out=Dat_L1;
by time; RUN;

/*show the first 6 observations*/
PROC PRINT data= Dat_L1(obs=6); RUN;

/*fit linear regression model for 40 patients and
                    extract intercept and slope*/
PROC REG data= Dat_L outest= coef;
by Subject;
model DBP= Time; RUN;

/*print out the coefficient:
```

```
  subject #1-20 are A and the others are B*/
PROC PRINT data= coef; RUN;

/*add column "Trt" into table coefficient*/
PROC SQL;
CREATE TABLE dat_coef AS
SELECT dat.Subject, dat.TRT, coef.Intercept, coef.time
FROM dat FULL JOIN coef
ON dat.subject= coef.subject;
QUIT;

/*model the slope and intercept relationship by linear
  regression*/
/*fit model 1 with interaction*/
PROC GLM data= dat_coef;
class TRT(ref= "A");
model time= Intercept TRT Intercept*TRt/ solution; RUN;

/*fit model 2 without interaction*/
PROC GLM data= dat_coef;
class TRT(ref= "A");
model time= Intercept TRT / solution; RUN;

/*test difference of intercept and slope between two treatments*/
PROC TTEST data= dat_coef sides=2 alpha=0.05 h0=0;
class TRT;
var time; RUN;

PROC TTEST data= dat_coef sides=2 alpha=0.05 h0=0;
class TRT;
var Intercept; RUN;

/***** Section 6.3.1.2 ****************************************/
/*fit model 1(set both intercept and slope as random effect)*/
PROC MIXED data=Dat_L  method= ML;
class TRT(ref= "A");
model DBP= TRT Time TRT*Time / s;
random int time / type= un subject=Subject;
RUN;

/*fit model 2(set intercept as random effect)*/
PROC MIXED data= Dat_L method= ML;
class TRT(ref= "A");
model DBP= TRT Time TRT*Time / s;
random int / type= un subject= Subject;
```

```
RUN;

/*fit model 3*/
PROC MIXED data= Dat_L;
class TRT(ref= "A");
model DBP= TRT Time / s;
random int time/ type= un subject= Subject; RUN;

/*fit model 4*/
PROC MIXED data= Dat_L;
class TRT(ref= "A");
model DBP= TRT Time / s;
random int / type= un subject= Subject;
RUN;

/*model 5: fit model 3 include "Age" effect*/
PROC MIXED data= Dat_L method= ML;
class TRT(ref= "A");
model DBP= TRT Time Age / s;
random int time/ type= un subject= Subject; RUN;


/*model 6: fit model 3 include "Age" and "Sex" effect*/
PROC MIXED data= Dat_L method= ML;
class TRT(ref= "A") Sex(ref= "F");
model DBP= TRT Time Age Sex / s;
random int time/ type= un subject= Subject;
RUN;

/****** Section 6.3.2.1***************************/
/*read data from the path of dataset*/
Data dat5;
infile "your path/Ulcer.csv" delimiter="," firstobs=2;
input Subject TRT WeekH Time0 Time1 Time2 Time4;
RUN;

/*print the first 6 observations*/
PROC PRINT data= dat5(obs= 6); RUN;

/*summary information for the four treatment groups
        and four time points*/
PROC FREQ data= dat5;
tables TRT TRT*Time1 TRT*Time2 TRT*Time4;
RUN;
```

```
DATA Dat_L2;
set dat5;
array AT[3] Time1 Time2 Time4;   /*create an array*/
do i= 1 to 3;    /*set new variable (DBP) equal to the value of
                                   the array for the given time*/
if i= 3 then Time= i+1;
else Time= i;
Heal= AT(i);
output;                          /*output the results*/
end;
drop i Time0 Time1 Time2 Time4;   /*drop non-use variables*/
RUN;


PROC SORT data= Dat_L2 out= Dat_L3;
by Subject; RUN;

/******** Section 6.3.2.2 ******************************/
/*fit model 1: with interaction*/
PROC GENMOD data= Dat_L2 descending;
class Trt(ref="1") Time(ref="1");
model Heal= Trt Time Trt*Time/ dist= binomial link= logit;
RUN;

/*fit model 2: without interaction*/
PROC GENMOD data= Dat_L2 descending;
class Trt(ref="1") Time(ref="1");
model Heal= Trt Time/ dist= binomial link= logit; RUN;

/*multiple comparison using "Tukey" test*/
PROC GLM data= Dat_L2;
class Trt Time;
model Heal= Trt Time;
means TRT Time / Tukey;
run;

/******* Section 6.3.2.3 ***************************/
/*fit model 3: Generalized Linear Mixed Model!!!some problem*/
PROC GLIMMIX data= DAT_L2;
class Trt(ref="1") Time(ref="1");
model Heal= Trt/ dist=binomial link=logit solution;
random int / subject= Subject;
RUN;

/*fit model 4*/
```

```
PROC GENMOD data= Dat_L2 descending;
class Trt(ref="1") Time(ref="1");
model Heal= Trt/ dist= binomial link= logit;
RUN;

/*********** Section 6.3.2.4  ****************/
/*fit the gee model with independent patient effect*/
PROC GENMOD data= Dat_L2 descending;
class Trt(ref="1") Time(ref="1") Subject;
model Heal= Trt/ dist= binomial link= logit;
repeated subject= Subject/ corr=ind corrw;
RUN;

/*fit the gee model with independent patient effect*/
PROC GENMOD data= Dat_L2 descending;
class Trt(ref="1") Time(ref="1") Subject;
model Heal= Trt/ dist= binomial link= logit;
repeated subject= Subject/ corr=exch corrw;
RUN;
```

Chapter 7

Sample Size Determination and Power Calculations in Clinical Trials

In this chapter, we discuss sample size determination in clinical trials with implementation in R. We begin with a review of the prerequisites for sample size determination in Section 7.1. We then present sample size calculations for the comparison of two-treatment groups for continuous endpoints in Section 7.2 followed by the two-treatment comparison for proportions in Section 7.3. In Section 7.4, we investigate sample size and power calculations for clinical trials with time-to-event endpoints. In Section 7.5 we use the R library gsDesign to design group sequential trials including sample size calculation and stopping boundaries. Design and sample size calculation for trials with longitudinal data is discussed in Section 7.6. In Section 7.7, we discuss an atypical situation in sample size calculation where percent change and coefficient of variation are known and end the chapter with concluding remarks in Section 7.8.

Note: To run the R programs in this chapter, the analyst should install the following R packages first: *samplesize*, *pwr* and *gsDesign*.

7.1 Pre-requisites for Sample Size Determination

Clinical trials should be well designed. An aspect of good design of clinical trial protocols is determining the number of patients (sample size) required by the clinical investigation to adequately address the research question or objective.

The formal statistical basis for sample size determination requires: (i) the question or objective of the clinical investigation to be defined; (ii) the most relevant endpoints reflecting the objective to be identified; (iii) the specification of the difference δ (which embodies the question) between groups in terms of the endpoint that is clinically important to detect; (iv) specification of the magnitudes of the Type-I and Type-II decision errors; and (v) estimates of the mean and variability of the endpoint.

The **objective**, particularly for Phase III trials comparing the efficacy of drug D to a placebo control P, is translated as the alternative hypothesis (H_a)

in the hypothesis testing construct:

$$H_0 : \mu_1 - \mu_2 = 0 \text{ versus } H_a : \mu_1 - \mu_2 = \delta > 0. \qquad (7.1)$$

where μ_1 and μ_2 represent the means of the efficacy endpoint for drug D and placebo P, respectively, H_a reflects that the objective of the trial is to demonstrate that the efficacy of drug D exceeds that of the control P by at least δ. This enables one to interpret δ as the **expected minimal comparative treatment effect size** at the design stage. It is noted that the above formulation of H_a is one-sided, consistent with the a *priori* belief that drug D is effective as discussed in Peace (1991b).

But what is the endpoint? An **Endpoint** is the analysis unit on each individual patient that will be statistically analyzed to address the study objective. An endpoint may be the actual data collected or a function of the data. If D is a drug thought to have anti-hypertensive efficacy, actual data reflecting potential efficacy are supine diastolic blood pressure measurements. However, the endpoint may be defined as the change in supine diastolic blood pressure from baseline to the end of the treatment period.

What is the difference δ between D and P that is clinically important to detect? The choice of δ reflects what is reasonable to expect about the degree to which the efficacy of D exceeds that of P in the population of patients to be treated, as long as that degree is clinically important. A δ that is too large may lead to a trial with sample sizes too small to detect a small treatment effect; whereas, a δ that is too small may lead to a trial that is too large to be conducted with available financial resources. Even if financial resources were available, drugs for which the true comparative treatment effect size is small may have little or no clinical utility in the marketplace. The choice of δ should be a joint effort between the clinician and the biostatistician with input from other scientists who understand the mechanism of action and pharmacokinetics of drug D.

A Type-I error occurs if H_0 is rejected when it is true. A Type-II error occurs if H_0 is accepted when it is false. It is therefore desirable that the magnitudes of the Type-I (α) and Type-II (β) decision errors regarding H_0 are chosen to be small. Historically, α is chosen to be 0.05; whereas, β is usually chosen to be anywhere from 0.05 to 0.20.

Hypothesis testing (and confidence interval) methods require **estimates of endpoint means and variances** of the control group. These estimates may be obtained from the literature or from previous studies. It is good practice for the Biometrics or Biostatistics Department to develop a file of such information from all studies conducted. In obtaining such information, care should be taken to make sure that the information is on a population similar to the target population of the study protocol being designed. If no such information exists, it may still be possible, particularly for dichotomous endpoints, to determine sample sizes by using the worst case of the Bernoulli variance or utilizing the coefficient of variation.

The well known per group sample size (n) formula (refer to Equation (7.5)) for clinical trials utilizing a **parallel design**:

$$n \geq 2(s^2/\delta^2)[z_{1-\alpha} + z_{1-\beta}]^2 \qquad (7.2)$$

where s is an estimate of the standard deviation σ (assuming homogeneous variances), δ is the difference between groups which is clinically important to detect (i.e., the minimum expected treatment effect), and $z_{1-\alpha}$ and $z_{1-\beta}$ are the appropriate critical points of the standard normal distribution corresponding to the magnitudes of the Type-I and Type-II errors, respectively, explicitly reflects the pre-requisites for sample size determination. It is noted that if the alternative hypothesis is two-sided; i.e., $H_a : \delta \neq 0$, α in the above sample size formula should be replaced with $\alpha/2$.

The above formula also reflects the interplay between the design characteristics: α, $1 - \beta$, δ, s^2 and n. As δ decreases, n increases and vice versa; as power increases, n increases or vice versa; as s^2 increases, n increases; and as α decreases, n increases. The above formula derives from standardizing the difference between the observed sample means of the drug and control groups, using the standardized form as a test statistic for H_0, and applying the definitions of the magnitudes of the Type-I decision error and power (the complement of the magnitude of the Type-II decision error). The per group sample size n is interpreted as "the number of patients required to detect δ with a power of $1 - \beta$ and a one-sided Type-I error of α is at least $2(s^2/\delta^2)[z_{1-\alpha} + z_{1-\beta}]^2$." A graphical derivation appears in the next section.

7.2   Comparison of Two Treatment Groups with Continuous Endpoints

7.2.1   Fundamentals

The general objective of many clinical trials is to compare two treatment groups such as a new drug to placebo (or control) where the endpoint is continuous. Here, we are interested in investigating whether the new drug is better than placebo (i.e., that new drug is effective) and want to determine how many patients should be enrolled in each treatment group.

In statistical terms, the null hypothesis is $H_0 : \mu_1 = \mu_2$ where μ_1 and μ_2 are the true response or endpoint means for the new drug and placebo, respectively. The alternative hypothesis is then $H_a : \mu_1 > \mu_2$. The null and alternative hypotheses may be rewritten as $H_0 : \mu_1 - \mu_2 = 0$ and $H_a : \mu_1 - \mu_2 = \delta > 0$.

Other concepts associated with sample size determination are Type-I error, Type-II error and power and they are defined as follows:

- Type-I Error (α): Probability of rejecting the null hypothesis when it is true

- Type-II Error (β): Probability of not rejecting the null hypothesis when it is false

- Power $= 1 - \beta$: Probability of rejecting the null hypothesis when it is false

Figure 7.1 summarizes graphically the ingredients in sample size calculations. In this figure, the null hypothesis in the left normal curve provides the basis for determining the rejection region (the dark shadowed region) where the probability of a Type-I error is α and is the size of the test.

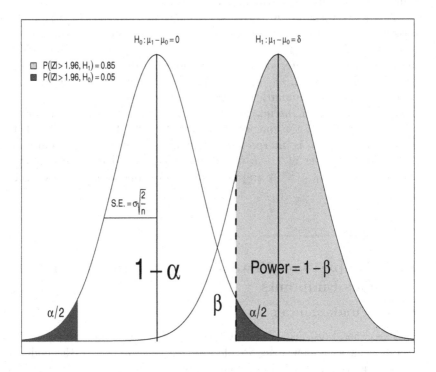

FIGURE 7.1: Graphical Features of Sample Size Determination

The rejection region is denoted by the dashed vertical line in the middle where the area on the right is $\alpha/2$. Here the magnitude of the Type-I decision error is halved to reflect the FDA convention of considering H_a to reflect $\neq$ rather than ">" even though drug is being compared to placebo in terms of efficacy. The alternative hypothesis in the right normal curve then defines the power (the light shadowed region on the right of the critical line) and the Type-

II error (β) (the region on the left side of the critical line). Notice that moving the curve associated with the alternative hypothesis to the right is equivalent to increasing the distance between the null and alternative hypotheses which in turn increases the area of the curve over the rejection region and thus increases the power.

In this hypothesis setting, the *critical value* defines the boundary between the rejection and non-rejection regions which should be the same under the null and alternative hypotheses. From the null hypothesis, this critical value can be calculated as $0 + z_{1-\alpha/2}\sigma\sqrt{\frac{2}{n}}$ and it is $\delta - z_{1-\beta}\sigma\sqrt{\frac{2}{n}}$ from the alternative hypothesis. Therefore, we have the fundamental equation for the two-sample situation as follows:

$$0 + z_{1-\alpha/2}\sigma\sqrt{\frac{2}{n}} = \delta - z_{1-\beta}\sigma\sqrt{\frac{2}{n}} \tag{7.3}$$

If the variances are not equal or the sample sizes are not equal, then Equation (7.3) has to be modified to reflect unequal variances of σ_1^2 and σ_2^2, and unequal sample sizes n_1 and n_2 as follows:

$$0 + z_{1-\alpha/2}\sigma_2\sqrt{\frac{1}{n_2} + \frac{1}{n_1}} = \delta - z_{1-\beta}\sqrt{\frac{\sigma_2^2}{n_2} + \frac{\sigma_1^2}{n_1}} \tag{7.4}$$

This formulation is the most general and is the basis for virtually all two-parallel group sample size calculations. In doing so, we assume a fixed total sample size or that $n_1 = k \times n_2$, where k is a scalar reflecting the ratio of the sample sizes.

7.2.2 Basic Formula for Sample Size Calculation

Based on the Equation (7.3), the required sample size to compare two population means μ_1 and μ_2 (against a 2-sided alternative: $H_a : \mu_1 - \mu_2 = \delta \neq 0$) with common variance σ^2 can be derived as

$$n \geq \frac{2(z_{1-\alpha/2} + z_{1-\beta})^2}{\left(\frac{\mu_1 - \mu_2}{\sigma}\right)^2} = \frac{2(z_{1-\alpha/2} + z_{1-\beta})^2}{\left(\frac{\delta}{\sigma}\right)^2} \tag{7.5}$$

From this Equation (7.5), we can see that the two key ingredients are the difference to be detected, $\delta = \mu_1 - \mu_2$, and the inherent variability in the observed data indicated by σ^2. The numerator can be calculated for other magnitudes of Type-I and Type-II errors.

For the common situation of Type-I error $\alpha = 0.05$ and 80% power [$\beta = 0.20$], the values of $z_{1-\alpha/2}$ and $z_{1-\beta}$ are 1.96 and 0.84, respectively. Then $2(z_{1-\alpha/2} + z_{1-\beta})^2 = 15.68$ which can be rounded up to 16. This produces the rule of thumb:

$$n = \frac{16}{\Delta^2} \tag{7.6}$$

where
$$\Delta = \frac{\mu_1 - \mu_2}{\sigma} = \frac{\delta}{\sigma} \tag{7.7}$$
is the treatment difference to be detected in units of the standard deviation - the standardized difference (or standardized design treatment effect).

Figure 7.2, which is produced in the following R code chunk, illustrates the values of the numerator (i.e., $2(z_{1-\alpha/2} + z_{1-\beta})^2$) for a Type-I error of $\alpha = 0.05$ and other values of power from 0.7 to 0.95 with the following R code. A power of 0.90 (as well as 0.95) is frequently used to evaluate new drugs in Phase III clinical trials (randomized, double blind, pivotal proof of efficacy comparisons of a new drug to placebo or a standard).

```
> # Type-I error
> alpha = 0.05
> # Type-II error
> beta   = c(0.05,0.1,0.15,0.2,0.25,0.3)
> # power
> pow    = 1-beta
> # numerator in the sample size
> num = 2*(qnorm(1-alpha/2)+qnorm(1-beta))^2
> # plot the power to the numerator
> plot(pow, num, xlab="Power",las=1, ylab="Numerator")
> lines(pow, num) # add the line to it
> # use arrows to show the values of numerator
> for(i in 1:length(pow))
 {
 arrows(pow[i],0, pow[i], num[i], length=0.13)
 arrows(pow[i],num[i], pow[length(beta)],num[i], length=0.13)
 }
```

7.2.3   R Function `power.t.test`

Suppose that a clinical trial is designed to detect a treatment difference of 0.5 with common standard deviation of 1, a power of 80% and a Type I error of 5%. Then the standardized difference of Δ in Equation (7.7) is 0.5, then $16/0.5^2 = 64$ subjects per treatment will be needed for a total of 128 subjects in the clinical trial for a total of 128 subjects in the clinical trial.

In R, this calculation is implemented (by Peter Dalgaard based on previous work from Claus Ekstrømin) in the R basic `Stats` package as a function call of `power.t.test`, which can be used to compute the statistical power of test, or to determine sample size and other parameters to obtain target power. The usage of `power.t.test` is illustrated with the following R code chunk:

```
power.t.test(n = NULL, delta = NULL, sd = 1, sig.level = 0.05,
   power = NULL, type = c("two.sample", "one.sample", "paired"),
   alternative = c("two.sided", "one.sided"), strict = FALSE)
```

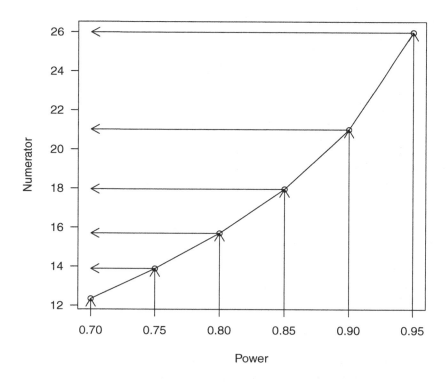

FIGURE 7.2: Numerator in Sample Size Calculation

where n is the number of subjects (per group), $delta = \delta = \mu_1 - \mu_2$ is the true difference in means, sd is the common standard deviation, $sig.level$ is the significance level (i.e., the Type-I error probability) with default value of 0.05, $power$ is the statistical power of test (i.e., 1 minus Type-II error probability), $type$ is the type of t-test with three choices of "two.sample" or "one.sample" or "paired", $alternative$ is to define the alternative hypothesis which can be one- or two-sided, and $strict$ is to use strict interpretation in two-sided case.

Detecting a treatment difference of 0.5 with common standard deviation of 1, can be implemented as:

```
> power.t.test(delta=0.5, sd=1, power=0.8)

    Two-sample t test power calculation

          n = 63.8
      delta = 0.5
```

```
            sd = 1
     sig.level = 0.05
         power = 0.8
   alternative = two.sided
```

NOTE: n is number in *each* group

This reproduces the sample size of 63.8 or 64 for each treatment. For a one-sided alternative, we use:

```
> power.t.test(delta=0.5, sd=1, power=0.8,
        alternative = c("one.sided"))
```

```
    Two-sample t test power calculation

            n = 50.2
        delta = 0.5
           sd = 1
    sig.level = 0.05
        power = 0.8
  alternative = one.sided
```

NOTE: n is number in *each* group

which gives a sample size 50 for each treatment group.

Not only can this **power.t.test** function be used for sample size calculation, it can be also used to calculate statistical power or other clinical trial characteristics, such as the power for a specific sample size or the minimum detectable treatment difference for a given sample size and power. For example, for a sample size 64 from each treatment group, we can calculate the associated statistical power as:

```
> power.t.test(n=64,delta=0.5, sd=1)
```

```
    Two-sample t test power calculation

            n = 64
        delta = 0.5
           sd = 1
    sig.level = 0.05
        power = 0.801
  alternative = two.sided
```

NOTE: n is number in *each* group

which is 0.801. For a fixed sample size of 64 and power of 80%, we can calculate the minimum detectable treatment difference as:

```
> power.t.test(n=64,sd=1,power=0.8)

      Two-sample t test power calculation

              n = 64
          delta = 0.499
             sd = 1
      sig.level = 0.05
          power = 0.8
    alternative = two.sided

NOTE: n is number in *each* group
```

which is 0.499. The sample size and statistical power are nonlinearly related as indicated in Equation (7.5). We can use `power.t.test` to illustrate this relationship with the following R code chunk as seen in Figure 7.3:

```
> # use pow from 0.2 to 0.9 by 0.05
> pow   = seq(0.2, 0.9, by=0.05)
> # keep track of the size using for-loop
> size = NULL
> for(i in 1:length(pow))
    size[i] = power.t.test(delta=0.5, sd=1, power=pow[i])$n
> # plot the size to power
> plot(pow, size, las=1,type="b", xlab="Power",
        ylab="Sample Size Required")
```

7.2.4 Unequal Variance: `samplesize` Package

When the treatment group sample sizes and variances are different, Equation (7.4) can be used to calculate the sample size along with other characteristics. In this situation, the so-called Welch approximation described in Equation (3.3) from Chapter 3 is used. A R package **samplesize** is created and maintained by Ralph Scherer (`scherer.ralph@mh-hannover.de`) with reference to Bock (1998). This package can be used to compute the sample size for Student's *t*-test, Student's *t*-test with Welch's approximation, and the Wilcoxon-Mann-Whitney test for ordinal data. In this package, there are several function calls for these purposes.

Specifically,

- *n.indep.t.test.eq* is used to calculate sample size for independent Student's t-test with equal group sizes;

- *n.indep.t.test.neq* is used to calculate sample size for independent Student's t-test with unequal group sizes;

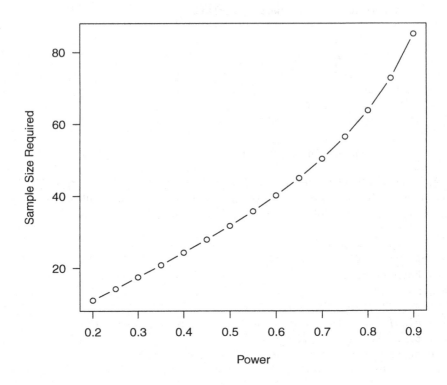

FIGURE 7.3: Nonlinear Relationship between Sample Size to Power

- *n.paired.t.test* is used to calculate sample size for the paired Student's t-test;

- *n.welch.test* is used to calculate sample size for Student's t-test with Welch's approximation;

- *n.wilcox.ord* is used to calculate sample size for the Wilcoxon-Mann-Whitney test for ordinal data with or without ties.

We illustrate some simple cases. Readers may use these function calls to design their own clinical trials.

For example, to design a clinical trial with two treatment groups to detect a mean difference (denoted by `mean.diff` in the function call) of 0.8 with standard deviation (denoted by `sd.est` in the function call) of 0.83, a two-sided Type-I error $\alpha=0.05$ expressed as $1-\alpha$ in this function, and 80% power, the required sample size for each group may be calculated by:

```
> # load the library
> library(samplesize)
> # sample size calculation
> n.indep.t.test.eq(power = 0.8, alpha = 0.95,
        mean.diff = 0.8, sd.est = 0.83)

[1] "sample.size:" "29"
```

which gives 29 patients for each group.

If we would like to have unbalanced randomization to the two treatment groups on the order of a 2 to 1 ratio, we can calculate the required sample size as:

```
> n.indep.t.test.neq(power = 0.8, alpha = 0.95,
        mean.diff = 0.8, sd.est = 0.83, k=0.5)

[1] "sample.size:"      "32"
[3] "sample.size n.1:" "21.3"
[5] "sample.size n.2:" "10.7"
```

which gives a total sample size of 32 with 21 randomized to treatment 1 and 11 randomized to treatment 2. To comply with the sample size ratio of 2 to 1, we would select 22 for treatment 1 and 11 for treatment 2 which increases the total sample size to 33. This number would increase the power to slightly above 80%.

In the design of a clinical trial if unequal treatment group variances were expected, the Welch approximation could be used. In this case, the n.welch.test can be used to calculate sample size for Student's t-test with Welch's approximation for unequal variances. Usage of this function is illustrated with the following code chunk:

```
n.welch.test(power = 0.8, alpha = 0.95,mean.diff = 2,
        sd.est1 = 1, sd.est2 = 2.65)
```

where power is the required power $= 1-\beta$, alpha is the required 2-sided Type-I error expressed as $1 - \alpha$ in this function, mean.diff is the required minimum difference between group means, sd.est1 is the standard deviation for treatment 1 and sd.est2 is the standard deviation for treatment 2. The output for this R function are values of the total sample size (i.e., total sample size N), and the sample sizes n_1 and n_2 for treatment groups 1 and 2. For example, to design a clinical trial with power of 80% and Type-I error rate of 0.05 to detect a mean difference of 4 between two treatment groups with standard deviations of 1 and 2, respectively, the required sample sizes may be calculated as:

```
> n.welch.test(power = 0.8, alpha = 0.95,
        mean.diff = 2, sd.est1 = 1, sd.est2 = 2)
```

```
sample.size: 16
sample.size n1: 6
sample.size n2: 11
```

which gives a total sample size of 16 with 6 for treatment group 1 and 11 for treatment group 2. Again to comply with the sample size ratio of 2 to 1, we would require 6 for treatment 1 and 12 for treatment 2 for a total of 18 subjects. This number of patients would increase the power slightly above 80%.

Another useful function in this package is to compute the sample size for the Wilcoxon-Mann-Whitney test for ordinal data with or without ties as described in Zhao et al. (2008). Use of this function is illustrated with the following code chunk:

```
n.wilcox.ord(beta, alpha, t, p, q)
```

where

- *beta* is the required Type-II error

- *alpha* is the required Type-I error

- t is the treatment fraction n/N and n is the sample size for treatment 2

- p is the vector of rates from treatment 1 in categories $1, \cdots, D$

- q is the vector of rates from treatment 2 in categories $1, \cdots, D$

The output of this function call is the value for total sample size. For example, in designing a clinical trial with power 80% and Type-I error rate of 0.05 to detect the rates from treatment 1 as $p = (0.66, 0.15, 0.19)$ and $q = (0.61, 0.23, 0.16)$ with $t = 0.5$, the required sample size would be:

```
> n.wilcox.ord(beta = 0.2, alpha = 0.05, t = 0.5,
        p = c(0.66, 0.15, 0.19), q = c(0.61, 0.23, 0.16))
```

```
$N
[1] 8341
```

which gives sample size of 8341.

7.3   Two Binomial Proportions

7.3.1   R Function `power.prop.test`

When the endpoints in clinical trials are proportions, the equations for sample size and power calculation in Equation (7.3) can be easily modified.

In this situation, we are assessing whether the proportion p_1 responding to a new treatment (D) exceeds the proportion p_2 responding to control treatment (P), such as a placebo or standard. This is equivalent to the null hypothesis $H_0 : p_1 - p_2 = 0$ versus $H_a : p_1 - p_2 = \delta > 0$.

The test statistic is constructed as:

$$z = \frac{p_1 - p_2}{\sqrt{\frac{p_1(1-p_1)}{n_1} + \frac{p_2(1-p_2)}{n_2}}} \tag{7.8}$$

which is asymptotically normally distributed and therefore the σ in Equation (7.3) can be replaced by

$$\sigma = \sqrt{\frac{p_1(1 - p_1)}{n_1} + \frac{p_2(1 - p_2)}{n_2}} \tag{7.9}$$

Based on this approximation, the sample size and statistical power can be calculated using the R function `power.prop.test` in the base package `Stats` by Peter Dalgaard based on previous work from Claus Ekstrøm. In addition to calculating the sample size, this function can also be used to compute the power of the test and to determine other parameters from target sample size and power. Use of this function is illustrated with the following code chunk:

```
power.prop.test(n=NULL, p1=NULL, p2=NULL, sig.level=0.05,
 power=NULL, alternative=c("two.sided", "one.sided"),
 strict = FALSE)
```

where

- *n* is the sample size for the number of subjects per treatment group,

- *p1* is the probability of responding in one treatment group D,

- *p2* is the probability of responding in the other treatment group P,

- *sig.level* is the significance level, i.e., the magnitude of the Type-I error, α, with default value of 0.05,

- *power* is the statistical power of the test $= 1$ - the magnitude of the Type-II error,

- *alternative* denotes one- or two-sided alternative hypothesis, and

- *strict* specifies whether the strict interpretation in two-sided alternative should be used.

Note that for the first five input parameters in `power.prop.test`, one can be determined from specification of the other four. This is accomplished with the univariate root finding function `uniroot`.

For example, to design a clinical trial with 80% power with Type-I error rate $\alpha = 0.05$ to detect a difference in the response proportions of $p_1 - p_2 = 0.75 - 0.50$ between treatment and placebo groups, the required sample size can be calculated as:

```
> power.prop.test(p1 = .75, p2 = .50, power = .80)

    Two-sample comparison of proportions power calculation

              n = 57.7
             p1 = 0.75
             p2 = 0.5
      sig.level = 0.05
          power = 0.8
    alternative = two.sided

NOTE: n is number in *each* group
```

This gives $n = 57.7$, which means that we would need at least 58 subjects in each treatment group to achieve the desired design characteristics.

Alternatively, suppose we want to know what the power is that 60 subjects per treatment group would have in detecting a difference in response proportions $p_1 - p_2 = 0.75 - 0.50$, at the Type-I error rate $\alpha = 0.05$. This statistical power may be calculated using the following R code chunk:

```
> power.prop.test(n = 60, p1 = .75, p2 = .5)

    Two-sample comparison of proportions power calculation

              n = 60
             p1 = 0.75
             p2 = 0.5
      sig.level = 0.05
          power = 0.816
    alternative = two.sided

NOTE: n is number in *each* group
```

which is 81.6%. Similar computations may be made to determine the proportions and the significance level from specifying other parameters and we leave this to interested readers.

With the `power.prop.test` function, we can easily illustrate relationships graphically among any of the parameters. For example, we know from statistical theory that the Type-I error rate α is nonlinearly related to the Type-II error rate β as indicated in Equation (7.3). Intuitively, we know that the Type-I error rate α increases when the Type-II error rate β decreases. Since the statistical power $= 1 - \beta$, power increases when the Type-I error rate increases and vice versa. We can show this nonlinear relationship using the example above for a sample size of 60, and $p_1 = 0.75$ and $p_2 = 0.5$. We generate a sequence of values of power from 0.5 to 0.9 by 0.05 and then calculate the Type-I error rate corresponding to each value of power to make Figure 7.4 using the following R code chunk, which shows the increasing nonlinear relationship between power and α. In this figure, the horizontal line denotes $\alpha = 0.05$ to point out the associated statistical power of 0.816 as calculated in the previous example.

```
> # set up the power range
> pow    = seq(0.5, 0.9, by=0.05)
> # a for-loop to calculate alpha
> alpha = NULL
> for(i in 1:length(pow)){
     alpha[i] = power.prop.test(n=60, p1=0.75, p2=0.5,
           power=pow[i], sig.level=NULL)$sig.level
 }
> # make the plot
> plot(pow, alpha, las=1,type="b", lwd=2, xlab="Power",
              ylab="Significance Level")
> # add a segment for alpha=0.05
> segments(pow[1], 0.05, 0.816,0.05, lwd=2)
> # point to the power=0.816 for alpha=0.05
> arrows(0.816,0.05, 0.816,0, lwd=2)
```

7.3.2   R Library: `pwr`

Since its publication, the seminal book by Cohen (1988) has been widely used and referenced in statistical power analysis. An R package `pwr` has been created and maintained by Stephane Champely (`champely@univ-lyon1.fr`) based on Cohen's book and is available in the R library. In this library, there are function calls to calculate the required sample size for given statistical power (and α, δ, and *standard deviations*) as well as to calculate the power for a given sample size (and α, δ, and *standard deviations*). These functions are:

1. *pwr.2p.test* is for power calculation for two proportions assuming equal sample sizes,

2. *pwr.2p2n.test* is for power calculation for two proportions assuming different sample sizes,

3. *pwr.anova.test* is for power calculations for balanced one-way analysis of variance tests,

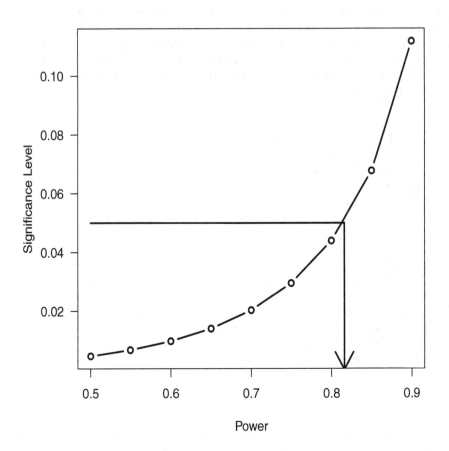

FIGURE 7.4: Nonlinear Relationship between Power and Significance Level

4. *pwr.chisq.test* is for power calculations for chi-squared tests,

5. *pwr.f2.test* is for power calculations for the general linear model,

6. *pwr.norm.test* is for power calculations for the mean of a normal distribution with known variance,

7. *pwr.p.test* is for power calculations for proportion tests (one sample),

8. *pwr.r.test* is for power calculations for correlation tests,

9. *pwr.t.test* is for power calculations for t-tests of means (one sample, two samples, and paired samples), and

10. *pwr.t2n.test* is for power calculations for two sample (of different sizes) t-tests of means.

Details about this library may be seen from the help menu using

```
> # load the library into R
> library(pwr)
> # display the help menu
> library(help=pwr)
```

These functions can be also used for sample size calculation. In doing so, the input parameters are based on the effect-size (**ES**) following the conventions in Cohen's book. For example, to calculate the sample size for a clinical trial with 80% power to detect a δ of 25% between $p_1 = 0.75$ and $p_0 = 0.5$ for a Type-I error rate of 0.05 using `pwr.2p.test`, we first need to calculate the ES from the two proportions as:

```
> h = ES.h(0.75,0.5)
> print(h)
```

```
[1] 0.524
```

which gives ES = 0.524. The ES for two proportions is defined as:

$$ES = 2 \times arcsin(\sqrt{p_1}) - 2 \times arcsin(\sqrt{p_2}) \tag{7.10}$$

With this ES, we call function `pwr.2p.test` to calculate the sample size for 80% power as:

```
> pwr.2p.test(h=h,power=0.8,sig.level=0.05)
```

```
     Difference of proportion power calculation for binomial
     distribution (arcsine transformation)

              h = 0.524
              n = 57.3
      sig.level = 0.05
          power = 0.8
    alternative = two.sided

NOTE: same sample sizes
```

This gives a sample size of 58.

We can check this with the result from `power.prop.test`:

```
> power.prop.test(p1=0.75, p2=0.5, power=0.8)
```

```
    Two-sample comparison of proportions power calculation

              n = 57.7
             p1 = 0.75
             p2 = 0.5
      sig.level = 0.05
          power = 0.8
    alternative = two.sided
```

NOTE: n is number in *each* group

We see that they are virtually the same.

Besides the traditional use of the t-test and proportion test, this package can be also used for sample size and power calculations for clinical trials with more than two-treatment groups using `pwr.anova.test`. This is equivalent to the R function `power.anova.test`, general linear regression model using `pwr.f2.test` and χ^2-test using `pwr.chisq.test`.

7.3.3   R Function nBinomial in gsDesign library

The library `gsDesign` was created by Keaven Anderson (`keaven_anderson@merck.com`) to provide a set of functions to design and analyze group sequential trials. The `Binomial` set provides statistical testing, confidence intervals, and sample size calculation for comparing two binomial proportions. This set also provides simulation for two-arm trials with a binary endpoint for fixed sample size and therefore this simulation is not for group sequential or adaptive trials.

The library can be loaded into R as:

```
> library(gsDesign)
```

and the help menu can be displayed as *library(help=gsDesign)*.

For this section to calculate sample size for comparing two binomial proportions, we can display the associated build-in functions as follows:

```
> help(nBinomial)
```

There are four functions associated with the `Binomial` set which are:

1. *nBinomial* uses the method of Farrington and Manning (1990) to compute the total sample sizes needed for comparing two binomial event rates in terms of superiority or non-inferiority,

2. *testBinomial* uses the method of Miettinin and Nurminen (1980) to compute a Z- or χ^2-statistic for comparing two binomial event rates,

3. *ciBinomial* is used to compute confidence intervals on the difference between two rates or on the risk-ratio of two rates or on the odds-ratio of two rates, and

4. *simBinomial* is used to conduct simulations to estimate the power for the Miettinin and Nurminen (1980) test comparing two binomial rates for superiority or non-inferiority.

The common usage of sample size is as follows:

```
nBinomial(p1, p2, alpha=.025, beta=0.1, delta0=0, ratio=1,
          sided=1, outtype=1, scale="Difference")
```

where

- *p1* is the event rate in treatment group 1 (i.e., D) under the alternative hypothesis,

- *p2* is the event rate in treatment group 2 (i.e., P) under the alternative hypothesis,

- *alpha* is the Type-I error rate for either a one-sided or two-sided test as noted in *sided*,

- *beta* is the Type-II error rate,

- *delta0* is a parameter associated with the null hypothesis. The default 0 represents no difference between treatment groups under the null hypothesis. If *scale* = "Difference" (the default), then $delta0 = p_{10} - p_{20}$ under H_0. If *scale* = "RR", then $delta0 = log\left(\frac{p_{10}}{p_{20}}\right)$. If *scale* = "LNOR", then $delta0 = log\left(\frac{p_{10}}{1-p_{10}}\right) - log\left(\frac{p_{20}}{1-p_{20}}\right)$,

- *ratio* is the ratio of sample size of treatment 2 divided by the sample size of treatment 1,

- *sided* is 2 for two-sided and 1 for one-sided alternatives,

- *outtype* specifies the output type; default = total sample size, 2 provides sample size for each group (n_1, n_2), 3 and delta0=0 provides a list with total sample size (n), sample size for each group (n_1, n_2), null and alternate hypothesis variance (sigma0, sigma1), input event rates (p_1, p_2) and null hypothesis event rates (p_{10}, p_{20}), and

- *scale* denotes the functional form of the comparison of the groups; i.e., "Difference", "RR" or "OR".

The sample size of 58 per treatment calculated in the previous section using

```
> power.prop.test(p1=0.75,p2=0.5, power=0.8)
```

can be reproduced using nBinomial as:

```
> nBinomial(p1=0.75, p2=0.5, alpha=.05, beta=0.2, sided=2)
```

[1] 115

which gives total sample size of 115. With equal sample size in both treatments, we would need to round 115/2=57.5 to 58 to have a total sample size of 116.

We now illustrate some calculations for sample size. Suppose we are designing a clinical trial whose **objective** is to demonstrate that a new drug is effective when compared to placebo in terms of the **endpoint**: proportion of patients showing marked improvement by the end of the treatment period, and we need to determine the number of patients needed to be randomized to the drug and placebo treated groups to have a power of 80% to detect a 15% difference (δ) between drug and placebo groups in terms of proportions of patients markedly improving given a false positive rate of 5%.

Suppose further that a search of the literature reveals that the proportion of patients randomized to placebo from reported trials of other drugs treating the same condition who showed marked improvement was 20%, and that for the trial we are designing, we wish to randomize twice as many patients to the drug group as to the placebo group.

From the information given and the literature search, we know that the proportion showing marked improvement in the placebo group is expected to be p2 $= 0.20$; p1 $=$ p2 $+ \delta = 0.35$, $\alpha = 0.05$ one-sided (the alternative hypothesis is the research objective which is to demonstrate that drug is better than placebo; i.e., is effective), $\beta = 1 - 0.80 = 0.20$, and that we want twice as many patients randomized to the drug group as the placebo group. Therefore, the desired sample size would be calculated as:

```
> nBinomial(p1=.35, p2=.2, beta=.2, ratio=0.5,outtype=2,
            alpha=.05, sided=1)
```

```
$n1
[1] 165
$n2
[1] 82.6
```

where *outtype*=2 to print the sample size for each treatment. We can see that the desired sample size is 165 and 83 (round 82.6 to 83), respectively with total of 165 + 83 = 248 subjects.

If we are to use 1-1 randomization, the total sample size is calculated as

```
> nBinomial(p1=.35, p2=.2, beta=.2, alpha=.05, sided=1)
```

```
[1] 217
```

More calculations may be performed under various other scenarios (two-sided, power of 90% and 95%, etc.) and the reader is encouraged to pursue these.

We again take advantage of the R graphical capabilities to plot the sample

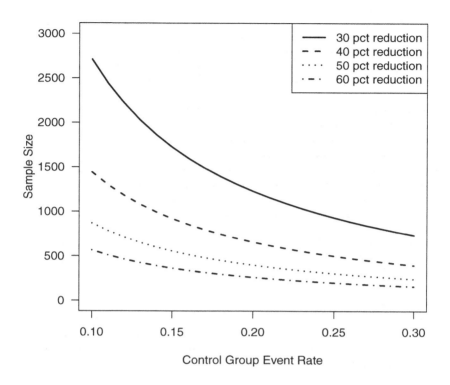

FIGURE 7.5: Sample Size Calculations for 80% Power

size required under different control rates with four types of risk reduction for the new treatment. This is illustrated in Figure 7.5:

This figure is produced with the R code chunk below. In this figure, all the sample size calculations are based on 80% power with Type-I error rate of 0.025 for one-sided binomial test.

```
> # sequence of control event rate
> p1  =  seq(.1, .3, .01)
> # reduce by 30%  to calculate the sample size required
> p2 <- p1 *.7
> y1 <- nBinomial(p1, p2, beta=.2, outtype=1, alpha=.025, sided=1)
> # reduce by 40%  to calculate the sample size required
> p2 <- p1 * .6
> y2 <- nBinomial(p1, p2, beta=.2, outtype=1, alpha=.025, sided=1)
> # reduce by 50%  to calculate the sample size required
> p2 <- p1 * .5
> y3 <- nBinomial(p1, p2, beta=.2, outtype=1, alpha=.025, sided=1)
```

```
> # reduce by 60%  to calculate the sample size required
> p2 <- p1 * .4
> y4 <- nBinomial(p1, p2, beta=.2, outtype=1, alpha=.025, sided=1)
> # make the plot for 30% reduction
> plot(p1, y1, type="l", las=1,ylab="Sample Size",
        xlab="Control Group Event Rate", ylim=c(0, 3000), lwd=2)
> # add a line for 40% reduction
> lines(p1, y2, lty=2, lwd=2)
> # add a line for 50% reduction
> lines(p1, y3, lty=3, lwd=2)
> # add a line for 60% reduction
> lines(p1, y4, lty=4, lwd=2)
> # add a legend
> legend("topright",lty=c(1,2, 3, 4), lwd=2,
      legend=c("30 pct reduction", "40 pct reduction",
      "50 pct reduction", "60 pct reduction"))
```

It can be seen from Figure 7.5 that the required sample size decreases when the event probability in the control group increases in all four situations. This is intuitively true since the absolute differences between p_1 and p_2 are increasing even though the values in the vector of p_2 are all reduced by the same amount. Theoretically, it takes larger sample sizes to detect smaller differences which explains why the required sample size decreases along with the p_1 since the absolute difference between p_1 and p_2 is increasing. This also explains why a smaller sample size is required for a higher percent reduction as depicted in this figure.

7.4   Time-to-Event Endpoint

In many clinical trials, the primary endpoint is time-to-some-critical-event (Peace (2009)). This is especially true in the clinical development of drugs for the treatment of cancer where the endpoint of primary interest is time-to-death, or survival time. Chapter 5 discussed methods for analysis of clinical trials with time-to-event data and in this section, we discuss design aspects of such trials, including sample size determination using R function nSurvival in gsDesign Library.

Similar to nBinomial, there is a function nSurvival in the gsDesign library which can be used to determine sample sizes for clinical trials where the primary endpoint is time-to-some-critical event. The function nSurvival uses the method described in Lachin and Foulkes (1986), which assumes known distributions for:

1. the time-to-event of primary interest in each treatment group,

2. the time until dropout in each group,

3. enrollment over time.

The Lachin-Foulkes method allows different distributional assumptions in different strata.

In nSurvival, time-to-enrollment, time-to-dropout, and time-to-the-primary event, are assumed to follow exponential distributions with no strat-ification. The number of patients and the number of events necessary to meet design characteristics are then calculable. It is well known that the cumulative distribution function for an exponential distribution with failure rate λ has the following form:

$$F(t) = 1 - e^{\lambda t} \tag{7.11}$$

Therefore, if we know the cumulative failure rate p_0 at time t_0, λ can be estimated as:

$$\hat{\lambda} = -\frac{ln(1 - p_0)}{t_0} \tag{7.12}$$

A detailed explanation and usage of this function can be obtained from *help(nSurvival)*. We briefly describe it here within the context of designing a trial comparing a drug treatment to placebo in terms of improving survival. The function call is as follows:

```
nSurvival(lambda1, lambda2, Ts, Tr, eta = 0, rand.ratio = 1,
    alpha = 0.05, beta = 0.10, sided = 2, approx = FALSE,
    type = c("rr", "rd"), entry = c("unif", "expo"), gamma = NA)
```

where

- *lambda1, lambda2* are the primary event hazard rates for the placebo and treatment groups, respectively;

- *Ts* is the maximum study duration;

- *Tr* is the accrual (recruitment) duration;

- *eta* is the dropout hazard rate for both groups. Default is eta $= 0$;

- *rand.ratio* is the randomization ratio between the placebo and treatment groups. Default is a balanced design, i.e., randomization ratio is 1;

- *alpha* is the Type-I error rate. Default is 0.05;

- *beta* is the Type-II error rate. Default is 0.10 (90% power);

- *sided* denotes one- or two-sided test. Default is two-sided;

- *approx* is a logical indicator. If TRUE, the approximation sample size formula for risk difference is used;

- *type* is the type of sample size calculation [i.e., based on the risk ratio ("rr") or the risk difference ("rd")];

- *entry* is the type of patient entry, whether uniform ("unif") or exponential ("expo");

- *gamma* is the rate parameter for exponential entry, which has a value of NA if entry type is "unif" (uniform); and a user supplied non-zero value if entry type is "expo" (exponential).

The outputs from this function include the total sample size (n) and the number of events (*Events*) required along with all inputs.

We now consider some examples of sample size calculations. Consider designing a clinical trial where the general objective is to demonstrate that a new drug treatment can reduce the constant, hazard death rate by 1/3 as compared to placebo.

Suppose that it is known from previous studies of the disease that the constant rate of death among untreated patients is 0.30 and that on average 10% of patients drop out prior to study completion. Further, suppose that the trial being designed will have uniform patient enrollment over 1 year, and that the maximum study duration from the time of enrollment of the first patient will be 3 years.

The sample size question is: How many patients should be enrolled and of those how many deaths are required to detect a reduction of 1/3 in the constant rate of death among treated patients compared to patients randomized to the placebo group, with a power of 80% and a Type-I (1-sided) error rate of 2.5%?

In terms of the difference in hazard rates, the objective of the trial is the alternative hypothesis H_a in the following:

$$H_0 : \lambda_1 - \lambda_2 = 0 \text{ versus } H_a : \lambda_1 - \lambda_2 = \delta < 0 \qquad (7.13)$$

where δ = -0.10 (1/3 of 0.30).

In terms of the ratio of hazard rates, the objective of the trial is the alternative hypothesis H_a in the following:

$$H_0 : \lambda_1/\lambda_2 = 1 \text{ versus } H_a : \lambda_1/\lambda_2 = 1 - \delta, \qquad (7.14)$$

where $\delta = 1/3$.

The required numbers of patients to be enrolled and of those the number of deaths required [to have an 80% power ($\beta = 0.20$) to detect the stated reduction in hazard rates with $\alpha = .025$] may be calculated as:

```
> # calculate sample size (denoted by ss1)
```

```
> ss1 = nSurvival(lambda1=.3,lambda2=.2,
        eta =.1,Ts=3,Tr=1,sided=1,alpha=.025,beta=0.2)
> # print the required ss
> print(ss1)



Fixed design, two-arm trial with time-to-event
outcome (Lachin and Foulkes, 1986).
Study duration (fixed):          Ts=3
Accrual duration (fixed):        Tr=1
Uniform accrual:                   entry="unif"
Control median:       log(2)/lambda1=2.3
Experimental median: log(2)/lambda2=3.5
Censoring only at study end (eta=0)
Control failure rate:        lambda1=0.3
Experimental failure rate:   lambda2=0.2
Censoring rate:                  eta=0.1
Power:                    100*(1-beta)=80%
Type I error (1-sided):    100*alpha=2.5%
Equal randomization:             ratio=1
Sample size based on hazard ratio=0.667 (type="rr")
Sample size (computed):             n=466
Events required (computed): nEvents=192
```

which gives the required number of patients to be 466 and the number of deaths to be 192 in order to achieve 80% power to detect a reduction of $1/3$ in λ_1/λ_2 with a 2.5% one-sided Type-I error.

Readers may change the inputs and use the function **nSurvival** to determine sample sizes for their own clinical trials where the primary endpoint is time-to-some-critical event.

There is an excellent example in Section 1.6 of the **gsDesign** manual and we re-produce it here. In this example, the general objective is to compare the efficacy of an experimental treatment to the standard treatment in terms of the primary endpoint: progression-free survival (PFS).

Here PFS is defined as the time from randomization until disease progression or death. Patients on the standard treatment (denoted by C) are assumed to have an exponential failure (return of the disease) rate with median PFS = 6 months. Based on Equation (7.12), the failure rate for standard treatment is estimated as $\lambda_C = -ln(.5)/6 = .1155$, with time measured in months.

The specific objective of the trial is to demonstrate that the experimental treatment (denoted by E) will reduce the hazard rate (of PFS) by 30% as compared to standard treatment (C).

The reduction stated in the objective enables us to estimate the experimental group hazard rate as $\lambda_E = 0.7 \times \lambda_C = .0809$. Patients are assumed to drop out at a rate of 5% per year of followup which implies an exponential dropout rate $\eta = -ln(.95)/12 = .00427$.

Enrollment of patients is assumed to be uniform over 30 months with patients followed for a minimum of 6 months, yielding a total study time duration of 36 months.

The design question is: How many patients should be enrolled and of those how many deaths are required to detect a reduction of 30% in the constant rate of failure among patients treated with the experimental regimen (E) as compared to patients treated with the standard regimen (C), with a power of 90% and a Type-I (1-sided) error rate of 2.5%?

The required sample size and number of events may be calculated using the following R code chunk:

```
> # call nSurvival to calculate sample size
> ss2 =  nSurvival(lambda1=-log(.5) / 6,
        lambda2=-log(.5) / 6 *.7, eta=-log(.95)/12,
        Tr=30 ,Ts=36, type="rr", entry="unif")
> # print the required sample size
> print(ss2$n)
```

416

```
> # print the required number of events
> print(ss2$nEvents)
```

329

This shows that 418 patients and 330 events (disease progression) are required to have a power of 90% to detect a 30% reduction in hazards with a one-sided Type-I error of 2.5%.

7.5   Design of Group Sequential Trials

7.5.1   Introduction

So far, we have presented applications of R functions: nBinomial and nSurvival, from the gsDesign library for sample size and power calculations. In fact, the primary use of the library gsDesign by Keaven M. Anderson from Merck Research Laboratories is to design group sequential clinical trials using α- and β-spending functions, Wang-Tsiatis designs including O'Brien-Fleming and Pocock designs. This package is based on the statistical theory developed for group sequential designs as seen in Jennison and Turnbull (2000) and Proschan et al. (2006). Detailed explanations about this package can be found from its manual (called *gsDesign: An R Package for Designing Group Sequential Clinical Trials*) which is available as a PDF file from the library subdirectories. As a further promotion to use this package, we briefly describe some of its functionalities and some of its applications.

The package can be loaded into R as follows:

```
> library(gsDesign)
```

All subroutines and functions can be found from the help manual using `library(help=gsDesign)`. As listed in the manual, three primary functions are provided for basic computations related to the design and evaluation of group sequential clinical trials:

1. *gsDesign* function "provides sample size and boundaries for a group sequential design based on treatment effect, spending functions for boundary crossing probabilities, and relative timing of each analysis. Standard and user-specified spending functions may be used. In addition to spending function designs, the family of Wang-Tsiatis designs, including O'Brien-Fleming and Pocock designs, are also available";

2. *gsProbability* "function computes boundary crossing probabilities and expected sample size of a design for arbitrary user-specified treatment effects, bounds, and interim analysis sample sizes";

3. *gsCP* "function computes the conditional probability of future boundary crossing given a result at an interim analysis. The *gsCP* function returns a value of the same type as *gsProbability*".

Besides these primary functions, there are several supporting functions to evaluate trials with binomial endpoints and trials with time-to-event endpoints, such as `nBinomial` in Section 7.3.3 and `nSurvival` in Section 7.4. The function set of **Binomial** provides sample size and power calculations, hypothesis testing, confidence intervals, and simulation, especially for designing noninferiority trials as well as superiority trials.

7.5.2 gsDesign

We further illustrate the use of **gsDesign** to develop boundaries and trial size required for a group sequential design. Other functions may be found from the manual. The default group sequential design is one with:

1. two interim analyses equally spaced at $1/3$ and $2/3$ of the way through the trial plus the final analysis (i.e., $k=3$);

2. two-sided, asymmetric, beta-spending with non-binding lower bound (i.e., *test.type*=4);

3. overall Type-I error $\alpha = 0.025$ (one-sided);

4. overall Type-II error $\beta = 0.1$ with power = 90%;

5. asymmetric boundaries, which means we may stop the trial for futility or superiority at an interim analysis;

6. β-spending is used to set the lower stopping boundary. This means that the spending function controls the incremental amount of the Type-II error at each analysis, $\beta(\delta), i = 1, 2, \cdots, K$;

7. non-binding lower bound. Lower bounds are sometimes considered as guidelines, which may be ignored during the course of the trial;

8. Hwang-Shih-DeCani spending functions with γ= -4 for the upper bound and γ=-2 for the lower bound. This provides a conservative, O'Brien-Fleming-like superiority bound and a less conservative lower bound.

This default design is specified by the default inputs in the usage of gsDesign as follows:

```
gsDesign(k = 3, test.type = 4, alpha = 0.025, beta = 0.1,
astar=0,delta=0,n.fix=1,timing = 1, sfu = sfHSD,
sfupar = -4, sfl = sfHSD, sflpar = -2, tol = 0.000001,
r = 18, n.I = 0, maxn.IPlan = 0)
```

It is noted that all the input parameters in the above function gsDesign, may be changed to fit the reader's specific design. For example, we can simply change $k = 5$ for a 5-interim stage group sequential design.

The default design can be illustrated with the following R code chunk:

```
> # load the default gsDesign
> x = gsDesign()
> # print the output
> x
```

Asymmetric two-sided group sequential design with
90 % power and 2.5 % Type I Error.
Upper bound spending computations assume
trial continues if lower bound is crossed.

	Sample Size		----Lower bounds----			----Upper bounds-----		
Analysis	Ratio*	Z	Nominal p	Spend+	Z	Nominal p	Spend++
1	0.357	-0.24	0.406	0.0148	3.01	0.0013	0.0013
2	0.713	0.94	0.827	0.0289	2.55	0.0054	0.0049
3	1.070	2.00	0.977	0.0563	2.00	0.0228	0.0188
Total				0.1000			0.0250

+ lower bound beta spending (under H1):

```
Hwang-Shih-DeCani spending function with gamma = -2
++ alpha spending:
Hwang-Shih-DeCani spending function with gamma = -4
* Sample size ratio compared to fixed design with no interim
```

```
Boundary crossing probabilities and expected sample size
assume any cross stops the trial
```

```
Upper boundary (power or Type I Error)
        Analysis
  Theta      1      2      3  Total  E{N}
  0.00 0.0013 0.0049 0.0171 0.0233 0.625
  3.24 0.1412 0.4403 0.3185 0.9000 0.791
```

```
Lower boundary (futility or Type II Error)
        Analysis
  Theta      1      2      3 Total
  0.00 0.4057 0.4290 0.1420 0.977
  3.24 0.0148 0.0289 0.0563 0.100
```

From the output of this default design, the total Type-I error is 0.025 and the total probability of crossing the upper boundary at any analysis when the lower bound stops the trial is 0.0233. Further, we can extract components from the output for specific usage. For example, the sample size ratio compared to fixed non-group sequential design can be extracted as:

```
> x$n.I
```

```
[1] 0.357 0.713 1.070
```

which is the column just before "Lower bounds" and shows 0.357, 0.713, and 1.070 for interim analyses 1, 2 and 3, respectively. Note that the sample size is inflated by 7% at the end of the trial which is expected since the purpose of group sequential designs is to permit interim analyses for stopping the trial before its end.

Suppose that we design a clinical trial with a binomial endpoint where we wish to detect an increase in the cure rate from 15% in the control group to 30% in the new treatment group with a power of 90% and a one-sided Type-I error rate of 2.5%. The fixed non-group sequential design required total sample size is computed as:

```
> # calculate the sample size for non-group sequential design
> n.fix = nBinomial(p1=0.3, p2=0.15)
> # print the fixed sample size
> n.fix
```

```
[1] 322
```

which shows that 322 is the required total sample size. For a group sequential design, the sample size would be

```
> # Calculate GS sample sizes at each interim
> n.GS = n.fix*x$n.I
> # print them
> n.GS
```

[1] 115 229 344

Rounding up to an even number, we would need 116 and 230 patients at interim stages 1 and 2. The total sample size required is now inflated to 344 using the default group sequential design. The total sample size for the group sequential design can be directly calculated by:

```
> # direct calculation of GS design
> x.new = gsDesign(n.fix=n.fix)
> # print the design
> x.new
```

```
Asymmetric two-sided group sequential design with
90 % power and 2.5 % Type I Error.
Upper bound spending computations assume
trial continues if lower bound is crossed.
```

| | | | ----Lower bounds---- | | ----Upper bounds----- | | |
Analysis	N	Z	Nominal p	Spend+	Z	Nominal p	Spend++
1	115	-0.24	0.406	0.0148	3.01	0.0013	0.0013
2	230	0.94	0.827	0.0289	2.55	0.0054	0.0049
3	345	2.00	0.977	0.0563	2.00	0.0228	0.0188
Total				0.1000			0.0250

```
+ lower bound beta spending (under H1):
 Hwang-Shih-DeCani spending function with gamma = -2
++ alpha spending:
 Hwang-Shih-DeCani spending function with gamma = -4
```

```
Boundary crossing probabilities and expected sample size
assume any cross stops the trial
```

```
Upper boundary (power or Type I Error)
          Analysis
```

Theta	1	2	3	Total	E{N}
0.000	0.0013	0.0049	0.0171	0.0233	201
0.181	0.1412	0.4403	0.3185	0.9000	254

```
Lower boundary (futility or Type II Error)
          Analysis
```

```
Theta        1       2       3 Total
0.000  0.4057  0.4290  0.1420  0.977
0.181  0.0148  0.0289  0.0563  0.100
```

Comparing the output object from *x* to *x.new*, we can see that the *Sample Size Ratio* is now replaced by the required sample size *N* and the rest remains the same.

Additional useful information in this output is the *Upper bounds* and *Lower bounds*. Both contain multiple variables for the upper and lower boundaries as well as boundary crossing probabilities. The boundaries can be plotted by calling `plot` as follows to produce the boundary plot as in Figure 7.6:

```
> # call "plot" to make the boundary plot
> print(plot(x, plottype=1))
```

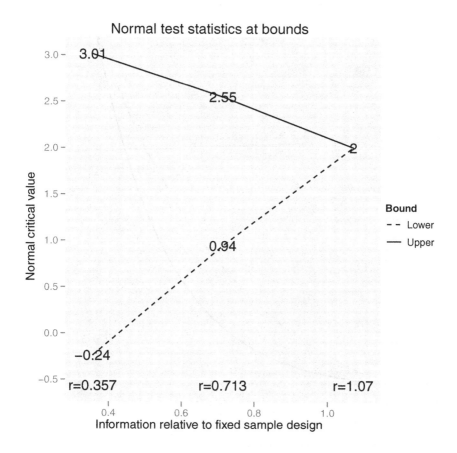

FIGURE 7.6: Default Plot for *gsDesign* Boundaries

In the `plot`, the `plottype` allows seven choices with *plottype* = *1* to be specified for the boundary plot (default for gsDesign) as seen in Figure 7.6. And *plottype* = *2* provides the power plot (default for *gsProbability*), *plottype* = *3* provides the estimated treatment effect at the boundaries, *plottype* = *4* provides the conditional power at boundaries, *plottype* = *5* provides the spending function plot, *plottype* = *6* provides the expected sample size plot, and *plottype* = *7* provides the B-values at the boundaries.

For example, we can plot the spending functions using *plottype* = *5* to produce Figure 7.7 for both α and β-spending functions as follows.

```
> # plot the alpha and beta spending function
> print(plot(x, plottype=5))
```

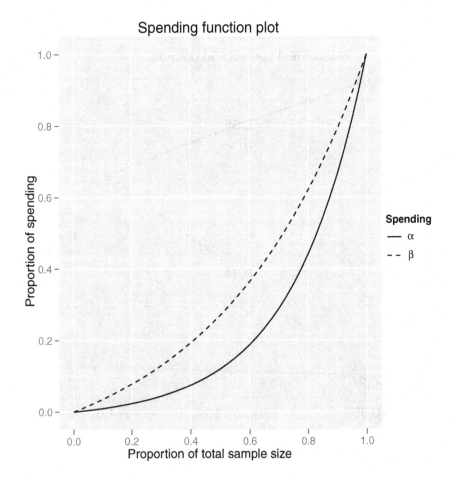

FIGURE 7.7: Spending Function Plot for *gsDesign*

A similar illustration using `gsDesign` can be generated for clinical trials with time-to-event endpoints as described in Section 5.3.2 in the manual. In the package, we can define different spending functions to fit the trial requirements as well investigate different spending functions to optimize design characteristics. This package is flexible and we encourage readers to become familiar with using it to design group sequential trials.

7.6   Longitudinal Trials

Chapter 6 discussed the analysis of data from longitudinal clinical trials. In this subsection, our focus is on designing longitudinal trials. In their Chapter 15, Fitzmaurice et al. (2004) described methods for sample size calculation for longitudinal studies which can be used in designing longitudinal trials. We program these methods in R and illustrate their application. Therefore, we use the same notation as in Fitzmaurice et al. (2004).

7.6.1   Longitudinal Trial with Continuous Endpoint

7.6.1.1   The Model Setting

Suppose a trial is designed to compare two treatments such as a new drug to control in terms of their effect on changes in mean response over time. We assume equal numbers of subjects, denoted by N, are randomized to both treatments with n repeated measurements on each subject. At the end of the trial, we are to compare the changes in mean response over the duration of trial, as typically seen in longitudinal studies such as the diastolic blood pressure (DBP) trial in Chapter 6. As is typically done in longitudinal studies, the changes in mean response are expressed as a linear trend and the treatment effect is expressed as the difference in slopes or rates of change denoted by δ. Therefore, the null hypothesis of no treatment difference, i.e., there is no treatment by linear trend interaction, can be denoted by $H_0 : \delta = 0$.

A two-stage model is used to describe the longitudinal trial. In the first stage, it is assumed that a simple parametric linear trend in time can be fit to the observed clinical response data for each subject. In the second stage, these subject-specific parameters are then linked to covariates that describe the different treatments as well as other covariates. Specifically,

- *Stage 1*: In this stage, we assume that the repeated measurements for each subject follow a time-trend regression line with the same set of covariates, with coefficients for each subject as in:

$$Y_{ij} = \beta_{1i} + \beta_{2i}t_j + e_{ij} \qquad (7.15)$$

where the error, e_{ij} are assumed to be independently and identically

normally distributed with mean 0 and homogeneous variance of σ_e^2; i.e.,
$e \sim N(0, \sigma_e^2)$,

- *Stage 2*: In this stage, we assume the subject-specific effects $\beta_i = (\beta_{1i}, \beta_{2i})'$ are random in order to describe population level parameters; i.e.,

$$
\begin{aligned}
E(\beta_{1i}) &= \beta_1 + \beta_2 \times Treatment_i \\
E(\beta_{2i}) &= \beta_3 + \beta_4 \times Treatment_i
\end{aligned} \tag{7.16}
$$

where $Treatment_i$ is an indicator variable denoting treatment group; i.e., $Treatment_i = 1$ if the ith subject was assigned to the new drug and $Treatment_i = 0$ if the ith subject was assigned to control. It can be seen in the model (7.16) that β_3 is the mean slope used to describe the population rates of change in mean response over time for the control group and $\beta_3 + \beta_4$ is the mean slope in the new drug treatment group. Therefore, β_4 describes the population mean difference between new drug treatment and control in mean slope or the rates of change in the repeated measurements, which corresponds to the definition of δ. Thus the null hypothesis can be expressed as $H_0 : \beta_4 = 0$.

Since the model (7.16) only describes the population mean response of β_i by treatment group, the residual between-subject variation in the β_i that cannot be explained by treatment group is expressed as:

$$
Cov(\beta_i) = G = \begin{pmatrix} g_{11} & g_{12} \\ g_{21} & g_{22} \end{pmatrix} \tag{7.17}
$$

where $g_{11} = var(\beta_{1i})$, $g_{22} = var(\beta_{2i})$ and $g_{12} = g_{21} = cov(\beta_{1i}, \beta_{2i})$.

7.6.1.2   Sample Size Calculations

Let $\hat{\beta}_{2i}$ denote the ordinary least squares (OLS) estimate of the slope for the ith subject. The variability of $\hat{\beta}_{2i}$ can be derived as:

$$
\sigma^2 = Var(\hat{\beta}_{2i}) = \frac{\sigma_e^2}{\sum_{j=1}^{n}(t_j - \bar{t})^2} + g_{22} \tag{7.18}
$$

where $\bar{t} = \frac{1}{n}\sum_{j=1}^{n} t_j$ which means that the variability of $\hat{\beta}_{2i}$ consists of two components: one from the within-subject variance of $\frac{\sigma_e^2}{\sum_{j=1}^{n}(t_j - \bar{t})^2}$ and the other from the between-subject variance of $g_{22} = Var(\beta_{2i})$. Therefore, to test the null hypothesis $H_0 : \delta = 0$ of equal mean changes over time of the two treatment groups, we can construct a z-test based on $\hat{\beta}_{2i}$ as:

$$
Z = \frac{\bar{\beta}_2^T - \bar{\beta}_2^C}{\sigma\sqrt{1/N + 1/N}} = \frac{\bar{\beta}_2^T - \bar{\beta}_2^C}{\sigma\sqrt{2/N}} \tag{7.19}
$$

where $\bar{\beta}_2^T$ and $\bar{\beta}_2^C$ are the sample means of $\hat{\beta}_{2i}$ in the new drug treatment (T) and control (C) groups, respectively. Given estimates of g_{22} and σ_e^2, the required sample size can be determined from the standard formula in Equation (7.5) as:

$$N = \frac{2(z_{1-\alpha/2} + z_{1-\beta})^2}{\left(\frac{\delta}{\sigma}\right)^2} \tag{7.20}$$

where σ is the estimate defined in Equation (7.18) and δ is the treatment effect. Notice that the sample size formula in Equation (7.20) is identical to Equation (7.5) except that variance of σ has two components: the within-subject and between-subject variances. It should be emphasized that the sample size formula in Equation (7.20) includes the length of the study (denoted by $\tau = t_n$), the number of repeated measures (n) and the spacing of the repeated measures of $(t_1, t_2, \cdots, t_n)$.

In a typical equal-spaced longitudinal trial with study duration τ, the n repeated measurements are to be taken at $t_1 = 0$, $t_2 = \frac{\tau}{n-1}$, $t_3 = \frac{2\tau}{n-1}$, $\cdots$, $t_n = \tau$. In this case, it is easily shown that:

$$\sum_{j=1}^{n}(t_j - \bar{t})^2 = \frac{\tau^2 n(n+1)}{12(n-1)} \tag{7.21}$$

7.6.1.3 Power Calculation

The sample size formula in Equation (7.20) may be used to calculate the statistical power for a specified sample size. Re-arranging Equation (7.20) as:

$$z_{1-\beta} = \sqrt{\frac{N\delta^2}{2\sigma^2}} - z_{1-\alpha/2}, \tag{7.22}$$

the statistical power $1 - \beta$ can be calculated as $\Phi(z_{1-\beta})$ where Φ denotes the cumulative standard normal distribution function.

7.6.1.4 Example and R Illustration

Following the example in Fitzmaurice et al. (2004), suppose we are planning a longitudinal trial to compare two treatments: new drug treatment versus control, say, in terms of the mean response over time. We plan to randomize equal numbers of patients (N) to both treatment groups. The trial is expected to require $\tau = 2$ years to complete, and a total of 5 $(= n)$ repeated measurements are to be taken, with one at baseline and the remaining four at 6-month intervals until trial completion. The response is assumed to be approximately normally distributed and we assume that change in response is linear over time and that the treatment effect can be expressed in term of the slopes (denoted by δ).

Suppose further that we want to enroll enough subjects to detect a minimum treatment effect of $\delta = 1.2$ in the annual rates of change between the new drug treatment and control. Based on historical data, suppose that the between-subject variability in the rate of change is $Var(\beta_{2i}) \approx 2$ and the within-subject variability $\sigma_e^2 \approx 7$. We want to determine the number of trial subjects required to have 90% power to detect $\delta = 1.2$ with a two-sided 5% false positive rate (i.e., $\alpha = 0.05$ and $\beta = 0.1$).

Based on these specifications, we first compute the variability of $\hat{\beta}_{2i}$ in Equation (7.18) using the Equation in (7.21) as:

$$\sigma^2 = \frac{\sigma_e^2}{\sum_{j=1}^{n}(t_j - \bar{t})^2} + g_{22}$$

$$= \frac{12(n-1)\sigma_e^2}{\tau^2 n(n+1)} = \frac{12 \times 4 \times 7}{4 \times 5} + 2 \qquad (7.23)$$

$$= 2.8 + 2 = 4.8 \qquad (7.24)$$

Then the required sample size may be calculated based on Equation (7.20) as:

$$N = \frac{2(z_{1-\alpha/2} + z_{1-\beta})^2}{\left(\frac{\delta}{\sigma}\right)^2}$$

$$= \frac{(1.96 + 1.282)^2 \times 2 \times 4.8}{1.44} = 70.1 \qquad (7.25)$$

The corresponding R code is as follows:

```
> # minimum treatment effect
> delta        = 1.2
> # number of repeated measurements
> n            = 5
> # trial duration
> tau          = 2
> # within-subject variability
> sig2within  = 7
> # between-subject variability
> sig2between = 2
> # significance level
> alpha        = 0.05
> # desired power
> pow          = 0.9
> # variance of slopes
> sig2        = 12*(n-1)*sig2within/(tau^2*n*(n+1))+sig2between
> print(sig2)

[1] 4.8

> # calculate sample size
> N            = (qnorm(1-alpha/2)+qnorm(pow))^2*2*sig2/delta^2
> cat("Sample size needed=",N, sep=" ","\n\n")
```

```
Sample size needed= 70
```

Therefore, 142 subjects should be randomized in balanced fashion (71 each) to both treatment groups to ensure the design characteristics.

For a given sample size, we can also calculate the power using the method described in Section 7.6.1.3. For example, for the same design characteristics with sample size $N = 40$ for each treatment, the statistical power is calculated to be 0.63 using following R code chunk:

```
> # sample size for each treatment
> N = 40;   n = 2 ; delta = 1.2; tau = 2
> sig2within  = 7; sig2between = 2; alpha      = 0.05
> sig2        = 12*(n-1)*sig2within/(tau^2*n*(n+1))+sig2between
> pow.get     = pnorm(sqrt( N*delta^2/(2*sig2))-qnorm(1-alpha/2))
> cat("Power obtained=", pow.get,sep=" ", "\n\n")
```

```
Power obtained= 0.629
```

The relationship among design characteristics (say, the number of repeated measurements n, sample size N and power) may be illustrated. To do so, we specify an R function called `pow.Long` to compute the statistical power from different design inputs as:

```
> pow.Long =
    function(N, n, delta, tau, sig2within, sig2between, alpha){
  sig2     = 12*(n-1)*sig2within/(tau^2*n*(n+1))+sig2between
  pow.get  = pnorm(sqrt( N*delta^2/(2*sig2))-qnorm(1-alpha/2))
  pow.get  } # end of function
```

We then call this function to calculate the power for sample size N from 20 to 100 by 20 and the number of repeated measurements n from 2 to 8 as follows:

```
> # the sample size inputs
> N = seq(20, 100, by=20)
> # the number of repeated measurements
> n = seq(2,10, by=2)
> # power matrix
> pow = matrix(0, ncol=length(N), nrow=length(n))
> colnames(pow) = n; rownames(pow) = N
> # loop to calculate the power
> for (i in 1:length(N)){
        for(j in 1:length(n)){
        pow[i,j] = pow.Long(N[i], n[j], delta, tau,
                    sig2within, sig2between, alpha)  } }
> # print the power matrix
> pow
```

	2	4	6	8	10
20	0.366	0.387	0.432	0.471	0.503
40	0.629	0.657	0.716	0.761	0.795
60	0.800	0.825	0.873	0.905	0.926
80	0.899	0.917	0.947	0.965	0.976
100	0.951	0.962	0.979	0.988	0.993

This reproduces Table 15.1 in Fitzmaurice et al. (2004). We can graphically display this relationship using the R plotting function `persp` in the following R code chunk to produce a perspective surface plot as seen in Figure 7.8.

```
> persp(N, n, pow, theta = 30, phi = 30, expand = 0.5,
col = "lightblue", xlab="Sample Size (N)",
ylab="# of Measurements (n)",  zlab="Power")
```

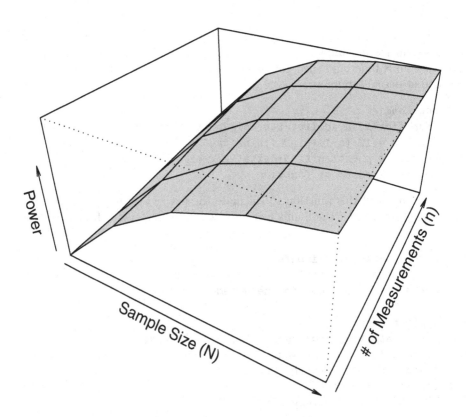

FIGURE 7.8: Perspective Surface for Power in Longitudinal Study

7.6.2 Longitudinal Binary Endpoint

7.6.2.1 Approximate Sample Size Calculation

Due to the underlying complications existing in logistic regression for its link function and dependence between mean and variance, Fitzmaurice et al. (2004) derived an approximate method to calculate sample size for longitudinal trials with binary response. The approximation is restricted to response probabilities ranging from 0.2 to 0.8 since in this range, the linearity on the log odds scale (the logit) or the probit scale coincides approximately to the linearity on the probability scale. Therefore, in this situation, the link function in the generalized linear model for response probabilities is:

$$g\left[E(Y_{ij}|X_{ij})\right] = X'_{ij}\beta \tag{7.26}$$

which can be well approximated by a linear relationship as

$$E(Y_{ij}|X_{ij}) = X'_{ij}\beta^* \tag{7.27}$$

for some $\beta^* \neq \beta$, where β^* represents changes in the probabilities while β represents changes in the log odds providing $g(\cdot)$ has a logistic form.

In addition, the variance of the binary response:

$$Var(Y_{ij}) = E(Y_{ij}) \times [1 - E(Y_{ij})], \tag{7.28}$$

will change more slowly when the response probabilities are in the range of 0.2 to 0.8 with maximum value of 0.25 when $E(Y_{ij}) = 0.5$. Therefore, the sample size formula in Equation (7.5) may be expressed as:

$$N = \frac{2\sigma^2(z_{1-\alpha/2} + z_{1-\beta})^2}{\delta^2}, \tag{7.29}$$

where δ is the linear contrast of response probabilities to denote the comparison of the two treatment groups.

Now,

$$\sigma^2 = Var(Y_{ij})(1-\rho)\left[\sum_{j=1}^{n}(t_j - \bar{t})^2\right] \approx 0.25 \times (1-\rho)\left[\sum_{j=1}^{n}(t_j - \bar{t})^2\right], \tag{7.30}$$

where $Var(Y_{ij})$ is approximated by the maximum possible value of 0.25 and $\rho = Corr(Y_{ij}, Y_{ik})$.

In the special case with study duration τ and n equally repeated measurements:

$$\sigma^2 = 0.25 \times (1-\rho)\left[\sum_{j=1}^{n}(t_j - \bar{t})^2\right] = \frac{3(n-1)(1-\rho)}{\tau^2 n(n+1)}. \tag{7.31}$$

It should be noted that the above formulation yields an over-estimate of sample size since the maximum value of the variance is used.

7.6.2.2   Example and R Implementation

Consider the design settings in Section 7.6.1.4 and suppose this is a cancer trial to investigate whether a new drug can reduce the mortality rate as compared to standard treatment. In this case, response is the change in the probability of the binary response over time which we assume is approximated by a linear trend. Suppose further that past experience indicates that the mortality rate of standard treatment is 30%. We want to be able to detect a reduction in the mortality rate of 15% at 2 years, which means $\delta = 0.15/\tau = 0.15/2 = 0.075$. Based on historical trials, the correlation among pairs of responses is approximately 0.5 (i.e., $\rho = 0.5$). Then

$$\sigma^2 \approx \frac{3(n-1)(1-\rho)}{\tau^2 n(n+1)} = \frac{3 \times 4 \times 0.5}{4 \times 5 \times 6} = 0.05 \qquad (7.32)$$

The required sample size for a power of 90% and a two-sided false positive rate of 5% is calculated as follows:

$$N = \frac{2\sigma^2(z_{1-\alpha/2} + z_{1-\beta})^2}{\delta^2} = \frac{(1.96 + 1.282)^2 \times 2 \times 0.05}{0.075^2} = 186.9, \qquad (7.33)$$

which means the required number of subjects needed to achieve the design specifications is 374 ($=187 \times 2$).

This method is implemented in R with the following code chunk:

```
> # the treatment effect
> delta  = 0.075
> # number of repeated measurements
> n       = 5
> # study duration
> tau     = 2
> # correlation
> rho     =  0.5
> # significance level
> alpha = 0.05
> # Type-II error
> beta  = 0.1
> # associated power
> pow  = 1-beta
> # sigma calculation
> sig2 = 3*(n-1)*(1-rho)/(tau^2*n*(n+1))
> # sample size calculation
> N = (qnorm(1-alpha/2)+qnorm(pow))^2*2*sig2/delta^2
> cat("Sample size needed=",N, sep=" ","\n\n")

Sample size needed= 187
```

This again reproduces the results from Fitzmaurice et al. (2004).

7.7 Relative Changes and Coefficient of Variation

7.7.1 Introduction

Often clinical trial practitioners (e.g., the biostatistician and the clinician) are unable to find estimates of treatment means, standard deviations, etc. in order to apply sample size formulae. Let's consider the following dialogue in a planning meeting for a clinical trial comparing a new drug treatment to a control:

The biostatistician: "What kind of treatment effect are you expecting?"

The clinician: "I'm looking for a 20% change in the mean."

The biostatistician again: "And how much variability is there in your observations?"

The clinician: "About 30%."

This dialogue reflects that clinicians (and other substantive researchers) frequently think of relative treatment effects and variability as percentages, and often think of standard deviation relative to the mean. The question now is how to calculate the required sample size? The answer is illustrated in the following:

7.7.2 Sample Size Calculation Formula

Recall that the coefficient of variation is defined as standard deviation divided by the mean; i.e., $CV = \sigma/\mu$. CV is unitless but is usually expressed as a percentage. A $CV = 50\%$ means that the magnitude of the standard deviation is one-half that of the mean.

The dialogue above implies the clinician is thinking about the treatment effect (as the difference in the means of new drug treatment and control) as being 20% of the control mean and variability as relative to the treatment effect. Since relative variability described as the coefficient of variation (CV) is intrinsically a constant, this implies that the variances of the two populations are not the same.

The variance σ^2 in Equation (7.5) is then replaced by the average of the two population variances:

$$\sigma^2 = \frac{\sigma_1^2 + \sigma_2^2}{2} \qquad (7.34)$$

Replacing σ_i by $\mu_i CV$ for $i = 1, 2$ and simplifying the algebra in Equation (7.5), we have the sample size formula as:

$$n = \frac{8(CV)^2}{(PC)^2} \left[1 + (1 - PC)^2\right] \qquad (7.35)$$

where PC is the proportion change in means defined as $PC = \frac{\mu_1 - \mu_2}{\mu_1}$ and CV is the usual coefficient of variation which is $CV = \frac{\sigma_1}{\mu_1} = \frac{\sigma_2}{\mu_2}$.

7.7.3   Example and R Implementation

For the clinical trial being planned as described in the dialogue session, the sample size can be calculated as

$$n = \frac{8(0.30)^2}{(0.20)^2}[1 + (1 - 0.2)^2] = 29.52 = 30 \qquad (7.36)$$

which means that at least 30 subjects per treatment group would be needed to achieve a 20% change in the mean with a CV of 30%. The R implementation is straightforward and we use this formulation to look into a series of CVs and PCs. Suppose we want to see the required sample size for CVs ranging from 0.1 to 0.7 and PCs ranging from 0.1 to 0.5. We may calculate them using the following R code chunk:

```
> # CV range
> CV =seq(0.1, 0.7, by=0.1)
> CV

[1] 0.1 0.2 0.3 0.4 0.5 0.6 0.7

> # PC range
> PC =  seq(0.1, 0.5, by=0.05)
> PC

[1] 0.10 0.15 0.20 0.25 0.30 0.35 0.40 0.45 0.50

> # Sample size calculation
> SS = matrix(0, ncol=length(PC), nrow=length(CV))
> colnames(SS) = PC
> rownames(SS)= CV
> # for-loop to calculate the sample size for each PC and CV
    combination
> for (i in 1:length(CV)){
        for(j in 1:length(PC)){
        SS[i,j] = ceiling(8*CV[i]^2/PC[j]^2*(1+(1-PC[j])^2))
                        }
                }
> # print out the table
> SS
```

	0.1	0.15	0.2	0.25	0.3	0.35	0.4	0.45	0.5
0.1	15	7	4	3	2	1	1	1	1
0.2	58	25	14	9	6	4	3	3	2
0.3	131	56	30	19	12	9	7	5	4
0.4	232	98	53	33	22	15	11	9	7
0.5	362	154	82	50	34	24	17	13	10
0.6	522	221	119	72	48	34	25	19	15
0.7	710	301	161	98	65	46	34	26	20

From this calculation, we see that the sample size required increases dramatically when CV increases and PC decreases which is intuitively true since one needs a larger sample size to detect a higher variation (CV) and a smaller effect size (PC). This feature can be seen from Figure 7.9.

```
> persp(CV, PC, SS, theta = 30, phi = 30, expand = 0.5,
  col = "lightblue", xlab="CV", ylab="PC", zlab="Sample Size")
```

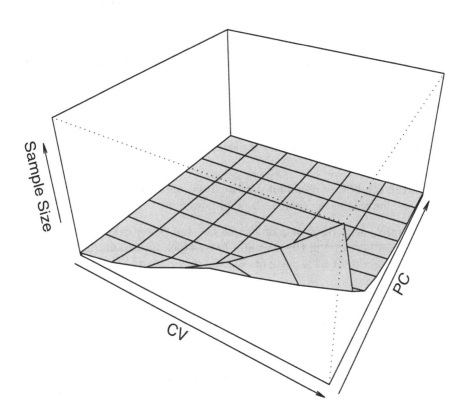

FIGURE 7.9: Perspective Surface for Sample Size

7.8   Concluding Remarks

In this chapter, we summarized the basic theory for sample size and power calculations. In addition we provided several examples illustrating sample size determination and power calculations using available R libraries and functions.

There are more libraries in R. We list a few of them for reference:

1. `samplingbook` is a library for survey sampling procedures by Juliane Manitz and others,

2. `SampleSizeProportions` is a library for calculating sample size requirements when estimating the difference between two binomial proportions based on a Bayesian approach,

3. `SampleSizeMeans` is a library for sample size calculations for normal means using Bayesian criteria,

4. `powerMediation` is a library for sample size and power calculations for mediation analysis,

5. `Hmisc` is a library useful for data analysis, high-level graphics and functions for computing sample size and power, etc.

A comprehensive discussion of sample size and power calculations in clinical trials can be found in Chow et al. (2008) which focuses on the statistical procedures for almost all aspects of clinical trials research.

7.9   Appendix: SAS Programs

The SAS program below corresponds to the R program in this chapter.

```
/*********************************************************
    Section 7.2.2
*********************************************************/
DATA dat6;
input alpha beta; /*alpha is Type-I error and beta is Type-II
                error*/
pow= 1-beta;
numberator= 2*(quantile("NORMAL",1-alpha/2,0,1)
        +quantile("NORMAL",1-beta,0,1))**2;
datalines;
0.05 0.05
```

```
0.05 0.1
0.05 0.15
0.05 0.2
0.05 0.25
0.05 0.3
;
RUN;


/***************************************************************
    Section 7.2.3
    *************************************************/
/*Determine the sample size with two-sided alternative*/
PROC POWER;
twosamplemeans
meandiff= 0.5
stddev= 1
power= 0.8
npergroup= .; RUN;

/*Determine the sample size with one-sided alternative*/
PROC POWER;
twosamplemeans sides= 1
meandiff= 0.5
stddev= 1
power= 0.8
npergroup= .;
RUN;

/*calculate the statistical power*/
PROC POWER;
twosamplemeans
meandiff= 0.5
stddev= 1
npergroup= 64
power=.;
RUN;

/*calculate the minimum detectable treatment difference*/
PROC POWER;
twosamplemeans
stddev= 1
npergroup= 64
power= 0.8
meandiff= .;
ods output Output= pwout;
```

```
RUN;

/*relationship between sample size and statistical power*/
PROC POWER;
twosamplemeans
meandiff= 0.5
stddev= 1
power= 0.2 to 0.9 by 0.05   /*use power from 0.2 to 0.9 by 0.05*/
npergroup= .;
plot x= power min=0.2 max=0.9;
RUN;

/**************************************************
    Section 7.2.4
    **********************************************/
/*equal group size*/
PROC POWER;
twosamplemeans
meandiff= 0.8
stddev= 0.83
power= 0.8
npergroup= .;
RUN;

/*two groups on the order of 2 to 1 ratio*/
PROC POWER;
twosamplemeans
meandiff= 0.8
stddev= 0.83
power= 0.8
groupweights= (2 1)
ntotal= .;
RUN;

/*calculate sample size for unequal variance */
PROC POWER;
twosamplemeans test=diff_satt
meandiff= 2
groupstddevs= 1|2
power= 0.8
ntotal= .
groupweights =(1 2);
RUN;

/*calculate sample size for unequal variance
```

```
                  using Wilcoxon test!!!*/
PROC POWER;
twosamplewilcoxon test=wmw
alpha= 0.05
vardist("myordinal1")= ordinal ((0 1 2) : (0.66 0.15 0.19))
vardist("myordinal2")= ordinal ((0 1 2) : (0.61 0.23 0.16))
variables= "myordinal1"|"myordinal2"
power= 0.8
ntotal= .;
RUN;


/**************************************************
    Section 7.3.1
    **********************************************/
/*calculate sample size for two independent proportion*/
PROC POWER;
twosamplefreq test=pchi
groupproportions= (0.75 0.5)
power= 0.8
npergroup= .;
RUN;


/*calculate power for two independent proportion*/
PROC POWER;
twosamplefreq test=pchi
groupproportions= (0.75 0.5)
npergroup= 60
power= .;
RUN;


/*relationship between power and significance level*/
PROC POWER;
twosamplefreq test=pchi
groupproportions= (0.75 0.5)
npergroup= 60
alpha= 0.02 to 0.12 by 0.02
power=. ;
RUN;


/***********************************************
    Section 7.3.3
    *********************************************/
/*calculate sample size*/
PROC POWER;
twosamplefreq test=FM
```

```
groupproportions= (0.75 0.5)
power= 0.8
npergroup= .;
RUN;


/*calculate sample size with unbalanced group*/
PROC POWER;
twosamplefreq test=FM
sides=1
groupproportions= (0.35 0.2)
groupweights= (2 1)
power= 0.8
ntotal= .;
RUN;


PROC POWER;
twosamplefreq test=FM
sides=1
groupproportions= (0.35 0.2)
power= 0.8
ntotal= .;
RUN;


/****************************************
    Section 7.4
    *****************************************/
PROC POWER;
twosamplesurvival test=logrank
sides=1
gexphs= 0.3|0.2
grouplossexphazards= (0.1 0.1)
accrualtime = 1
followuptime= 2
alpha=0.025
ntotal=.
/*or nevent= .*/
power = 0.8;
RUN;


/************************************************
    Section 7.6.1.4
    *************************************************/
Data Long_Trials;
delta= 1.2;           /*minimum treatment effect*/
n= 5;
```

```
n1= 2;                    /*number of repeated measurement*/
tau= 2;                   /*trial duration*/
sig2within= 7;            /*within-subject variability*/
sig2between= 2;           /*between subject variablity*/
alpha= 0.05;              /*significance level*/
pow= 0.9;                 /*desired power*/
S1= 40;
/*variance of slope*/
sig2   = 12*(n-1)*sig2within/(tau**2*n*(n+1))+sig2between;
sig2_1 = 12*(n1-1)*sig2within/(tau**2*n1*(n1+1))
            +sig2between;
S      = ceil((quantile("NORMAL",1-alpha/2,0,1)
            +quantile("NORMAL",pow,0,1))**2*2*sig2/delta**2);
pow_get= probnorm(sqrt(S1*delta**2/(2*sig2_1))
            -quantile("NORMAL",1-alpha/2,0,1));
RUN;


/*print result*/
PROC PRINT data= Long_Trials;
var sig2 S pow_get;
RUN;


/*****************************************
    Section 7.6.2.2
    ****************************************/
Data Long_Trials1;
delta= 1.2;
tau= 2;
sig2within= 7;
sig2between= 2;
alpha= 0.05;
do S= 20 to 100 by 20;
do n= 2 to 10 by 2;
sig2   = 12*(n-1)*sig2within/(tau**2*n*(n+1))
        +sig2between;
pow_get= round(probnorm(sqrt(S*delta**2/(2*sig2))
        -quantile("NORMAL",1-alpha/2,0,1)),0.001);
output;
end; end; RUN;


/*print the power matrix*/
PROC Transpose data= Long_Trials1;
by S;
id n;
var pow_get;
```

```
RUN;

/**********************************************
    Section 7.6.2.2
    *******************************************/
DATA Long_Trials2;
delta= 0.075;          /*the treatment effect*/
n= 5;                  /*number of repeated measurement*/
tau= 2;                /*trial duration*/
rho=0.5;                /*correlation*/
alpha= 0.05;           /*significance level*/
beta=0.1;              /*Type-II error*/
pow= 1-beta;           /*associated power*/
sig2= 3*(n-1)*(1-rho)/(tau**2*n*(n+1));
S= round(((quantile("NORMAL",1-alpha/2,0,1)
        +quantile("NORMAL",pow,0,1))**2*2*sig2/delta**2);
RUN;

/*print result*/
PROC PRINT data= Long_Trials2;
var sig2 S;
RUN;

/***************************************************************
    Section 7.7.3
    ************************************************/
DATA Long_Trials3;
do CV= 0.1 to 0.7 by 0.1;                 /*cv range*/
do PC= 0.1 to 0.5 by 0.05;                /*pv range*/
S= ceil(8*CV**2/PC**2*(1+(1-PC)**2));/*sample size calculation*/
output;
end;
end;
RUN;

/*print out the result*/
PROC TRANSPOSE data= Long_Trials3;
by CV;
id PC;
var S;
RUN;
```

Chapter 8

Meta-Analysis of Clinical Trials

Clinical trials conducted of new drugs prior to regulatory approval are usually categorized as Phase I, Phase II or Phase III. Phase I trials are almost always conducted at a single investigational site. Many Phase II trials are conducted at two or more investigational sites or centers. Virtually all Phase III clinical trials have to be conducted at several investigational sites in order to accrue the number of patients required by the protocol. Statistical analyses of multi-center clinical trials pose challenges in terms of what are the most appropriate analyses of the data collected. Chapter 8 of Peace and Chen (2010) discusses the importance of planning, conducting, and statistically analyzing multi-center clinical trials. Analysis methods in that chapter are restricted to the usual linear models appropriate for a completely randomized block (centers) design (CRBD).

In this chapter, we present meta-analysis methods for clinical trials using the R system. Meta-analysis methods may be used to combine estimates of treatment effects at individual centers across centers in a multi-center clinical trial as well as overall treatment effects for individual clinical trials across clinical trials. Three datasets are presented in Section 8.1.

The first dataset is the 22 multi-center betablocker trial to reduce mortality after myocardial infarction that was analyzed in Chapter 4 to illustrate logistic regression. We re-analyze the dataset using meta-analysis models.

The second dataset is the classical and famous data from Cochrane Collaboration logo that resulted from systematic reviews of the entire, pre-1980 clinical trial literature of corticosteroid therapy in premature labor and its effect on neonatal death. The meta-analysis figure is part of the logo of the Cochrane Collaboration (http://www.cochrane.org). We present meta-analyses of this dataset using the R system. The response measure in the first and second datasets is binary.

The response measure in the third dataset is continuous (work capacity). The third dataset contains estimates of treatment effect from eight randomized controlled trials of the effectiveness of amlodipine as compared to placebo in improving work capacity in patients with angina.

Section 8.2 presents useful meta-analysis models including the weighted mean method known as fixed-effects model and the DerSimonian-Laird random-effects model implemented in R libraries **rmeta** (Author: Thomas Lumley from the Department of Biostatistics at the University of Washington, USA) and **meta** (Author: Guido Schwarzer from the Institute for Medical

Biometry and Medical Informatics at the University Hospital Freiburg, Germany). The library `rmete` is used mainly for binary data, whereas the library `meta` may be used for both binary and continuous data. In Section 8.3, we demonstrate how to use R and the R functionalities from both libraries to analyze the three datasets in this chapter. Discussion and recommendations appear in Section 8.4.

Due to vast applications and demands on meta-analysis in clinical trials, this chapter has been expanded to a book as in Chen and Peace (2013).

8.1   Data from Clinical Trials

8.1.1   Clinical Trials for Betablockers: Binary Data

We again use the data presented in Table 4.1 of Chapter 4. These data derive from a 22-center clinical trial in which betablockers were used to reduce mortality after myocardial infarction. From Chapter 4, we note that treatment is marginally statistically significant in reducing mortality. We re-analyze these data using meta-analysis models. Parenthetically, although McLachlan and Peel (2000) interpret the data as deriving from a 22-center clinical trial, the numbers of patients in each center argue that the data derive from 22 separate clinical trials which may have used different betablockers. In either case, the methodology for combining the individual summary results across centers or trials would be the same.

8.1.2   Data for Cochrane Collaboration Logo: Binary Data

Data from seven randomized trials conducted prior to 1980 of corticosteroid therapy in premature labor and its effect on neonatal death were meta-analyzed. These data are included in R meta-analysis library `rmeta` and are reproduced in Table 8.1 for easy reference.

TABLE 8.1: Data for Cochrane Collaboration Logo

name	ev.trt	n.trt	ev.ctrl	n.ctrl
Auckland	36	532	60	538
Block	1	69	5	61
Doran	4	81	11	63
Gamsu	14	131	20	137
Morrison	3	67	7	59
Papageorgiou	1	71	7	75
Tauesch	8	56	10	71

This data frame contains five columns. Column 1 contains the "name" as an identifier for the study. Column 2 contains the number ("ev.trt") of deaths among patients in the treated group. Column 3 contains the total number of patients ("n.trt") in the treated group. Column 4 contains the number of deaths ("ev.ctrl") in the control group. Column 5 contains the total number of patients ("n.ctrl") in the control group.

8.1.3 Clinical Trials on Amlodipine: Continuous Data

Eight randomized controlled trials of the effectiveness of the calcium channel blocker amlodipine as compared to placebo in improving work capacity in patients with angina are summarized in Table 8.2. These data are used in Li et al. (1994) to illustrate potential bias in meta-analysis. The data are reproduced further in Hartung et al. (2008). The change in work capacity is defined as the ratio of exercise time after the patient receives the intervention (i.e., drug or placebo) to the exercise time at baseline (before receiving the intervention). It is assumed that the logarithms of these ratios are normally distributed. Table 8.2 lists the observed sample size, mean, and variance for both treatment and placebo groups. We meta-analyze these data to illustrate application of (meta-analysis) methods for continuous data.

TABLE 8.2: Angina Trial Data

Protocol	nE	meanE	varE	nC	meanC	varC
154	46	0.2316	0.2254	48	-0.0027	0.0007
156	30	0.2811	0.1441	26	0.0270	0.1139
157	75	0.1894	0.1981	72	0.0443	0.4972
162	12	0.0930	0.1389	12	0.2277	0.0488
163	32	0.1622	0.0961	34	0.0056	0.0955
166	31	0.1837	0.1246	31	0.0943	0.1734
303	27	0.6612	0.7060	27	-0.0057	0.9891
306	46	0.1366	0.1211	47	-0.0057	0.1291

8.2 Statistical Models for Meta-Analysis

Hedges and Olkin (1985) regard meta-analysis as a rubric used to describe quantitative methods for combining evidence across experiments. DerSimonian and Laird (1986) define meta-analysis as the statistical analysis of a collection of analytic results for the purpose of integrating the findings. Although neither Cochran (1937), Cochran (1943), Cochran (1954), nor Yates and Cochran (1938) used the rubric, their methods for combining results from a series of experiments are clearly meta-analysis methods. In fact, many refer to the Dersimonian-Laird procedure as the Cochran-Dersimonian-Laird procedure.

Meta-analysis methods require the identification of a common response measure reflecting a common experimental objective across the experiments to be combined, which has been estimated from the data collected in the individual experiments. Depending on the response measure, its variance may need to be estimated and the sample sizes specified.

As described in Wikipedia, "In statistics, a meta-analysis combines the results of several studies that address a set of related research hypotheses. This is normally done by identification of a common measure of *effect size*, which is modeled using a form of meta-regression. Resulting overall averages when controlling for study characteristics can be considered meta-effect sizes, which are more powerful estimates of the true effect size than those derived in a single study under a given single set of assumptions and conditions". This *effect size* will be detailed in Section 8.2.1.

8.2.1   Clinical Hypotheses and Effect Size

The fundamental objective for conducting a clinical trial of the efficacy of a new drug (D) in the treatment of some disease is to demonstrate that the new drug is effective in treating the disease. Translating into the statistical hypothesis framework, the objective becomes the alternative hypothesis in contrast to the null hypothesis of inefficacy given by:

H_0 : Effect of D is no different from that of control (placebo = P)

H_a : Effect of D is better than that of P

Treatment effect size is a comparative function of the efficacy response measure in each treatment group. The comparative function may be the difference in means if response is continuous, or the difference in proportions if response in dichotomous or binary. Other comparative functions of effect size for binary data are the log-odds ratio or relative risk. The treatment effect size is denoted by δ to be compatible with the notations used in Peace and Chen (2010). Then H_0 and H_a above become:

$$H_0 : \delta = 0$$
$$H_a : \delta > 0$$

For a multi-center trial under a common protocol, H_0 and H_a are the same for each center. Randomization of patients to treatment groups within centers and conducting the trial in a blinded and quality manner guarantees valid, unbiased estimates of treatment effect within centers.

A design-based analysis strategy for a multi-center clinical trial begins with combining the estimates of treatment effect across centers in a manner consistent with the design of the trial and behavior of the data. Fundamentally, a design-based analysis strategy is no different than a meta-analysis of the treatment effect estimates across the centers. That is, first compute the estimates of treatment effect $\hat{\delta}_i$ and the within variance $\hat{\sigma}^2$ of treatment effect at each center $i(i = 1, \cdots, C)$, and then meta-analyze the $\hat{\delta}_i$ across centers. There are typically two analysis approaches in this direction with one as *fixed-effects* and the other as *random-effects*.

In fixed-effects meta-analysis, we assume that we have an estimate of *treatment effect* $\hat{\delta}_i$ and its (within) variability estimate $\hat{\sigma}_i^2$ from each clinical center i. Each $\hat{\delta}_i$ is an estimate of the underlying global overall effect of δ across all centers. To meta-analyze this set of $\hat{\delta}_i$ means we combine them using some weighting scheme.

However, for the random-effects meta-analysis model, we assume that each $\hat{\delta}_i$ is an estimate of its own underlying true effect δ_i which is one realization from the overall global effect δ. Therefore, the random-effects meta-analysis model can incorporate both within-center variability and between-center variability, which is an important source of heterogeneity for multi-center clinical trials.

8.2.2 Fixed-Effects Meta-Analysis Model: The Weighted Average

In the fixed-effects model, each $\hat{\delta}_i$ is assumed to be an estimate of the underlying global overall effect δ as:

$$\hat{\delta}_i = \delta + \epsilon_i \qquad (8.1)$$

where ϵ_i is assumed to be normally distributed by $N(0, \hat{\sigma}_i^2)$. That is

$$\hat{\delta}_i \sim N(\delta, \hat{\sigma}_i^2) \qquad (8.2)$$

The global δ is then estimated by combining the individual estimates by some weighting scheme. That is, we weigh $\hat{\delta}_i$ at each center i with an appropriate weight w_i, then compute the weighted mean or pooled estimate $\hat{\delta}$ of treatment effect as well as its variance $\hat{\sigma}^2$, where

$$\hat{\delta} \;=\; \sum_{i=1}^{C} w_i \hat{\delta}_i \qquad (8.3)$$

$$\hat{\sigma}^2 \;=\; Var(\hat{\delta}) = \sum_{i=1}^{C} w_i^2 \hat{\sigma}_i^2 \text{ (under independence of centers)} \qquad (8.4)$$

Using the weighted-mean in Equation 8.3 and its variance in Equation 8.4, an approximate 95% confidence interval (CI) for δ is:

$$\hat{\delta} \pm 1.96 \times \sqrt{\hat{\sigma}^2} \tag{8.5}$$

In addition, we may formulate a t-type of test as:

$$T = \frac{\hat{\delta} - \delta}{\sqrt{\hat{\sigma}^2}} \tag{8.6}$$

to be used to test $H_0 : \delta = 0$. Based on the test statistic in Equation 8.6, we construct confidence intervals on the overall global effect of δ in the usual manner.

The weighted mean in Equation (8.3) requires $\sum_{i=1}^{C} w_i = 1$. Typical choices of w_i are:

1. Weighting by the number of centers as

$$w_i = \frac{1}{C} \tag{8.7}$$

   where C is the number of centers (fixed);

2. Weighting by the number of patients in each center as:

$$w_i = \frac{N_i}{N} \tag{8.8}$$

   where N_i is the number of patients at center i, and N is the total number of patients as $N = \sum_{i=1}^{C} N_i$;

3. Weighting by the number of patients from each center and each treatment as:

$$w_i = \frac{N_{iD} N_{iP}}{N_{iD} + N_{iP}} \times \frac{1}{w} \tag{8.9}$$

   where $w = \sum_{i=1}^{C} w_i$ and N_{iD} and N_{iP} are the numbers of patients in the new drug treatment (D) and Placebo (P) groups, respectively, at center i;

4. Weighting by the inverse variance

$$w_i = \frac{1}{\hat{\sigma}_i^2} \times \frac{1}{w} \tag{8.10}$$

   where $w = \sum_{i=1}^{C} w_i$.

The weighting scheme 1 in Equation 8.7 yields the unweighted mean or arithmetic average of the estimates of treatment effect across centers.

The weighting scheme 2 in Equation 8.8 yields the average of the estimates of treatment effect across centers weighted according to the number of patients at each center. Note that the weighting scheme 2 in Equation 8.8 reduces to weight scheme 1 in Equation 8.7 if there is balance across centers.

The weighting scheme 3 in Equation 8.9 yields the average of the estimates of treatment effect across centers weighted to allow treatment group imbalance at each center. Note that scheme 3 in Equation 8.9 reduces to scheme 2 in Equation 8.8 if treatment groups are balanced across centers.

The weighting scheme 4 in Equation 8.10 yields the average of the estimates of treatment effect across centers weighting the estimates inversely to their variance which is used in almost all the fixed-effects models and we will use this weighting hereafter. Note that scheme 4 in Equation 8.10 reduces to scheme 1 in Equation 8.7 if the $\hat{\sigma}_i^2$ are the same (homogeneous) across centers.

It should be noted that for dichotomous response data, the data at each center may be summarized by a two-by-two table with responders versus non-responders as columns and treatment groups as rows. Let O_i denote the number of responders in the pivotal cell of the two-by-two table at each center, and $E(O_i)$ and $Var(O_i)$, denote the expected value and variance of O_i, respectively, computed from the hypergeometric distribution. The square of Equation 8.6 becomes the Mantel-Haenszel statistic proposed by Mantel and Haenszel (1959) for addressing association between treatment and response across centers. For this reason, the weighted mean estimate in 8.3 with its variance in 8.4 using weighting scheme 4 is implemented in R library `rmeta` as function `meta.MH` for *"Fixed effects (Mantel-Haenszel) meta-analysis"*. This R library is created by Professor Thomas Lumley at the University of Washington with functions for simple fixed and random-effects meta-analysis for two-sample comparisons and cumulative meta-analyses as well as drawing standard summary plots, funnel plots, and computing summaries and tests for association and heterogeneity.

8.2.3 Random-Effects Meta-Analysis Model: DerSimonian-Laird

In the random-effects meta-analysis model, we assume the treatment effect $\hat{\delta}_i$ from each center i is an estimate of its own underlying true treatment effect δ_i with variance σ_i^2, and further that the δ_i from all the C centers follow some overall global distribution denoted by $N(\delta, \tau^2)$. This random-effects meta-model can be written as:

$$
\begin{aligned}
\hat{\delta}_i &\sim N(\delta_i, \sigma_i^2) \\
\delta_i &\sim N(\delta, \tau^2)
\end{aligned}
\tag{8.11}
$$

This random-effects model can be described as an extension of the fixed-effects model in Equation 8.1 as:

$$\hat{\delta}_i = \delta + \nu_i + \epsilon_i \tag{8.12}$$

where $\nu_i \sim N(0, \tau^2)$ describes the between-center variation.

We make an assumption that ν_i and ϵ_i are independent and, therefore, the random-effects model in Equation 8.11 can be re-written as:

$$\hat{\delta}_i \sim N(\delta, \sigma_i^2 + \tau^2) \tag{8.13}$$

In this formulation, the extra parameter τ^2 represents the between-center variability around the underlying global treatment effect δ. It is easy to show in this formulation that the global δ is also estimated by the weighted mean similar to the fixed-effects meta-model as given in Equation 8.3 as:

$$\hat{\delta}^* = \frac{\sum_{i=1}^{C} w_i^* \hat{\delta}_i}{\sum_{i=1}^{C} w_i^*} \tag{8.14}$$

with standard error estimated as:

$$se\left(\hat{\delta}^*\right) = \sqrt{\frac{1}{\sum_{i=1}^{C} w_i^*}} \tag{8.15}$$

where the weights now are given by:

$$\hat{w}_i^* = \frac{1}{\hat{\sigma}_i^2 + \hat{\tau}^2} \tag{8.16}$$

$$se\left(\hat{\delta}^*\right) = \sqrt{\frac{1}{\sum_{i=1}^{C} w_i^*}} \tag{8.17}$$

Therefore, a 95% CI may be formulated to provide statistical inference similar to the fixed-effects model.

There are several methods to estimate the $\hat{\tau}^2$. The most commonly used one is from DerSimonian and Laird (1986) and is derived using the method of moments (which does not involve iterative search algorithms as do likelihood-based ones). This estimate is given as:

$$\hat{\tau}^2 = \frac{Q - (C - 1)}{U} \tag{8.18}$$

if $Q > C - 1$, otherwise, $\hat{\tau}^2 = 0$ where

$$Q = \sum_{i=1}^{C} w_i(\hat{\delta}_i - \hat{\delta})^2$$

$$U = \sum_{i=1}^{C} w_i - \frac{\sum_{i=1}^{C} w_i^2}{\sum_{i=1}^{C} w_i}$$

Note that the statistic Q is used for testing heterogeneity across the centers. This random-effects meta-model is implemented in the R library `rmeta` as function `meta.DSL` for "*Random-effects (DerSimonian-Laird) meta-analysis*". It is also implemented as `metabin` and `metacont` in library `meta`.

Therefore, the random-effects meta-analysis model can incorporate both within-center and between-center variability which is an important source of heterogeneity for multi-center clinical trials. In this sense, the random-effects meta-analysis model is more conservative since $w_i^* \leq w_i$, which leads to

$$se(\hat{\delta}^*) = \sqrt{\frac{1}{\sum_{i=1}^{C} w_i^*}} \geq \sqrt{\frac{1}{\sum_{i=1}^{C} w_i}} = se(\hat{\delta}). \tag{8.19}$$

8.2.4 Publication Bias

Publication bias is sometimes referred as "selection bias". The studies selected to be included in the meta-analysis are vital to the inferential conclusion. Publication bias could arise when only the positive studies (those that demonstrate statistical significance or if not statistically significant do not reflect qualitative interaction) of a drug are published. Therefore, even though all published studies of a drug for the treatment of some disease may be selected for a meta-analysis, the resulting inferential results may be biased (may over-estimate the effectiveness of the drug). The bias may be particularly significant when meta-analyses are conducted or are sponsored by a group with a vested interest in the results.

In meta-analysis, Begg's *funnel plot* or Egger's plot is used to graphically display the existence of publication bias. Statistical tests for publication bias are usually based on the fact that clinical studies with small sample sizes (and therefore large variances) may be more prone to publication bias in contrast to large clinical studies. Therefore, when estimates from all studies are plotted against their variances (sample size), a symmetrical funnel should be seen when there is no publication bias, while a skewed asymmetrical funnel is a signal of potential publication bias. We illustrate this funnel plot along with the data analysis using the R system.

8.3 Data Analysis in R

8.3.1 Analysis of Betablocker Trials

We read the data into R using `read.csv` and create a new dataframe named `betablocker`. For this dataset, we use the library `rmeta`. First, we load this library as:

```
> library(rmeta)
```

8.3.1.1   Fitting the Fixed-Effects Model

We first fit the fixed-effects model as described in Section 8.2.2 using the R function `meta.MH` to compute the individual odds ratios or relative risks, the Mantel-Haenszel weighted mean estimate and Woolf's test for heterogeneity. The R implementation is illustrated by the following R code chunk:

```
> # Get the data from the ``beta"
> n.trt   = betablocker[betablocker$Treatment=="Treated",]$Total
> n.ctrl  = betablocker[betablocker$Treatment=="Control",]$Total
> ev.trt  = betablocker[betablocker$Treatment=="Treated",]$Deaths
> ev.ctrl = betablocker[betablocker$Treatment=="Control",]$Deaths
> # call the meta.MH for calculations
> betaOR  = meta.MH(n.trt,n.ctrl,ev.trt,ev.ctrl,
          names=paste("Center",1:22,sep=" "))
> # print the summary from meta.MH
> summary(betaOR)

Fixed effects ( Mantel-Haenszel ) meta-analysis
Call: meta.MH(ntrt = n.trt, nctrl = n.ctrl, ptrt = ev.trt,
     pctrl = ev.ctrl,names=paste("Center",1:22,sep = " "))
------------------------------------
            OR (lower  95% upper)
Center 1   1.03    0.19       5.45
Center 2   0.48    0.18       1.23
Center 3   0.58    0.19       1.76
Center 4   0.78    0.60       1.03
Center 5   1.07    0.62       1.86
Center 6   0.56    0.15       2.10
Center 7   0.60    0.46       0.79
Center 8   0.92    0.62       1.38
Center 9   0.65    0.38       1.12
Center 10  0.72    0.57       0.90
Center 11  0.81    0.55       1.18
Center 12  0.96    0.61       1.51
Center 13  0.55    0.24       1.27
Center 14  1.33    0.89       1.98
Center 15  0.73    0.40       1.30
Center 16  0.87    0.52       1.46
Center 17  1.15    0.56       2.35
Center 18  1.38    0.47       4.08
Center 19  1.56    0.38       6.35
Center 20  0.80    0.48       1.34
Center 21  0.55    0.33       0.92
Center 22  0.54    0.32       0.93
------------------------------------
Mantel-Haenszel OR =0.77 95% CI ( 0.7,0.85 )
Test for heterogeneity: X^2( 21 ) = 23.26 ( p-value 0.3301 )
```

From the summary, we observe the odds-ratios (OR) comparing treatment to placebo with associated 95% confidence intervals for all centers. These are very variable with the smallest OR = 0.48 from center 2 and largest OR = 1.56 from center 19. There are a few ORs which are significantly different from 1, but most are not. From the meta-analysis point of view, those ORs are the estimates for the global OR as indicated by Mantel-Haenszel OR = 0.77 with 95% CI of (0.70, 0.85) indicating global statistical significance. The χ^2 test for heterogeneity gave *p*-value of 0.3301 indicating heterogeneity is not statistically significant.

This meta-analysis is shown graphically in Figure 8.1 using R function `plot` as follows:

```
> plot(betaOR, ylab="Center")
```

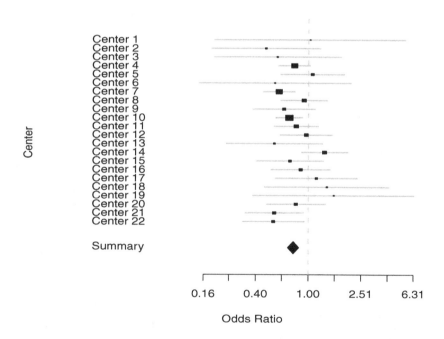

FIGURE 8.1: Forest Plot for the Betablockers Trial with 95% CIs from Fixed-Effects Meta-Analysis

This is the so-called "forest plot" in meta-analysis; i.e., a plot of the estimates and their associated 95% CIs for each center (or trial), as well as the global (summary or combined) estimate. The 95% CI intervals are the lines, the squares in the middle of the lines represent the point estimates. The global estimate or "Summary" is the diamond whose width associated 95% CI.

To assess potential publication bias, we create the funnel plot for this dataset as illustrated in Figure 8.2 with the following R code chunk:

```
> funnelplot(betaOR)
```

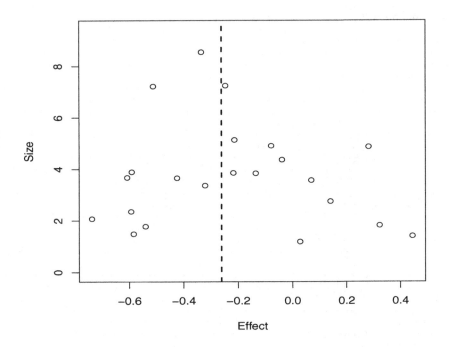

FIGURE 8.2: Funnel Plot for the Betablocker Trial

The basic idea for funnel plot is based on the fact that the smaller studies with larger variations should have greater spread around the mean effect. Therefore, a plot of a measure of precision (such as the sample size or inverse standard error, etc.) from all studies to their treatment effect would look like a funnel if there is no publication bias. For these data, the funnel plot in Figure 8.2 demonstrates symmetry about the mean effect suggesting no strong evidence of publication bias. We will illustrate a statistical test in the analysis of the angina trial using R library `meta`.

8.3.1.2 Fitting the Random-Effects Model

Similarly, the random-effects model as described in Section 8.2.3 can be implemented using R function `meta.DSL` to compute the individual odds ratios or relative risks, the Mantel-Haenszel weighted mean estimate and Woolf's test for heterogeneity along with the estimate of the random-effects variance. The R implementation is illustrated by the following R code chunk:

```
> # Call the meta.DSL for calculations
> betaDSL  = meta.DSL(n.trt,n.ctrl,ev.trt,ev.ctrl,
        names=paste("Center",1:22,sep=" "))
> # Print the summary from meta.DSL
> summary(betaDSL)

Random effects ( DerSimonian-Laird ) meta-analysis
Call: meta.DSL(ntrt = n.trt, nctrl = n.ctrl, ptrt = ev.trt,
    pctrl = ev.ctrl, names = paste("Center", 1:22, sep = " "))
------------------------------------
          OR (lower  95% upper)
Center 1   1.03    0.19      5.45
Center 2   0.48    0.18      1.23
Center 3   0.58    0.19      1.76
Center 4   0.78    0.60      1.03
Center 5   1.07    0.62      1.86
Center 6   0.56    0.15      2.10
Center 7   0.60    0.46      0.79
Center 8   0.92    0.62      1.38
Center 9   0.65    0.38      1.12
Center 10  0.72    0.57      0.90
Center 11  0.81    0.55      1.18
Center 12  0.96    0.61      1.51
Center 13  0.55    0.24      1.27
Center 14  1.33    0.89      1.98
Center 15  0.73    0.40      1.30
Center 16  0.87    0.52      1.46
Center 17  1.15    0.56      2.35
Center 18  1.38    0.47      4.08
Center 19  1.56    0.38      6.35
Center 20  0.80    0.48      1.34
Center 21  0.55    0.33      0.92
Center 22  0.54    0.32      0.93
------------------------------------
SummaryOR= 0.78  95% CI ( 0.7,0.87 )
Test for heterogeneity: X^2( 21 ) = 23.26 ( p-value 0.3302 )
Estimated random effects variance: 0.01
```

From the summary, we see that the estimated between-center variance = 0.01 and the global OR = 0.78 with 95% CI of (0.70, 0.87). Because of the estimated non-zero between-center variance, the 95% CIs from individual centers and the one based on the global estimate are slightly wider than those from the fixed-effects meta-analysis, which is consistent with the theory described in Section 8.2.3. Both fixed-effects and random-effects models indicated that betablocker treatment was effective.

Similarly, the random-effects meta-analysis is shown graphically in Figure 8.3.

```
> plot(betaDSL, ylab="Center")
```

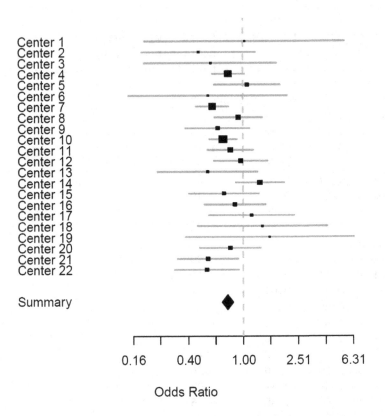

FIGURE 8.3: Forest Plot for the Betablocker Trial with 95% CIs from Random-Effects Meta-Analysis

Both Figure 8.1 for the fixed-effects model and Figure 8.3 for the random-effects model are produced using the default `plot` to call the `forestplot`. These figures may be re-produced with more options directly by using `forestplot` with the following R code chunk:

```
> # Create the ``text" to include all the outputs
> text = cbind(c("","Center",betaOR$names,NA,"Summary"),
            c("Deaths","(Betablockers)",ev.trt,NA,NA),
            c("Deaths","(Placebo)", ev.ctrl, NA,NA),
            c("","OR",format(exp(betaOR$logOR),digits=2),
                    NA,format(exp(betaOR$logMH),digits=2)))
> # Generate the OR and 95\% CI
> mean   = c(NA,NA,betaOR$logOR,NA,betaOR$logMH)
> sterr  = c(NA,NA,betaOR$selogOR,NA,betaOR$selogMH)
> l      = mean-1.96*sterr
> u      = mean+1.96*sterr
> # Call forestplot with a few options
> forestplot(text,mean,l,u,zero=0,is.summary=c(TRUE,TRUE,
    rep(FALSE,22),TRUE),clip=c(log(0.1),log(2.5)), xlog=TRUE)
```

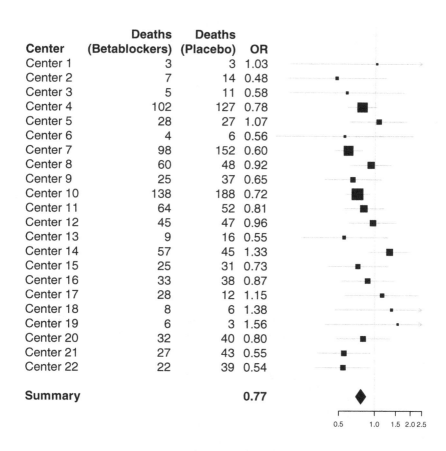

Center	Deaths (Betablockers)	Deaths (Placebo)	OR
Center 1	3	3	1.03
Center 2	7	14	0.48
Center 3	5	11	0.58
Center 4	102	127	0.78
Center 5	28	27	1.07
Center 6	4	6	0.56
Center 7	98	152	0.60
Center 8	60	48	0.92
Center 9	25	37	0.65
Center 10	138	188	0.72
Center 11	64	52	0.81
Center 12	45	47	0.96
Center 13	9	16	0.55
Center 14	57	45	1.33
Center 15	25	31	0.73
Center 16	33	38	0.87
Center 17	28	12	1.15
Center 18	8	6	1.38
Center 19	6	3	1.56
Center 20	32	40	0.80
Center 21	27	43	0.55
Center 22	22	39	0.54
Summary			**0.77**

0.5   1.0   1.5 2.0 2.5

FIGURE 8.4: Forestplot with More Options

We illustrate this using the fixed-effects model output. We encourage readers to try different settings and options for `forestplot`. In generating the forest plot, we first make `text` to list all the "Deaths", ("OR" or any other information the analyst would like to include for all centers). Then, "forestplot" is called to place the detailed trial information along with the forest plots in Figure 8.1. This produces Figure 8.4 with a few options. The reader may wish to use "col" to add more colors.

8.3.2   Meta-Analysis for Cochrane Collaboration Logo

We first load the "Cochrane" data from `rmeta` library as:

```
> # Load the data
> data(cochrane)
> # print it
> cochrane
```

	name	ev.trt	n.trt	ev.ctrl	n.ctrl
1	Auckland	36	532	60	538
2	Block	1	69	5	61
3	Doran	4	81	11	63
4	Gamsu	14	131	20	137
5	Morrison	3	67	7	59
6	Papageorgiou	1	71	7	75
7	Tauesch	8	56	10	71

This gives the data in Table 8.1. With this dataframe, we fit the fixed-effects model in Section 8.2.2 as follows:

```
> # Fit the fixed-effects model
> steroid = meta.MH(n.trt, n.ctrl, ev.trt, ev.ctrl,
                        names=name, data=cochrane)
> # Print the model fit
> summary(steroid)

Fixed effects ( Mantel-Haenszel ) meta-analysis
Call: meta.MH(ntrt = n.trt, nctrl = n.ctrl, ptrt = ev.trt,
      pctrl = ev.ctrl,names = name, data = cochrane)
------------------------------------
```

	OR	(lower	95% upper)
Auckland	0.58	0.38	0.89
Block	0.16	0.02	1.45
Doran	0.25	0.07	0.81
Gamsu	0.70	0.34	1.45
Morrison	0.35	0.09	1.41
Papageorgiou	0.14	0.02	1.16

```
Tauesch      1.02    0.37       2.77
------------------------------------
Mantel-Haenszel OR =0.53 95% CI ( 0.39,0.73 )
Test for heterogeneity: X^2( 6 ) = 6.9 ( p-value 0.3303 )
```

It is observed from the model fit that the overall OR is 0.53 with 95% CI of (0.39, 0.73), indicating significant overall effect for steroid treatment in reducing neonatal death. However, if analyzed individually, in only two ("Auckland" and "Doran") of the seven studies was steroid treatment statistically significant. In addition, the χ^2 test for heterogeneity yielded a p-value of 0.3303 indicating non-statistically significant heterogeneity.

We could call the default function `plot` to plot the meta-analysis, but we can produce a more comprehensive figure for this analysis by calling the `forestplot` using the following R code chunk which gives Figure 8.5:

```
> # Create the ``tabletext" to include all the outputs
> tabletext = cbind(c("","Study",steroid$names,NA,"Summary"),
              c("Deaths","(Steroid)",cochrane$ev.trt,NA,NA),
              c("Deaths","(Placebo)",cochrane$ev.ctrl, NA,NA),
              c("","OR",format(exp(steroid$logOR),digits=2),
                NA,format(exp(steroid$logMH),digits=2)))
> # Generate the CI
> mean   = c(NA,NA,steroid$logOR,NA,steroid$logMH)
> stderr = c(NA,NA,steroid$selogOR,NA,steroid$selogMH)
> l      = mean-1.96*stderr
> u      = mean+1.96*stderr
> # Call forestplot
> forestplot(tabletext,mean,l,u,zero=0,
          is.summary=c(TRUE,TRUE,rep(FALSE,8),TRUE),
          clip=c(log(0.1),log(2.5)), xlog=TRUE)
```

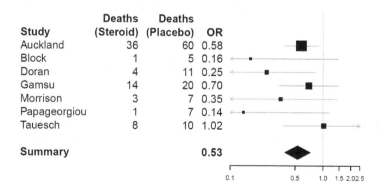

FIGURE 8.5: Forestplot for Cochrane Data

8.3.3   Analysis of Amlodipine Trial Data

8.3.3.1   Load the Library and Data

For this data, we illustrate the application of the R library meta for its functionalities in meta-analysis. We load the library as:

```
> library(meta)
```

The functions associated with this library may be seen using:

```
> library(help=meta)
```

This library may be used also for fixed- and random-effects meta-analysis. In addition, there are functions that can be used for tests of bias, and for producing forest and funnel plots. We load the data in Table 8.2 into R as follows:

```
> angina = read.csv("angina.csv",header=T)
> # Print the data
> angina
```

```
  Protocol nE meanE  varE nC   meanC   varC
1      154 46 0.232 0.2254 48 -0.0027 0.0007
2      156 30 0.281 0.1441 26  0.0270 0.1139
3      157 75 0.189 0.1981 72  0.0443 0.4972
4      162 12 0.093 0.1389 12  0.2277 0.0488
5      163 32 0.162 0.0961 34  0.0056 0.0955
6      166 31 0.184 0.1246 31  0.0943 0.1734
7      303 27 0.661 0.7060 27 -0.0057 0.9891
8      306 46 0.137 0.1211 47 -0.0057 0.1291
```

We see that there are eight protocols, each with the number of observations, mean, and variance for treatment and control groups.

8.3.3.2   Fit the Fixed-Effects Model

This is a dataset with continuous response data and we use the metacont to model the data with the following R chunk:

```
> # Fit fixed-effect model
> fixed.angina=metacont(nE,meanE,sqrt(varE),nC,meanC,sqrt(varC),
        data=angina,studlab=Protocol,comb.random=FALSE)
> # Print the fitted model
> fixed.angina
```

```
        MD         95%-CI %W(fixed)
154 0.2343 [ 0.0969; 0.3717]      21.2
156 0.2541 [ 0.0663; 0.4419]      11.4
```

```
157   0.1451 [-0.0464;  0.3366]      10.9
162  -0.1347 [-0.3798;  0.1104]       6.7
163   0.1566 [ 0.0072;  0.3060]      17.9
166   0.0894 [-0.1028;  0.2816]      10.8
303   0.6669 [ 0.1758;  1.1580]       1.7
306   0.1423 [-0.0015;  0.2861]      19.4


Number of studies combined: k = 8


                        MD         95%-CI     z  p-value
Fixed effect model 0.162 [0.0986; 0.2252] 5.01  < 0.0001


Quantifying heterogeneity:
tau^2=0.0066; H=1.33[1.00;2.00]; I^2=43.2%[0.0%; 74.9%]


Test of heterogeneity:
     Q d.f.  p-value
 12.33    7   0.0902
```

From this fixed-effect model fitting, we note from the 95% CI's that amlodipine treatment is not statistically significant in four of the eight protocols. However, the overall effect of amlopidine from the fixed-effects model is 0.1619 with corresponding 95% CI of [0.0986; 0.2252] and p-value < 0.001 – indicating a statistically significant treatment effect. The test of heterogeneity gave a p-value of 0.09 from $Q = 12.33$ with degrees of freedom of 7 indicating that there is no strong evidence against homogeneity.

A simple forest plot can be generated by calling the **plot**. However, a better presentation can be produced using R function **forest** in the following R code chunk:

```
> # Round to 2-digit
> fixed.angina$mean.e = round(fixed.angina$mean.e,2)
> fixed.angina$sd.e   = round(fixed.angina$sd.e,2)
> fixed.angina$mean.c = round(fixed.angina$mean.c,2)
> fixed.angina$sd.c   = round(fixed.angina$sd.c,2)
> # Call forest to make plot
> forest(fixed.angina)
```

This produces Figure 8.6. Note that we first use **round** to "round" the number of digits to the right of the decimal to 2 for better display purposes.

To assess potential publication bias informally, we generate the funnel plot as seen in Figure 8.7 and visually assess whether it is symmetric. This funnel plot can be generated using the following R code code:

```
> funnel(fixed.angina)
```

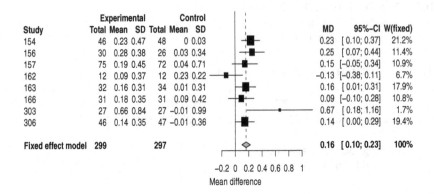

FIGURE 8.6: A Detailed Forest Plot for the Angina Trial with 95% CIs

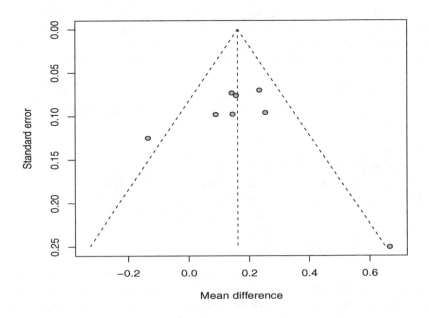

FIGURE 8.7: Funnel Plot for the Angina Trial

From this figure, we note that protocol 303 has the largest mean difference of 0.6669 on the right and protocol 162 has the smallest mean difference of -0.1347 on the left. The remaining are quite symmetric. A statistical significance test can be performed using `metabias`. This test is based on the rank correlation between standardized treatment estimates and variance estimates of estimated treatment effects where Kendall's tau is used as the correlation measure (see from Begg and Mazumdar (1994)). Other tests may be performed and may be seen in the library `meta`.

By calling `metabias` for this model fitting as follows:

```
> metabias(fixed.angina)
```

we see the *p*-value associated with this test is 0.4579 indicating symmetry of the funnel plot.

8.3.3.3 Fit the Random-Effects Model

Similar to the fixed-effects model in Section 8.3.3.2, we can fit the random-effects model as follows:

```
> # fit random-effects model
> random.angina = metacont(nE, meanE, sqrt(varE),nC,meanC,sqrt(varC),
            data=angina,studlab=Protocol,comb.random=T)
> # print the summary fit
> random.angina
```

	MD	95%-CI	%W(fixed)	%W(random)
154	0.2343	[0.0969; 0.3717]	21.2	17.5
156	0.2541	[0.0663; 0.4419]	11.4	12.7
157	0.1451	[-0.0464; 0.3366]	10.9	12.5
162	-0.1347	[-0.3798; 0.1104]	6.7	9.0
163	0.1566	[0.0072; 0.3060]	17.9	16.2
166	0.0894	[-0.1028; 0.2816]	10.8	12.4
303	0.6669	[0.1758; 1.1580]	1.7	2.9
306	0.1423	[-0.0015; 0.2861]	19.4	16.8

```
Number of studies combined: k = 8
```

	MD	95%-CI	z
Fixed effect model	0.162	[0.0986; 0.2252]	5.01
Random effects model	0.159	[0.0710; 0.2467]	3.54

	p-value
Fixed effect model	< 0.0001
Random effects model	0.0004

```
Quantifying heterogeneity:
tau^2 = 0.0066; H = 1.33 [1.00; 2.00]; I^2 = 43.2% [0.0%; 74.9%]
```

```
Test of heterogeneity:
    Q d.f.  p-value
 12.33    7   0.0902
```

```
Details on meta-analytical method:
- Inverse variance method
- DerSimonian-Laird estimator for tau^2
```

This gives the model fitting for random-effects as well as for fixed-effects. We note from the output that the estimated between-protocol variance $\hat{\tau}^2 = 0.0066$ and that the mean difference is estimated as 0.159 from the random-effects model as compared to 0.162 from the fixed-effects model. The 95% CI from the random-effects model is (0.071, 0.247) as compared to (0.098, 0.225) from fixed-effects model. Again the 95% CI from the random-effects model is wider than that for the fixed-effects model. We leave the forest plot as an exercise for interested readers.

8.4   Summary and Conclusions

In this chapter, we illustrated meta-analysis methods for multi-center clinical trials using publicly available datasets with both fixed-effects and random-effects models. Woolf's test was used to test for lack of homogeneity.

Lack of homogeneity among centers in a multi-center clinical trial can demonstrably impact the statistical detection of treatment effects as indicated by Peace (1992). A goal of a quality designed and quality conducted multi-center clinical trial is to strive for homogeneity among centers. In order to accomplish or come close to accomplishing this goal requires ownership and commitment from all personnel having some responsibility in the design, conduct, monitoring, data management, statistical analysis and reporting of the trial.

It may be that modifying the typical design of multi-center trials to account for biological variation in terms of how patients metabolize the drug may lead to greater homogeneity of treatment effect across centers. For example, after patients qualify for the protocol, but prior to randomization, give them a single dose of the drug; obtain sufficient blood samples to estimate the maximum concentration (i.e., CMAX); and then stratify before randomization on levels of CMAX as recommended in Chapter 8 of Peace and Chen (2010).

Readers of this chapter may use the models and associated R code contained herein to analyze their own clinical trials by combining treatment effects across centers, or to synthesize trial estimates of treatment effects across trials. For further reading, we recommend Hedges and Olkin (1985), Whitehead (2003) and Hartung et al. (2008). For R application, we recommend the reader become more familiar with the `rmeta` and `meta` libraries. There are other R libraries, such as `metacor` for meta-analysis of correlation coefficients and another library of `metafor` for meta-analysis. Chapter 12 (Meta-Analysis) in Everitt and Hothorn (2006) is again an excellent reference on the subject. We also extended this chapter to an extensive book as in Chen and Peace (2013) to cover several topics in meta-analysis.

Fundamental to the validity of inference from a meta-analysis as a research synthesis of a collection of trials is the selection of individual trials in the collection. If the results of meta-analyses are to be credible, then the analysis methods must be only part of an investigative research process reflecting good science. Simply put, a protocol should be developed prior to beginning any meta-analysis that reflects the process. Attention should be given to the objective of the investigation, endpoints reflecting the objective, how the studies are to be identified and included, procedures for investigating bias, and statistical methods as presented in Peace (1991a), Chalmers et al. (1981), Chalmers (1987), Chalmers et al. (1987a) and Chalmers et al. (1987b) are excellent references regarding a meta-analytic scientific process.

8.5   Appendix: SAS Programs

There is no SAS procedure for statistical meta-analysis and in this section; we programmed the meta-analysis in Section 8.3.3 using SAS `proc iml` for illustration purposes. We recommend that interested readers use R for their meta-analysis due to its extensive functionalities and ease of use. We also recommend our book (Chen and Peace (2013)) for meta-analyses using R.

```
/*****************************************************
Section 8.3.3: Amlodipine Data (Continuous data)
*****************************************************/
/* Section 8.3.3.1*/
Data Angina;
infile "Your file path/angina.csv" delimiter="," firstobs=2;
input Protocol nE meanE varE  nC meanC varC;
RUN;
proc iml;
* Read data into IML ;
  use angina;
  read all ;

/* Protocol-specific Analysis*/
```

```
/* mean difference*/
iMD = meanE-meanC;
/* var for iMD*/
ivar4MD = (varE/nE+varC/nC);
/* 95% CI for each Study*/
ilowCI  = iMD-1.96*sqrt(ivar4MD);
iupCI   = iMD+1.96*sqrt(ivar4MD);
/* inverse variance for weight Calculation */
iwt     = 1/ivar4MD;
pctwt   = iwt/sum(iwt);
print "Protocol-Specific Summary";
iout    = Protocol||iMD||ilowCI||iupCI||pctwt;
print iout;

/*Section 8.3.3.2. Fixed-Effects Meta-Analysis*/
/* MA estimate */
MD    = iMD`*pctwt;
/* variance of MD*/
varMD = 1/sum(iwt);
lowCI = MD-1.96*sqrt(varMD);
upCI  = MD+1.96*sqrt(varMD);
/* z-value and p-value*/
z     = MD/sqrt(varMD);
pval  = 2*(1-probnorm(z));
print "Summary of Fixed-Effects MA";
MA4FE = MD||lowCI||upCI||z||pval;
print MA4FE;

/* Section 8.3.3.3: Random-Effects MA*/
/* calculate the Q, U and Tau-sq*/
C     = 8; /* 8 studies*/
U     = sum(iwt) - sum(iwt`*iwt)/sum(iwt);
Q     = sum(iwt`*(iMD-MD)##2);print Q;
tau2 = (Q-(C-1))/U;
if Q <= C-1 then tau2=0; print tau2;
/*  with tau2, recalculate the weights*/
REiwt   = 1/(ivar4MD+tau2);
REpctwt = REiwt/sum(REiwt);print REpctwt;
/* MA estimate */
REMD = iMD`*REpctwt;
/* variance of MD*/
REvarMD = 1/sum(REiwt);
RElowCI = REMD-1.96*sqrt(REvarMD);
REupCI  = REMD+1.96*sqrt(REvarMD);
/* z-value and p-value*/
```

```
z    = REMD/sqrt(REvarMD);
pval = 2*(1-probnorm(z));
print "Summary of Random-Effects MA";
Re4FE = REMD||RElowCI||REupCI||z||pval;
print RE4FE;
```

Chapter 9

Bayesian Methods in Clinical Trials

Bayesian methods are increasingly being used in the design and analysis of clinical trials. Chen and Kim (2009) presented Bayesian analyses of melanoma data from a clinical trial conducted by Eastern Cooperative Oncology Group (ECOG) and of prostate cancer data from a clinical trial conducted at St. Anne's Hospital in Fall River, MA utilizing cure rate models. Tan et al. (2002) explored a Bayesian approach to the design, analysis, and interpretation of Phase II clinical trials conducted at the National Cancer Centre in Singapore on the activity of Gemcitabine in patients with metastatic nasopharyngeal carcinoma. Connor and Berry (2005) used Bayesian methods to analyze adverse event data from medical device clinical trials.

In this chapter we introduce relevant Bayesian models, applications of R packages, and simulation of some commonly known distributions that are useful in the Bayesian analysis of clinical trial data. Bayesian models are discussed in Section 9.1. Applications of the R package `MCMCpack` appear in Section 9.2. Simulations of distributions are provided in Section 9.3.

In addition, data from clinical trials analyzed earlier in the book using frequentist based methods are re-analyzed using Bayesian methods. We re-analyze the duodenal ulcer clinical trial data from Chapter 3 in Subsection 9.3.2 and in Subsection 9.4.4. In Section 9.4 we re-analyze the diastolic blood pressure clinical trial data from Chapter 4 using Bayesian MCMC algorithms. In Subsection 9.4.3, we re-analyze the familial andenomatous polyposis clinical trial data from Section 4.3.3 using Bayesian Poisson regression. A brief summary and discussion is provided in Section 9.5.

9.1 Bayesian Models

9.1.1 Bayes' Theorem

The most elemental beginning of a discussion of Bayesian methods is Bayes' Theorem, named after Thomas Bayes, an eighteenth century English mathematician and Presbyterian minister. Bayes' Theorem relates the conditional probability $P(H|E)$ to its inverse $P(E|H)$ for any two events E and H as follows:

$$P(H|E) = \frac{P(E|H)P(H)}{P(E)} = \frac{P(E|H)P(H)}{P(E|H)P(H) + P(E|H^c)P(H^c)} \tag{9.1}$$

where H^c is the complementary event of H.

To illustrate use of Bayes' Theorem, suppose that H denotes the event of a patient having breast cancer and E denotes the event of the patient having a positive mammogram. From Equation 9.1 the conditional probability $P(H|E)$ of the patient having breast cancer (H) given the patient has a positive mammogram (E) may be calculated from (prior) knowledge of the unconditional probabilities $P(E)$ and $P(H)$, as well as the conditional probability of $P(E|H)$. $P(E)$ could be estimated as the proportion of patients with a positive mammogram; $P(H)$ could be estimated as the proportion of patients having breast cancer; and $P(E|H)$ could be estimated as the proportion of patients having breast cancer in whom the mammogram is positive.

For instance, suppose a mammogram is 95% accurate in detecting breast cancer among patients with known breast cancer (i.e., the **sensitivity** of the mammogram $P(E|H)$=0.95), and is 99% accurate in failing to detect breast cancer among patients not having breast cancer (i.e., the **specificity** of the mammogram $P(E^c|H^c) = 0.99$). Further suppose 1% of subjects will have breast cancer (i.e., the **prevalence** of breast cancer $P(H) = 0.01$). Bayes' Theorem enables one to calculate the probability that a patient actually has breast cancer, given the mammogram was positive (i.e., the **precision** of the mammogram $P(H|E)$); e.g.,

$$
\begin{aligned}
P(H|E) &= \frac{P(E|H)P(H)}{P(E|H)P(H) + P(E|H^c)P(H^c)} \\
&= \frac{0.95 \times 0.01}{0.95 \times 0.01 + (1-0.99) \times (1-0.01)} = 0.49
\end{aligned}
$$

which is surprisingly small.

We can also calculate the probability that a patient does not have breast cancer given the mammogram was negative (i.e., the **negative predictive probability** of the mammogram $P(H^c|E^c)$); e.g.,

$$
\begin{aligned}
P(H^c|E^c) &= \frac{P(E^c|H^c)P(H^c)}{P(E^c|H^c)P(H^c) + P(E^c|H)P(H)} \\
&= \frac{0.99 \times (1-0.01)}{0.99 \times (1-0.01) + (1-0.95) \times 0.01} = 0.999
\end{aligned}
$$

which is quite high, particularly in comparison to the precision (0.49).

More technically, Bayes' Theorem expresses the posterior probability for a hypothesis H of having breast cancer after a positive mammogram E is observed – in terms of the prior probabilities of H and E, and the probability of E given H. In more general statistical terms, if E represents an observed data event y and H is described in terms of a hypothetical parameter θ, then the probability $P(E|H)$ is the **likelihood function** $L(\theta) = L(\theta|y)$ and $P(H) = \pi(\theta)$ is the **prior distribution** about the parameter θ. In this setting, Bayes' Theorem becomes:

$$p(\theta|y) = \frac{L(\theta)\pi(\theta)}{\int L(\theta)\pi(\theta)d\theta} \propto L(\theta)\pi(\theta) \qquad (9.2)$$

which may be used for providing statistical inference about an unknown parameter θ based on the data y. In above formulation, $\propto$ is the notation for "proportional to" and $p(\theta|y)$ is called the **posterior** probability distribution in Bayesian statistics.

Therefore in Bayesian statistics, the observed data y and our prior knowledge about θ are combined to form the corresponding posterior distribution $[y, \pi(\theta)] \to p(\theta|y)$ via Bayes' Theorem.

Note in Equation 9.2, the denominator $\int L(\theta)\pi(\theta)d\theta$ is a constant independent of the parameter θ and is usually difficult to obtain especially for higher dimensional parameter vectors. This constant is sometimes called a **normalization constant**.

9.1.2 Posterior Distributions for Some Standard Distributions

The computation of the posterior distribution in Equation 9.2 is then the next step in Bayesian modeling. In this section, we illustrate posterior distributions without detailed proof for some standard distributions commonly used in Bayesian statistics and clinical trials. The detailed mathematical derivation may be found in Gelman et al. (2009) and other Bayesian statistics textbooks.

There are different types of prior distributions which are being used in Bayesian modeling. Two of the most commonly used are a noninformative or reference prior and another is a conjugate prior. A noninformative prior is used when no prior information is available about the parameter of interest. A conjugate prior leads to the same distribution family when combined with the likelihood. We illustrate these two types of priors in this section.

9.1.2.1 Normal Distribution with Known Variance

Consider a set of i.i.d. observations y_i with $i = 1, 2, \cdots, n$ on some random variable Y and let $y = (y_1, \cdots, y_n)$ represent all n observations. Assume that $Y_i \sim N(\theta, \sigma)$ with σ **known**.

1. *Noninformative or reference prior.* The noninformative or reference prior is $\pi(\theta) = 1$, representing that no prior information is available. For this prior, the posterior distribution is easily shown to be:

$$p(\theta|y) = N(\bar{y}, \sigma^2/n) \qquad (9.3)$$

which is the usual normal distribution. Therefore, a $1-\alpha$ credible interval is $\bar{y} \pm z_{\alpha/2}\frac{\sigma}{\sqrt{n}}$ which is the usual $100(1-\alpha)\%$ confidence interval under the Bayesian framework. For clarification, by a $(1-\alpha)\%$ **credible interval** for a parameter we mean that the posterior probability of the parameter lying in the interval is a $(1-\alpha)\%$.

2. *The conjugate prior.* The so-called conjugate prior is a prior distribution when combined with the likelihood leads to the same distribution. In the normal case, the conjugate prior is $\pi(\theta) = N(\theta_0, \tau^2)$ where θ_0 and τ^2 are the prior mean and variance which leads to the posterior normal distribution. We can easily show this as:

$$p(\theta|y) \propto N(\mu_P, \sigma_P^2) \qquad (9.4)$$

where $\mu_P = w\bar{y} + (1-w)\theta_0$ is the posterior mean and $\sigma_P^2 = \frac{1}{\frac{n}{\sigma^2} + \frac{1}{\tau^2}}$ is the posterior variance.

It is noted that μ_P is the weighted average of the prior mean θ_0 and data mean $\bar{y}$ with the weight w depending on the prior and the data variances; i.e., $w = \frac{n/\sigma^2}{(1/\tau^2 + n/\sigma^2)}$. The posterior variance σ_P^2 incorporates variances from both the data and the prior distribution and is less than $\frac{\sigma^2}{n}$, representing a shrinkage to the posterior mean.

9.1.2.2   Normal Distribution with Unknown Variance

Now more realistically we assume that $Y_i \sim N(\theta, \sigma)$ with σ **unknown**. In this situation, the usual noninformative or reference prior is $\pi(\mu, \sigma) \propto 1/\sigma$. The posterior distribution can be shown to be:

$$p(\mu, \sigma|y) = p(\sigma|y)p(\mu|\sigma, y) \qquad (9.5)$$

where $\sigma|y \sim (n-1)s^2/\chi_{n-1}^2$ which is the so-called inverse-χ^2 distribution and $\mu|\sigma, y \sim N(\bar{y}, \sigma^2/n)$. For statistical inference on the mean μ, the marginal posterior distribution for μ can be obtained by integrating out the σ from the joint posterior distribution in Equation 9.5 and can be expressed as:

$$\mu = \bar{y} + \frac{s}{\sqrt{n}}T_{n-1} \qquad (9.6)$$

where $T_{n-1} \sim t_{n-1}$. Therefore, a $1-\alpha$ credible interval for μ is $\bar{y} \pm t_{n-1,\alpha/2}\frac{s}{\sqrt{n}}$, which is the usual $100(1-\alpha)\%$ confidence interval on μ based on the t-distribution.

9.1.2.3   Normal Regression

We now consider the typical simple linear regression model:

$$y_i = \beta_0 + x_{1i}\beta_1 + \cdots + \beta_p x_{pi} + \epsilon_i \qquad (9.7)$$

where $\epsilon_i \sim N(0, \sigma^2)$ with observed data $(y_i, x_{1i}, \cdots, x_{pi})$. From the theory of linear regression, the regression parameter vector $\beta = (\beta_0, \beta_1, \cdots, \beta_p)$ can be estimated by least squares as $\hat{\beta} = (X^T X)^{-1} X^T Y$ with variance estimated as $\hat{\sigma}^2 = s^2 = \frac{SSR}{n-p-1}$, where SSR is the residual sum of squares and X^T is the transpose matrix of X.

For Bayesian inference, let's assume the noninformative or usual reference prior to be $\pi(\beta, \sigma) \propto \sigma^{-1}$. We can show that the posterior distribution for σ^2 is $\sigma^2 | data \sim (n-p-1)s^2 / \chi^2_{n-p-1}$ (i.e., the inverse-χ^2 distribution) and that the posterior for β_i is $\beta_i \sim \hat{\beta}_i + s_i T_{n-p-1}$, where $s_i^2 = s^2 (X^T X)^{-1}_{ii}$ (i.e., the iith element of matrix $(X^T X)^{-1}$). Therefore, a $1 - \alpha$ credible interval for β_i is $\hat{\beta}_i \pm t_{\alpha/2} s_i$, which again is equivalent to the traditional $100(1-\alpha)\%$ confidence interval based on the t-distribution in the Bayesian framework.

9.1.2.4 Binomial Distribution

When the observations are binomially distributed as $y \sim Bin(n, \theta)$, where θ is the binomial proportion parameter, using the usual noninformative or reference prior $\pi(\theta) = 1$, leads to the well-known beta-binomial as the posterior distribution. This posterior distribution can be shown to be $p(\theta|y) = Beta(y + 1, n - y + 1)$ where $Beta(a, b)$; a beta distribution with parameters a and b with functional form given by: $Beta(a, b) = \frac{\Gamma(a+b)}{\Gamma(a)\Gamma(b)} x^{a-1} (1-x)^{b-1} dx$. If we use the conjugate prior $Beta(a, b)$ as $\pi(\theta) \propto \theta^{a-1}(1 - \theta)^{b-1}$, the posterior distribution can be shown to be $p(\theta|y) = Beta(a + y, b + n - y)$. This beta-binomial distribution is commonly used in clinical trials with binomial observations.

9.1.2.5 Multinomial Distribution

If $y \sim Multinomial(n, \theta)$ where $y = (y_1, \cdots, y_p)$ and $\theta = (\theta_1, \cdots, \theta_p)$, the noninformative or reference prior $\pi(\theta) \propto 1$ leads to the multinomial posterior distribution $p(\theta|y) \propto \theta_1^{y_1} \cdots \theta_p^{y_p}$.

The conjugate prior for multinomial distribution is the Dirichlet distribution $Dirichlet(\alpha_1, \cdots, \alpha_p)$; i.e.,

$$\pi(\theta) \propto \theta_1^{\alpha_1 - 1} \cdots \theta_p^{\alpha_p - 1}.$$

The posterior distribution is $\theta|y \sim Dir(\alpha_1 + y_1, \cdots, \alpha_p + y_p)$. The multinomial distribution is used the analysis of clinical trial frequency data with multiple categories.

9.1.3 Simulation from the Posterior Distribution

From Equation 9.2 in Section 9.1.2, we note that the posterior distribution can easily become intractable and lead to an unrecognizable distribution. This created a burden in the early development stages of Bayesian modeling. With the availability of high-speed computers, we can make statistical inferences from a posterior distribution through simulation. To do so, we draw random samples of size N as $\theta_1, \cdots, \theta_N$ from the posterior distribution $p(\theta|y)$. From these samples, for any function of the parameter θ of g, the mean of $E[g(\theta)|y]$ can be estimated by $\frac{\sum_i g(\theta_i)}{N}$ and the posterior distribution for $g(\theta)$ can be approximated by a histogram of the values $g(\theta_1), \cdots, g(\theta_N)$. Then, statistical inferences can be made from this sample.

The challenge for this simulation approach is to find a viable way to draw samples from $p(\theta|y)$. There are many methods to do so and we briefly describe four of the more common ones used in Bayesian modeling. These are direct simulation, importance sampling, Gibbs sampling, and Metropolis-Hastings sampling.

9.1.3.1   Direct Simulation

The direct simulation method is to "directly simulate" from the posterior distribution provided it can be linked to known distributions that can be *easily* simulated. The term *easily* is very relative depending on the readers' analytical background.

Consider a simple two-treatment randomized clinical trial setting with n patients from treatment 1 and m from treatment 2, where the data from treatment 1 are $X_1, \cdots, X_n \sim N(\mu_X, \sigma_X^2)$ and the data from treatment 2 are $Y_1, \cdots, Y_m \sim N(\mu_Y, \sigma_Y^2)$. For simplicity, assume that the noninformative prior is $\pi(\mu_X, \mu_Y, \sigma_X, \sigma_Y) \propto \frac{1}{\sigma_X \sigma_Y}$. Typically in a clinical trial, we are interested in the mean treatment difference denoted by $\delta = \mu_X - \mu_Y$ and its posterior distribution $\pi(\delta|data)$.

The marginal posterior distribution $p(\mu_X, \mu_Y|data)$ for μ_X and μ_Y can be derived by multiplying the likelihood by the prior distribution and integrating out σ_X and σ_Y. It can be shown that μ_X and μ_Y are independent with posterior distributions:

$$\mu_X \sim \bar{x} + \frac{s_x}{\sqrt{n}}T_{n-1}$$

$$\mu_Y \sim \bar{y} + \frac{s_y}{\sqrt{m}}T_{m-1}$$

where T_k denotes a random variable having a Student's-t distribution with k degrees of freedom, $\bar{x}$ and $\bar{y}$ are the sample means, and s_X and s_Y are the sample standard deviations for samples X_i's and Y_i's.

Since Student's t-distribution is common and can be easily simulated, a direct simulation can be performed as follows:

- Step 1: Randomly draw samples $T_X^1, \cdots, T_X^N$ from t_{n-1} and $T_Y^1, \cdots, T_Y^N$ from t_{m-1},

- Step 2: Calculate $\mu_X^i = \bar{x} + \frac{s_x}{\sqrt{n}}T_X^i$ and $\mu_Y^i = \bar{y} + \frac{s_y}{\sqrt{m}}T_Y^i$,

- Step 3: Calculate $\delta_i = \mu_X^i - \mu_Y^i, i = 1, \cdots, N$.

The δ_i from Step 3 are samples from the posterior distribution $\pi(\delta|data)$ which can be used to estimate the posterior mean and a credible interval and to provide any other Bayesian inference.

9.1.3.2 Importance Sampling

In the case that direct simulation is not feasible, importance sampling with Monte Carlo simulation may be used. It is often used as the first method for sampling from intractable posterior distributions.

Consider a posterior density function $f(z)$ and suppose we are interested in the expectation of a function $g(z)$ which can be approximated by $E(g(Z)) = \int g(z)f(z)dz \approx \frac{1}{N}\sum_i g(Z_i)$, where $z_1, \cdots, z_n$ is a random sample from the density $f(z)$. But suppose it is too difficult to directly simulate from f.

Let $s(z)$ be another density function (called the *importance function*) which is close to f in form and is easy to simulate. Simulate $z_1, \cdots, z_n$ from $s(z)$. Then

$$
\begin{aligned}
E(g(Z)) &= \int g(z)f(z)dz \\
&= \int \frac{g(z)f(z)}{s(z)}s(z)dz \\
&\approx \frac{1}{N}\sum_i \frac{g(z_i)f(z_i)}{s(z_i)}
\end{aligned}
$$

So if the posterior distribution $f(\theta) = p(\theta|y) \propto L(\theta)\pi(\theta)$ is not amenable to direct simulation, we randomly draw samples instead from an *importance* density s. Similarly,

$$
E[g(\theta)|y] \approx \frac{\frac{\sum_i g(\theta_i) \times L(\theta_i)\pi(\theta_i)}{s(\theta_i)}}{\frac{\sum_i L(\theta_i)\pi(\theta_i)}{s(\theta_i)}} \tag{9.8}
$$

Importance sampling is an obvious improvement to direct sampling and both are useful when the number of parameters is small. However, both sampling methods have limitations when the number of parameters is large. When the dimension of parameter space is large, sampling from the importance density also becomes intractable. In such cases, recent developments in Gibbs sampling and Metropolis-Hastings sampling can be used.

9.1.3.3 Gibbs Sampling

Gibbs sampling was proposed in the landmark paper by Geman and Geman (1984) and popularized by Gelfand and Smith (1990) in Bayesian methods and statistical computing.

The basic idea in Gibbs sampling is to randomly sample from the conditional distributions. As an example, let $f(x, y)$ be a bivariate density function from which we wish to randomly draw samples. Gibbs sampling starts by obtaining x_0 and y_0, and proceeds iteratively in the following fashion. At the tth iteration we randomly draw

$$
\begin{aligned}
x_t &\sim f(x|y_{t-1}) \\
y_t &\sim f(y|x_t)
\end{aligned}
$$

Repeating N times, the sample $(x_1, y_1), \cdots, (x_N, y_N)$ may be regarded as an approximate sample from $f(x, y)$. Since the sample pairs are dependent especially in the beginning, the common practice is to discard the first m pairs, referred to as "burn-in".

With this sample, the estimation of $f(x)$ proceeds as follows:

$$
\begin{aligned}
f(x) &= \int f(x, y) dy \\
&= \int f(x|y) f(y) dy \\
&\approx \frac{\sum_i f(x|y_i)}{N}.
\end{aligned}
\tag{9.9}
$$

To use Gibbs sampling in Bayesian modeling, we choose $f(\theta_1, \theta_2)$ as the posterior distribution; i.e., $f(\theta_1, \theta_2) = p(\theta_1, \theta_2|y)$. Gibbs sampling easily generalizes to any number of parameters as long as their conditional distributions are available.

9.1.3.4   Metropolis-Hastings Algorithm

Similar to Gibbs sampling, the Metropolis-Hastings (MH) algorithm utilizes a Markov-chain (MC) to generate correlated Monte-Carlo (MC) samples and is therefore referred to as one of the general Markov-chain Monte-Carlo (MCMC) algorithms. Proposed initially by Metropolis et al. (1953) and later generated by Hastings (1970), the Metropolis-Hastings (MH) algorithm is very general. It may be used to generate samples from a distribution $p(\theta)$, where $p(\theta)$ is only known up to a constant, such as $p(\theta) = h(\theta)/C$ and $C = \int h(\theta) d\theta$. This links immediately to Bayesian modeling where $p(\theta)$ is a posterior distribution and $h(\theta) = L(\theta)\pi(\theta)$.

The essence of the MH algorithm is to choose a *working* Markov chain with easily simulated kernel $q(\psi|\theta)$ (the probability of jumping into state ψ from state θ), then modify the chain to approximate the posterior $p(\theta)$. This is done by starting the selected chain q at an arbitrary point $\theta^{(0)}$ and drawing a candidate value $\psi \sim q\left(\psi|\theta^{(i)}\right)$ from the selected arbitrary chain q. Then $\theta^{(i+1)}$ is obtained as:

$$
\theta^{(i+1)} = \begin{cases} \psi & \text{with probability } \alpha \\ \theta^{(i)} & \text{with probability } 1 - \alpha \end{cases}
$$

where

$$\alpha = min\left\{\frac{h(\psi)}{h(\theta^{(i)})}\frac{q(\theta^{(i)}|\psi)}{q(\psi|\theta^{(i)})}, 1\right\}$$

Note in the formula of the above α calculation, the constant C cancels out in the ratio so we do not need to evaluate the integral $\int h(\theta)d\theta$ which makes the MH algorithm especially useful in Bayesian modeling.

There are several MH algorithms depending on the choice of the initial MC $q(\psi|\theta)$ kernel. Two of the more commonly used are the independent and random walk as follows:

1. Independent MH: In the independent MH, the working MC is independent of the present state of the chain, i.e., $q(\psi|\theta) = q(\psi)$. In this situation, $\alpha = min\left\{\frac{h(\psi)}{h(\theta^{(i)})}\frac{q(\theta^{(i)})}{q(\psi)}, 1\right\}$

2. Random Walk: Different from the independent MH which ignores information from the previous state, the random-walk MH takes into account the MC value previously simulated in generating the next value in the chain. The random-walk MC can be expressed as:

$$\theta^{i+1} = \theta^i + \epsilon_i \tag{9.10}$$

where ϵ_i is a random perturbation. The most common choice of distributions for the Markov chain kernel is the standardized normal distribution; i.e., choose $\psi|\theta^{(i)} \sim N\left(\theta^{(i)}, \sigma_0^2\right)$ where σ_0 is some fixed number.

In this case, α can be simplified to $\alpha = min\left\{\frac{h(\psi)}{h(\theta^{(i)})}, 1\right\}$ which is independent of q. This MH algorithm is called a *normal random walk chain* and is one of the simplest MH algorithms. With this simplified MH, the candidate value ψ is drawn from a normal distribution with mean at the current value to compute α as $\alpha = min\left\{\frac{h(\psi)}{h(\theta^{(i)})}, 1\right\}$. The next value is equal to the candidate value with probability α and equal to the previous value with probability $1 - \alpha$.

9.2 R Packages in Bayesian Modeling

9.2.1 Introduction

Historically, Bayesian modeling has been heavily dependent on obtaining a suitable posterior distribution. In the early stage, from the introduction of Bayes' Theorem to the 1960s, conjugate priors were used to facilitate determining conjugate posterior distributions. Over the next two decades, a wide range of approaches was used to approximate posterior distributions, such as Gaussian quadrature, Expectation-Maximization algorithm, and Laplace's method. In the 1980s, simple Monte Carlo (MC) methods began to be used in Bayesian modeling, such as direct sampling in Section 9.1.3.1 and importance sampling in Section 9.1.3.2, which are referred to as non-iterative MC methods. Since the 1990s, due to the rapid development of computer technology, MCMC methods, such as the Gibbs sampling in Section 9.1.3.3 and the Metropolis-Hastings algorithm described in Section 9.1.3.4, have become widely used in Bayesian modeling.

The availability of R since the 1990s has greatly contributed to MCMC methods gaining wider use in Bayesian modeling. There are many R packages developed for Bayesian modeling using MCMC. We briefly outline some of the commonly used packages in R for Bayesian modeling.

9.2.2   R Packages using WinBUGS

As mentioned in the previous section, MCMC methods became useable in the 1990s. This is largely due to the development of WinBUGS, the Windows version of BUGS which stands for "**B**ayesian inference **U**sing **G**ibbs **S**ampling" as outlined in Spiegelhalter et al. (2003). WinBUGS incorporates Gibbs sampling and the Metropolis-Hastings algorithm to generate a Markov chain by sampling from full conditional distributions. It is freely available at http://www.mrc-bsu.cam.ac.uk/bugs/. Building on WinBUGS, there are several packages (commonly referred to as "libraries") in R to call the functions in WinBUGS.

9.2.2.1   R2WinBUGS

Based on the publicly available WinBUGS, the R2WinBUGS package was developed to provide functions to call WinBUGS from R by Sturtz et al. (2005). As described by the authors, "It automatically writes the data and scripts in a format readable by WinBUGS for processing in batch mode." "After the WinBUGS process has finished, it is possible either to read the resulting data into R by the package itself – which gives a compact graphical summary of inference and convergence diagnostics – or to use the facilities of the coda package for further analysis of the output. Examples are given to demonstrate the usage of this package."

This package can be downloaded from the R website and loaded into R as follows:

```
> library(R2WinBUGS)
```

If the analyst's computer is linked to the Internet, R2WinBUGS can be installed by typing install.packages("R2WinBUGS") from the R command prompt and then loading the library into R using the above R code chunk and using:

```
> library(help=R2WinBUGS)
```

to get the help manual for this package which can be viewed to see that this package is for running WinBUGS from R. Therefore WinBUGS should be installed in advance in order for R2WinBUGS to call the functions.

For further information on how to use this package step-by-step, readers are directed to the paper by Sturtz et al. (2005). The manual and some examples are given in the subdirectory of "/library/R2WinBUGS/doc" under the R home directory.

9.2.2.2 BRugs

BRugs is another R library for use in R to call OpenBUGS. The OpenBUGS is a newly revised version of WinBUGS as described in Spiegelhalter et al. (2004). Since OpenBUGS is still under development, it suffers frequent crashes. When OpenBUGS becomes more reliable, the development team will merge BRugs with R2WinBUGS into an R package. This package can be installed from R webpage and loaded into R.

Both usage and help information is available from library(help=BRugs). Interested readers may wish to explore this package.

9.2.2.3 rbugs

The R package rbugs was developed by Jun Yan (jyan@stat.uconn.edu) with part of the code modified from bugs.R (http://www.stat.columbia.edu/~gelman/bugsR/) by Andrew Gelman (gelman@stat.columbia.edu). As mentioned in the manual, the "design philosophy of rbugs is to take advantage of the universal MCMC sampler of BUGS through an interface as simple as possible, and return the MCMC samples in a format which can be fed into other R packages specializing in Bayesian output analysis, such as boa and coda".

Similarily, the package rbugs may be installed and loaded into R using following R code chunk:

```
> library(rbugs)
```

Both usage and help information may be accessed by "library(help=rbugs)". Again interested readers may wish to explore the functionalities of this package.

9.2.2.4 Typical Usage

Typical use of these packages is to call WinBUGS. Therefore, the model building steps in WinBUGS must be followed. Usually at a minimum, there are three files that need to be built beforehand to run the program. These are a model file, a data file, and an initial value file. The model file is written by the user with syntax from WinBUGS, which is basically R code. Therefore, the user needs to be good at programming in both R and WinBUGS. The data and initial files are built using R syntax. With these files, these packages will then use a function call to WinBUGS to run the program and output the results. The output can then be analyzed in R for convergence and relevant output analysis.

The flexibility of these packages to use WinBUGS language is an advantage for advanced users who want to build and fit advanced custom models.

9.2.3   MCMCpack

Different from the packages listed in Section 9.2.2 to call WinBUGS, MCMCpack is designed separately from WinBUGS. It is a standalone package developed by Andrew D. Martin (admartin@wustl.edu), Kevin M. Quinn (kevin_quinn@harvard.edu) and Jong Hee Park (jhp@uchicago.edu). This package implements MCMC algorithms, which is model-specific as is usually done by R function calls, therefore is easy to use even for a novice user of R.

The package can be downloaded from R and loaded into R using the following R code chunk:

```
> library(MCMCpack)
```

Details about this package may be found from the help manual using "library(help=MCMCpack)" which states "this package contains functions to perform Bayesian inference using posterior simulation for a number of statistical models. Most simulation is done in compiled C++ written in the Scythe Statistical Library Version 1.0.2. All models return CODA (i.e., Convergence Diagnostics and Output Analysis) MCMC objects that can then be summarized using the coda package. The *MCMCpack* also contains some useful utility functions, including some additional density functions and pseudo-random number generators for statistical distributions, a general purpose Metropolis-Hastings sampling algorithm, and tools for visualization."

A website at http://mcmcpack.wustl.edu is available for the *MCMCpack* project which contains a more detailed description. At the time of writing this chapter, MCMCpack can be used to fit an extensive list of statistical models. We list several commonly used models which may be used in the analysis of data from clinical trials: a linear regression (with Gaussian errors), a hierarchical longitudinal model with Gaussian errors, a probit model, a logistic regression model, a Poisson regression model, a tobit regression model, a multinomial logit model, and an ordered probit model. In addition, this package includes random number generators for several distributions that are not part of the standard distributions in R; e.g., a general purpose Metropolis-Hastings sampling algorithm and some utilities for visualization and data manipulation.

We use this package in Section 9.3 to illustrate applications in MCMC, and in Section 9.4 to re-analyze some of the clinical trial datasets in Chapter 4.

9.3 MCMC Simulations

9.3.1 Normal-Normal Model

We start with the simplest case as described in Section 9.1.2.1 for normally distributed data with known standard deviation σ. Suppose a pilot trial enrolled $n = 30$ patients and from the sample data collected, the sample mean and standard deviation are 3 and 2, respectively. We wish to simulate data from a population for which these data are representative; i.e., from a normal population mean $\mu = 3$ with known standard deviation $\sigma = 2$. The data are simulated directly as follows:

```
> # set seed to 123
> set.seed(123)
> # n=30 patients
> n  = 30
> # known mean and sigma
> sigma = 2; mu = 3
> # simulate data
> y  =  rnorm(n, mu,sigma)
> # print the data
> # the mean and variance of the simulated data
> mean(y)

[1] 2.91

> var(y)

[1] 3.85
```

Suppose from prior knowledge it is reasonable to assume that the prior distribution is normal with prior mean $\mu_0 = 2$ and prior standard deviation $\tau_0 = 0.5$. Then from Section 9.1.2.1, the posterior distribution is also normal with posterior mean $\mu_P = w\bar{y} + (1-w)\theta_0$ and posterior variance $\sigma_P^2 = \frac{1}{\frac{n}{\sigma^2} + \frac{1}{\tau^2}}$, where $w = \frac{\tau^2}{\tau^2 + \sigma^2/n}$. The direct simulation can be implemented in R as follows:

```
> # the prior parameters
> mu0 = 2; tau0 = .5
> # the weight
> w   =  tau0^2/(tau0^2+sigma^2/n)
> # the posterior mean
> muP =  w*mean(y) + (1-w)*mu0
> # the posterior standard deviation
```

```
> sigmaP = sqrt(1/(1/tau0^2+n/sigma^2))
> # direct simulation of posterior normal
> Bayes1.norm2norm = rnorm(10000, muP,sigmaP)
```

We simulate 10,000 samples and name the resulting dataset in Bayes1.norm2norm. The density plot of the sampling distribution is seen in Figure 9.1. The quantiles of this posterior distribution are determined from:

```
> quantile(Bayes1.norm2norm, c(0.025,0.25,0.5,0.75,0.975))
```

```
2.5%   25%   50%   75% 97.5%
2.01  2.39  2.59  2.79  3.17
```

We can also call the MCnormalnormal function in MCMCpack for this simulation as follows:

```
> # call the function
> Bayes2.norm2norm = MCnormalnormal(y, sigma^2, mu0, tau0^2, 10000)
> # print the summary
> summary(Bayes2.norm2norm)
```

```
Iterations        = 1:10000
Thinning interval = 1
Number of chains  = 1
Sample size per chain = 10000
```

```
1. Empirical mean and standard deviation for each variable,
   plus standard error of the mean:
     Mean       SD      Naive SE    Time-series SE
     2.58766  0.29548  0.00295       0.00295
2. Quantiles for each variable:
     2.5%   25%   50%   75% 97.5%
     2.01  2.39  2.59  2.79  3.17
```

We observe that the quantiles are identical to those from the direct simulation. The prior, likelihood, and the resulting posterior distributions are displayed in Figure 9.1 using following R code chunk.

```
> # Create x sequence
> x      = seq(0,6,0.01)
> # plot the densities
> plot(x, dnorm(x, mu0,tau0), type="l", lwd=1,las=1,
       ylim=c(0,1.4),    xlab="mu", ylab="density")
> lines(x, dnorm(x, mean(y), sigma/sqrt(n)), lty=8, lwd=1)
> lines(density(Bayes1.norm2norm), lty=8, lwd=3)
> legend("topright", c("Prior","Likelihood", "Posterior"),
       lwd=c(1,1,3), lty=c(1,8,4))
```

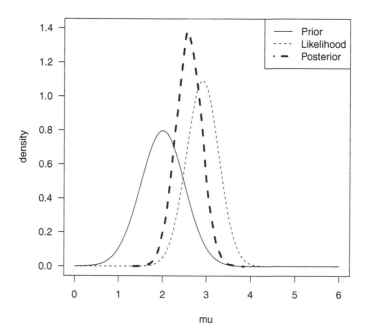

FIGURE 9.1: Distributions of Prior, Direct Simulation, and MCnormalnormal

9.3.2 Beta-Binomial Model

As described in Section 9.1.2.4, the beta-binomial distribution is commonly used in Bayesian analysis of clinical trial data. The beta-binomial distribution results from binomially distributed data with a beta conjugate prior on the binomial probability parameter leading to a new (posterior) beta distribution which can be directly simulated from the R function `rbeta`.

As an example, we re-visit the duodenal ulcer trial in Chapter 3 where we found that the 800 mg C treatment was clinically optimal among the four treatments. In this trial, a total of 168, 182, 165, and 188 patients were randomly entered in the 0 mg C, 400 mg C, 800 mg C, and 1600 mg C treatment groups, respectively. The corresponding cumulative numbers of patients whose ulcers healed by the end of week 4 were 69, 113, 120, and 145, respectively. These data are loaded into R as:

```
> # total patients for each treatment
> n  = c(168, 182, 165,188)
> # number healed
```

```
> x  = c(69, 113, 120, 145)
> # the observed proportion
> p  = x/n
> p
```

[1] 0.411 0.621 0.727 0.771

Consider first the 800 mg C treatment where we observed that $x_3=120$ of $n_3 = 165$ patients had their ulcers healed. x_3 is binomially distributed with the probability p_3 estimated as $\hat{p} = x_3/n_3 = 120/165 = 0.73$. The likelihood is

$$L(p) \propto p^{x_3}(1-p)^{n_3-x_3} \qquad (9.11)$$

For Bayesian inference, we need to identify a suitable prior for the cumulative 4-week healing rate p (which ranges from 0 to 1 since it is a probability). We could use the noninformative prior where the posterior distribution would be the same as the likelihood. However, we illustrate a simple approach to derive an informative prior.

Suppose that results from prior, smaller trials suggest that the median of the distribution of p is about 0.75 and the 95 percentile is 0.85 for this treatment. We can build a search algorithm to find values to be used for the prior parameters a and b as follows.

We first build an objective function with parameter input $parm = c(a, b)$ as:

```
> # the objective function
> obj = function(parm){
 a = parm[1]; b = parm[2]
 ( pbeta(0.50,a,b)  -0.75)^2 +( pbeta(0.95,a,b)- 0.85)^2
 }
```

Then we call the R function optim to optimize (more specifically minimize for this situation) the objective function to find (a, b) as:

```
> # call optim to search the root with initial values at (3,3)
> out = optim(c(3,3), obj)
> print(out)
```

$par
[1] 0.0621 0.1829

$value
[1] 2.57e-10

$counts
function gradient
      119   NA

```
$convergence
[1] 0

$message
NULL
```

It should be noted that this search is a local one and in fact there are many roots to be found depending on where the search is started. Anyway, we use $a = 0.062$ and $b = 0.183$ from this search as the prior parameters for our beta prior. We can check whether the median is 0.75 and the 95th percentile is 0.85 using following R code chunk:

```
> pbeta(0.5,out$par[1], out$par[2])

[1] 0.75

> pbeta(0.95,out$par[1], out$par[2])

[1] 0.85
```

Based on this prior, the posterior distribution for the cumulative 4-week healing rate is:

$$
\begin{aligned}
p(p|n_3, x_3) &\propto L(p) \times \pi(p) \\
&= p^{x_3}(1-p)^{n_3-x_3} \times p^{a-1}(1-p)^{b-1} \\
&= p^{x_3+a-1}(1-p)^{n_3-x_3+b-1}
\end{aligned}
\tag{9.12}
$$

which is $beta(x_3 + a, n_3 - x_3 + b) = beta(120 + 0.062, 165 - 120 + 0.183) = beta(120.062, 45.183)$. This posterior can be directly simulated in R for 10,000 simulations as follows:

```
> # direct simulation
> Bayes1.betabin = rbeta(10000, 120.062, 45.183)
> # print the quantiles
> quantile(Bayes1.betabin, c(0.025,0.25,0.5,0.75,0.975))

 2.5%   25%   50%   75% 97.5%
0.657 0.704 0.728 0.751 0.791
```

This shows that the simulated distribution of p has mean 0.728 and 95% credible interval of (0.656, 0.792).

We can employ the `MCbinomialbeta` function from the `MCMCpack` package for the same purpose. This function is for Monte Carlo simulation from a binomial likelihood with a beta prior and is called as follows:

```
> # keep the parameters
> x3 = 120; n3 =165; a = 0.062; b=0.183
> # call the MCbinomialbeta function for 10000 simulation
> Bayes2.betabin = MCbinomialbeta(x3, n3, a, b, mc=10000)
> # print the summary
> summary(Bayes2.betabin)

Iterations = 1:10000
Thinning interval = 1
Number of chains = 1
Sample size per chain = 10000

1. Empirical mean and standard deviation for each variable,
   plus standard error of the mean:

          Mean              SD        Naive SE  Time-series SE
       0.726215        0.034730      0.000347      0.000347

2. Quantiles for each variable:

  2.5%    25%    50%    75% 97.5%
 0.656 0.703 0.727 0.750 0.792
```

We see from this summary that the quantiles from this MC simulation are identical to those from the direct simulation. The reader may wish to plot this simulation and visualize the convergence and the MC sampling distribution using R code as plot(Bayes2.betabin).

We plot the prior and the simulation distributions from both direct simulation and from MCbinomialbeta in Figure 9.2 using the following code chunk:

```
> # create a sequence for p for plotting
> p = seq(0,1,0.01)
> # plot beta-density
> plot(p, dbeta(p,a, b),  lwd=3, type="l",ylim=c(0,13),
    xlab="Healing Rate", ylab="density")
> # Add lines to the density
> lines(density(Bayes1.betabin), lty=4, lwd=3)
> lines(density(Bayes2.betabin), lty=8, lwd=3)
> # add legend to the plot
> legend("topleft", c("Prior", "Direct Simulation",
    "MCbinomialbeta"), lwd=3, lty=c(1,4,8))
```

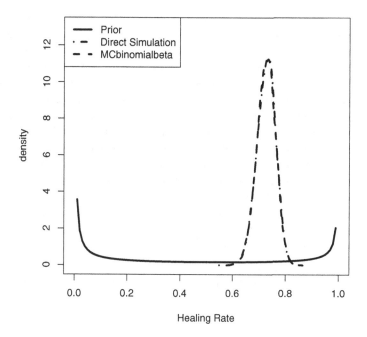

FIGURE 9.2: Distributions of Prior, Direct Simulation, and MCbinomial-beta

Note in this figure that both distributions from the direct simulation and from `MCbinomialbeta` are almost identical, and therefore it is difficult to distinguish one from the other.

9.4 Bayesian Data Analysis

In this section, we re-analyze the data from Chapter 4 taking a Bayesian modeling approach using the `MCMCpack`.

9.4.1 Blood Pressure Data: Bayesian Linear Regression

We start with the typical linear regression using the blood pressure data in Section 4.1 where we used the R function `lm` for ACNOVA. As was done in Section 4.1, we read in this data as:

```
> dat = read.csv("DBP.csv",header=T)
> # we are interested in the blood pressure change
> dat$diff = dat$DBP5-dat$DBP1
```

As summarized in Section 4.1 the lm fitting of the regression model revealed that both "TRT" and "Age" were statistically significant. We now use MCMCpack to re-analyze this data from a Bayesian perspective using MCMC algorithms.

Since the data are continuous, we can use the function MCMCregress in the MCMCpack package for this purpose. From the help file, this function is used to generate "a sample from the posterior distribution of a linear regression model with Gaussian errors using Gibbs sampling (with a multivariate Gaussian prior on the beta vector, and an inverse Gamma prior on the conditional error variance). The user supplies data and priors, and a sample from the posterior distribution is returned as an MCMC object, which can be subsequently analyzed with functions provided in the coda package".

This function uses the regression model:

$$y_i = x'_i\beta + \epsilon_i \tag{9.13}$$

where the errors ϵ_i are assumed to be normally distributed; i.e., $\epsilon_i \sim N(0, \sigma^2)$. For Bayesian modeling, the standard, semi-conjugate priors are assumed to be:

$$\beta \sim N(b_0, B_0^{-1})$$
$$\sigma^{-2} \sim Gamma(c_0/2, d_0/2)$$

It is noted that the Bayesian model with noninformative prior described in Section 9.1.2.3 is a special case when $B_0 = 0$. We fit this special model since we have no prior information about β.

To fit a linear regression model with this noninformative prior for the regression parameters and an inverse gamma prior with shape and scale parameters both equal to 0.0005 for the error variance, we call the function MCMCregress (which is identical in syntax to the lm function call using the default settings for the parameters in the MCMC) as follows:

```
> # fit the Bayes regression model with 1000 burn-in
> BayesMod  = MCMCregress(diff~TRT+Age, dat)
> # print the MCMC result
> summary(BayesMod)

Iterations = 1001:11000
Thinning interval = 1
Number of chains = 1
Sample size per chain = 10000
```

1. Empirical mean and standard deviation for each variable,
   plus standard error of the mean:

```
              Mean       SD  Naive SE  Time-series SE
(Intercept) -6.813  3.0402  0.030402       0.030772
TRTB        10.119  0.8108  0.008108       0.008108
Age         -0.173  0.0614  0.000614       0.000619
sigma2       6.484  1.6015  0.016015       0.017318
```

2. Quantiles for each variable:

```
              2.5%     25%     50%     75%    97.5%
(Intercept) -12.704 -8.838  -6.823 -4.792  -0.7915
TRTB          8.543  9.575  10.119 10.648  11.7387
Age          -0.295 -0.213  -0.172 -0.132  -0.0542
sigma2        4.086  5.329   6.225  7.329  10.2339
```

The summary function prints out summary information of the MCMC objects for various quantities of interest such as the posterior mean, standard deviation, and quantiles. We note from the MCMC output, that both "TRT" and "Age" are statistically significant based on the 95% quantiles where "TRT" is positive with 50% quantile = 10.12, which is close to the linear regression estimate of 10.13; again indicating that treatment is effective. The same conclusion is observed for the "Age" effect.

We can call plot to generate trace plots for convergence diagnostics and marginal posterior kernel density plots for the MCMC results (Figure 9.3) as follows:

```
> # make the margin
> par(mar = c(3,2,1.5,1))
> # make the MCMC plot
> plot(BayesMod)
```

Note from Figure 9.3 that the MCMC converged.

9.4.2 Binomial Data: Bayesian Logistic Regression

In Section 4.1, we analyzed data from the betablocker trial using logistic regression. We will re-use the data from center 1 for illustration since MCMCpack only takes binary data as input.

```
> # extract center 1
> beta1 = betablocker[betablocker$Center == 1,
                      c("Deaths","Total","Treatment")]
> # print the center 1 data
> beta1

   Deaths Total Treatment
1       3    39   Control
23      3    38   Treated
```

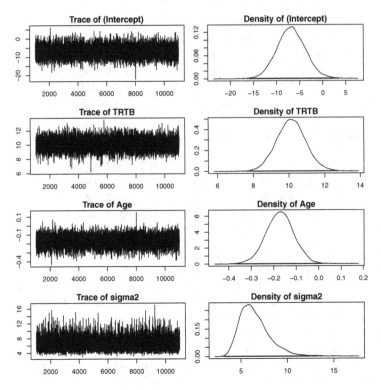

FIGURE 9.3: MCMC Plots

We note that there are 3 deaths from 39 patients in the control group and 3 deaths from 38 patients in the treatment group. We then convert these binomial count data into a dataframe with binary outcome as:

```
> # make a dataframe
> beta1 = data.frame(trt = c(rep("TRT", 38),rep("Cont",39)),
        death = c(rep(1,3), rep(0,38-3), rep(1,3), rep(0,39-3)))
> # print the first 6 observations
> head(beta1)

  trt death
1 TRT    1
2 TRT    1
3 TRT    1
4 TRT    0
5 TRT    0
6 TRT    0
```

We re-use `beta1` to name this new dataframe. In this dataframe, there are two columns. The first column represents "trt" and the second column represents the binary outcome, where "1" denotes death and "0" denotes alive.

We fit a logistic regression model to the data using `glm` as follows:

```
> # fit logistic regression
> glm.beta = glm(death ~trt,binomial,beta1)
> # print the result
> summary(glm.beta)

Call:
glm(formula = death ~ trt, family = binomial, data = beta1)

Deviance Residuals:
   Min      1Q   Median      3Q     Max
-0.406  -0.406  -0.400  -0.400   2.265

Coefficients:
            Estimate Std. Error z value Pr(>|z|)
(Intercept)  -2.4849     0.6009   -4.14 3.5e-05 ***
trtTRT        0.0282     0.8503    0.03    0.97

(Dispersion parameter for binomial family taken to be 1)

    Null deviance: 42.144  on 76  degrees of freedom
Residual deviance: 42.143  on 75  degrees of freedom
AIC: 46.14

Number of Fisher Scoring iterations: 5
```

From the logistic regression we note that the estimated parameter $\hat{\beta} = (-2.485, 0.028)$, that treatment effect is not statistically significant with p-value of 0.974 (which is expected since only 3 of 39 patients in the control group and 3 of 38 patients in treatment group died), and the observed proportions are almost the same.

For Bayesian modeling using MCMC for binary data, we make use of the `MCMClogit` function in `MCMCpack`. This function generates a sample from the posterior distribution of a logistic regression model using a random walk Metropolis-Hastings algorithm. In this function, the model is as follows:

$$y_i \sim Bernoulli(p_i) \tag{9.14}$$

with the logit link function as $p_i = \frac{exp(x_i'\beta)}{1+exp(x_i'\beta)}$. The multivariate normal prior is assumed for β as $\beta \sim N(b_0, B_0^{-1})$, where B_0 is the prior precision of β under a multivariate normal prior. The noninformative prior obtains if $B_0=0$. Other priors can be incorporated into this function call.

We now fit the Bayesian model using the noninformative prior distribution with the default setting using $B_0 = 0$ as follows:

```
>  ## Call MCMClogit with default
> Bayes1.beta = MCMClogit(death~trt, data=beta1)
> # print the summary for MCMC
> summary(Bayes1.beta)

Iterations = 1001:11000
Thinning interval = 1
Number of chains = 1
Sample size per chain = 10000
```

1. Empirical mean and standard deviation for each variable, plus standard error of the mean:

	Mean	SD	Naive SE	Time-series SE
(Intercept)	-2.6516	0.652	0.00652	0.0207
trtTRT	0.0422	0.909	0.00909	0.0283

2. Quantiles for each variable:

	2.5%	25%	50%	75%	97.5%
(Intercept)	-4.10	-3.043	-2.597	-2.194	-1.55
trtTRT	-1.75	-0.558	0.025	0.647	1.78

We note that the estimate of β is $\hat{\beta} = (-2.652, 0.042)$ and that the 95% credible interval for treatment effect is (-1.746, 1.784), which is not statistically significant.

Similarly we call `plot` to make traceplots for convergence diagnostics and marginal posterior kernel density plots for the MCMC results (Figure 9.4) using the following code chunk:

```
> plot(Bayes1.beta)
```

We note from Figure 9.4 that the MCMC algorithm converged. To further illustrate Bayesian robustness, we consider a vague multivariate normal prior using $B_0 = 0.001$, which means that the prior precision matrix is B_0 times the identity matrix. With this prior, we fit a Bayesian logistic regression model as follows:

```
> # Bayesian logistic regression with multivariate normal prior
> Bayes2.beta = MCMClogit(death~trt, B0=.001,data=beta1)
> # print the fit
> summary(Bayes2.beta)

Iterations = 1001:11000; Thinning interval = 1;
Number of chains = 1; Sample size per chain = 10000
```

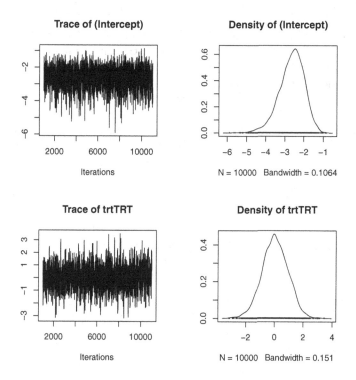

FIGURE 9.4: MCMC Plots for Betablocker

1. Empirical mean and standard deviation for each variable,
   plus standard error of the mean:

	Mean	SD	Naive SE	Time-series SE
(Intercept)	-2.6540	0.653	0.00653	0.0208
trtTRT	0.0437	0.906	0.00906	0.0282

2. Quantiles for each variable:

	2.5%	25%	50%	75%	97.5%
(Intercept)	-4.11	-3.04	-2.5944	-2.197	-1.54
trtTRT	-1.71	-0.57	0.0456	0.631	1.79

We note that the estimate of β is $\hat{\beta} = (-2.654, 0.044)$ and that the 95% credible interval for treatment effect is (-1.707, 1.790), which again is not statistically significant. A plot similar to that in Figure 9.4 can be made by plot(Bayes2.beta). The reader may wish to produce this plot.

9.4.3   Count Data: Bayesian Poisson Regression

In Section 4.1, we considered data from a placebo-controlled clinical trial of a non-steroidal anti-inflammatory drug in treating familial andenomatous polyposis (FAP). We analyzed these data in Section 4.3.3 using several methods and concluded that both treatment and "age" were statistically significant.

We re-use these data to illustrate the `MCMCpoisson` function in the `MCMCpack` package for Bayesian Poisson regression. According to its `help` manual, "this function generates a sample from the posterior distribution of a Poisson regression model using a random walk Metropolis-Hastings algorithm" programmed in compiled C++ code to maximize efficiency. The model for this function is as follows:

$$y_i \sim Poisson(\mu_i) \tag{9.15}$$

with log link function as $\mu_i = exp(x_i'\beta)$. The prior distribution for the parameter β is assumed to be multivariate normal; i.e., $\beta \sim N(b_0, B_0^{-1})$.

The Bayesian Poisson regression with noninformative prior can be easily performed with the default setting using $B_0 = 0$ as follows:

```
> ## Call MCMCpoissont with default
> Bayes.polyps <- MCMCpoisson(number ~ treat+age, polyps)
> # print the summary for MCMC
> summary(Bayes.polyps)

Iterations = 1001:11000
Thinning interval = 1; Number of chains = 1
Sample size per chain = 10000
```

1. Empirical mean and standard deviation for each variable,
   plus standard error of the mean:

	Mean	SD	Naive SE	Time-series SE
(Intercept)	4.5343	0.14788	1.48e-03	0.004794
treatdrug	-1.3612	0.12006	1.20e-03	0.003997
age	-0.0392	0.00604	6.04e-05	0.000196

2. Quantiles for each variable:

	2.5%	25%	50%	75%	97.5%
(Intercept)	4.2388	4.4372	4.5360	4.6307	4.8274
treatdrug	-1.6091	-1.4388	-1.3607	-1.2811	-1.1236
age	-0.0512	-0.0432	-0.0394	-0.0352	-0.0272

We note that the estimate of β is $\hat{\beta} = (4.534, -1.361, -0.039)$ and that the 95% credible intervals are (-1.609, -1.124) for treatment effect and (-0.051, -0.027) for age effect. This confirms that both treatment effect and age effect are statistically significant.

The diagnostics plot (Figure 9.5) for MCMC run can be generated using the following code chunk:

```
> # set a beta margin for plotting
> par(mar = c(3,2,1.5,1))
> # plot the MCMC
> plot(Bayes.polyps)
```

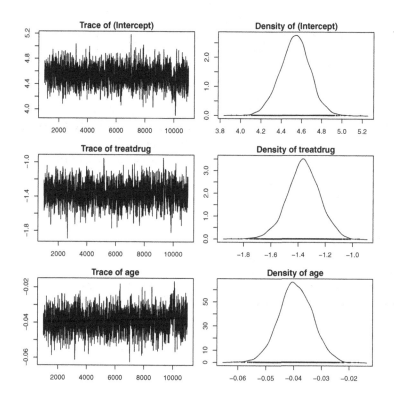

FIGURE 9.5: MCMC Plots for Polyps Data

We note from Figure 9.5 that the MCMC algorithm converged. Similarly, we may investigate the robustness of this Bayesian model for different priors by specifying different b_0 and B_0. We leave this as an exercise for the interested readers.

9.4.4 Comparing Two Treatments

We now consider applying the beta-binomial posterior distribution to compare and select superior treatments in clinical trials with a binomial endpoint from the Bayesian perspective. Specifically, we are interested in comparing two treatments denoted by X and Y and deciding which treatment is superior by calculating the probability $P(X > Y)$. If $P(X > Y)$ is greater than some threshold, say 0.95, we conclude treatment X is superior to treatment Y.

In clinical trials with binary/binomial endpoints, we typically use a beta prior as the conjugate prior which leads to the posterior distribution in the same beta family. Then, the posterior distributions of both treatments are also beta, which we denote as $X \sim Beta(u_X, v_X)$ and $Y \sim Beta(u_Y, v_Y)$. Then, it can be shown with some mathematical manipulations (see Cook (2005)) that:

$$
\begin{aligned}
P(X > Y) &= \int_0^1 \frac{x^{s_X-1}(1-x)^{t_X-1}}{B(s_X, t_X)} \left(\int_0^x \frac{y^{s_Y-1}(1-y)^{t_Y-1}}{B(s_Y, t_Y)} dy \right) dx \\
&= \frac{B(s_X + s_Y, t_X + t_Y)}{B(s_X, s_Y)B(s_Y, t_Y)s_Y} \, {}_3F_2 \left(\begin{matrix} s_X + s_Y, s_Y + t_Y, 1 \\ s_Y + 1, s_X + t_X + s_Y + t_Y \end{matrix} \middle| 1 \right)
\end{aligned}
$$

where $B(s, t)$ is the usual beta function defined as $B(s, t) = \frac{\Gamma(s)\Gamma(t)}{\Gamma(s+t)}$ and ${}_3F_2$ is the hypergeometric function with upper parameters $(s_X + s_Y, s_Y + t_Y, 1)$ and lower parameters $(s_Y + 1, s_X + t_X + s_Y + t_Y)$. The calculation of the probability $P(X > Y)$ can be easily implemented in R by calling the **hypergeo** library as follows:

```
> # call the hypergeo library
> library(hypergeo)
> # make a function call
> pXgtY = function(sx,tx,sy,ty){
tmp1 = beta(sx+sy,tx+ty)/(beta(sx,tx)*beta(sy,ty)*sy)
tmp2 = genhypergeo(U=c(sx+sy,sy+ty,1),L=c(sy+1,sx+tx+sy+ty),
         check_mod=FALSE,z=1)
#return
tmp1*tmp2
}
```

To illustrate, we re-use data from the duodenal ulcer trial with a noninformative prior. As previously noted, this leads to a beta posterior distribution which is the same as the likelihood. Therefore:

```
> # compare 800 mg C to 400 mg C
> p800to400 = pXgtY(x[3], n[3]-x[3], x[2],n[2]-x[2])
> p800to400

[1] 0.983

> # compare 800 mg C to 0 mg C
> p800to0 = pXgtY(x[3], n[3]-x[3], x[1],n[1]-x[1])
> p800to0

[1] 1
```

```
> # compare 1600 mg C to 800 mg C
> p1600to800 = pXgtY(x[4], n[4]-x[4], x[3],n[3]-x[3])
> p1600to800
```

[1] 0.83

```
> # compare 1600 mg C to 400 mg C
> p1600to400 = pXgtY(x[4], n[4]-x[4], x[2],n[2]-x[2])
> p1600to400
```

[1] 0.999

We note that: (1) the probability that the 800 mg C treatment is better than the 400 mg C treatment is 0.983; (2) the probability that the 800 mg C treatment is better than the 0 mg C treatment is 0.999; (3) the probability that the 1600 mg C treatment is better than the 800 mg C treatment is 0.830; and (4) the probability that the 1600 mg C treatment is better than the 400 mg C treatment is 0.999. In selecting the superior treatment, if we deem a probability of 0.95 as the required threshold, we conclude that the 800 mg C treatment is better than the 400 mg C treatment and the 0 mg C treatment and the 1600 mg C treatment is also better than 400 mg C treatment. However, the probability that the 1600 mg C treatment is better than the 800 mg C treatment is 0.83, which does not meet the threshold for concluding superiority. These results are consistent with those in Chapter 3 where it was concluded that the 800 mg C treatment was clinically optimal.

The reader may wish to modify the above code to include comparisons of the 400 mg C treatment to the 0 mg C treatment and of the 1600 mg C treatment to the 0 mg C treatment.

A graphical illustration for the four treatment groups and the prior distribution (the horizontal dashed line) appears in Figure 9.6. This figure is generated using the following R code chunk:

```
> #  make p from 0.3 to 0.9 by 100 points
> n.pts =100
> p      = seq(0.3,0.9,length=n.pts)
> # the prior and the distributions from 4 treatments
> pb0  = dbeta(p,1,1)
> pb1  = dbeta(p,x[1],n[1]-x[1])
> pb2  = dbeta(p,x[2],n[2]-x[2])
> pb3  = dbeta(p,x[3],n[3]-x[3])
> pb4  = dbeta(p,x[4],n[4]-x[4])
> # the maximum to set the yaxis limit
> ymax= max(pb1,pb2,pb3,pb4)
> # plot the prior and posterior
> plot(p,pb0, lwd=1, lty=8, las=1,type="l",xlab="Healing
    Probability", ylab="Density",ylim=c(0,ymax))
> lines(p,pb1, lwd=3, lty=1)
```

```
> lines(p,pb2, lwd=3, lty=2)
> lines(p,pb3, lwd=3, lty=3)
> lines(p,pb4, lwd=3, lty=4)
> legend("topleft", c("0 mg C","400 mg C", "800 mg C","1600 mg
    C"), lwd=c(3,3,3,3), lty=c(1,2,3,4))
```

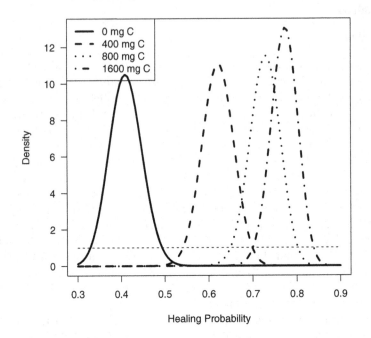

FIGURE 9.6: Distributions of Prior and the Four Treatments

From Figure 9.6, we observe that the 800 mg C and 1600 mg C treatment groups overlap; which illustrates graphically that the 1600 mg C treatment is not statistically superior to the 800 mg C treatment.

As noted above, this illustration used a noninformative prior. It can be easily modified to incorporate an informative prior.

It should be stressed that the probability that treatment X is better than treatment Y; i.e., $P(X > Y)$ and its calculation in Equation 9.16 are very important in clinical trials that incorporate a Bayesian adaptive randomization scheme to assign patients to treatment groups as discussed in Thall and Wathen (2007), Muss et al. (2009) and Giles et al. (2003). Further references on Bayesian adaptive clinical trials can be found from Berry et al. (2010).

9.5 Summary and Discussion

In this chapter, we discussed the application of Bayesian modeling using R. We reviewed relevant models and MCMC simulation as well as the most commonly used R packages. We recommend the MCMCpack package for applied Bayesian modeling for users without much programming experience in R. Advanced users will want to use WinBUGS to build more complex and more flexible models.

The reader may find the book by Ntzoufras (2009) on how to use WinBUGS for Bayesian modeling and the references contained therein helpful. The book by Albert (2007) gives an extensive implementation in R. Chapter 11 outlines how to use R to call RcmdWinBUGS. The book by Robert and Casella (2009) is an excellent textbook on the introduction of Monte Carlo methods using R.

Bayesian statistics is widely used in the biopharmaceutical industries and in government agencies, such as the U.S. Food and Drug Administration (FDA). The FDA issued a guidance on February 5, 2010 (http://www.fda.gov/MedicalDevices/DeviceRegulationandGuidance/GuidanceDocuments/ucm071072.htm) on the use of Bayesian statistical methods in the design and analysis of medical device clinical trials more efficiently and in a less costly way. This guidance described the use of Bayesian methods, design and analysis of medical device clinical trials, the benefits and difficulties with the Bayesian approach, and comparisons with standard statistical methods.

9.6 Appendix: SAS Programs

Bayesian analysis is common in SAS with procedure proc MCMC. Also, we can use the proc genmod with the option bayes to implement the Bayes modeling. We illustrate this implementation with the following SAS programs.

```
/****************************************************************
Section 9.3.1: Normal-Normal Model
****************************************************************/
/*simulated data*/
DATA S1(keep= y);
n= 30; sigma= 2; mu= 3;
call streaminit(123);
do i= 1 to 30;
y= mu+sigma*rand("Normal");
```

```
output;
end;
RUN;

/*the mean and variance of simulated data*/
PROC MEANS data=S1 mean var stddev;
var y;
output out=I1 mean= mean var=var stddev=sd;
RUN;

DATA S2(keep= bayes_norm2norm);
set I1;
n= 30; sigma= 2; mu= 3;
/*the prior parameter*/
mu0= 2; tau0= 0.5;
/*the weight*/
w= tau0**2/(tau0**2+sigma**2/n);
/*the posterior mean*/
muP =w*mean+(1-w)*mu0;
/*the posterior standard deviation*/
sigmaP =sqrt(1/(1/tau0**2+n/sigma**2));
/*set seed*/
call streaminit(123);
/*direct simulation of posterior normal*/
do i= 1 to 10000;
bayes_norm2norm= muP+sigmaP*rand("Normal");
output;
end;
RUN;

/*the quantiles of this posterior distribution*/
PROC UNIVARIATE data= S2;
var bayes_norm2norm;
output out= DS PCTLPTS= 2.5 25 50 75 97.5 PCTLPRE= p;
RUN;


PROC PRINT data=DS;
title "Posterior Quantile from Direct Simulation";
RUN;

/*direct simulate using proc*/
PROC MCMC data= S1 outpost= MCsimu seed= 123
    nmc= 10000 statistics= all;
parms mu0;
```

```
prior mu0 ~ normal(2,sd=0.5);
model y ~ normal(mu0, sd=2);
RUN;

PROC PRINT data=MCsimu;
RUN;

/*the quantiles of this posterior distribution*/
PROC UNIVARIATE data= MCSimu;
var mu0;
output out= MCq PCTLPTS= 2.5 25 50 75 97.5 PCTLPRE = q;
RUN;

PROC PRINT data=MCq;
RUN;


/***************************************************************
9.3.2 Beta-Binomial Model
***************************************************************/
DATA S4;
input n x;
p= x/n;
datalines;
168 69
182 113
165 120
188 145
RUN;

/*search the root with initial value at (3,3)*/
PROC NLP tech=nmsimp;
min y;
parms a= 3,b= 3;
y=(probbeta(0.5,a,b)-0.75)**2+(probbeta(0.95,a,b)-0.85)**2;
RUN;

/*check the optimization results*/
DATA check;
c1=probbeta(0.5,0.062366,0.183202);
c2=probbeta(0.95,0.062366,0.183202);
RUN;

/*direct simulation*/
DATA S5;
```

```
call streaminit(123);
do i= 1 to 10000;
bayes1_betabin= rand("Beta",120.062,45.183);
output;
end;
RUN;

/*print the quantiles*/
PROC UNIVARIATE data= S5;
var bayes1_betabin;
output out= q PCTLPTS= 2.5 25 50 75 97.5 PCTLPRE = q;
RUN;


/*****************************************************************
Section 9.4.1: Blood Pressure Data - Bayesian Linear Regression
*****************************************************************/
Data DBP;
infile "Your file path/DBP.csv" delimiter="," firstobs=2;
input Subject TRT$ DBP1 DBP2 DBP3 DBP4 DBP5 Age Sex$;
diff= DBP5-DBP1;
RUN;

/*fit the Bayes regression model with 1000 burn-in*/
PROC GENMOD data= DBP;
class TRT(ref= "A");
model diff= TRT Age / dist= normal;
bayes nbi=1000 seed= 123 outpost= postDBP ;
RUN;

/*****************************************************************
Section 9.4.2: Binomial Data - Bayesian Logistic Regression
*****************************************************************/
DATA Betablocker(where= (Center= 1));
infile "Your file path/betablocker.csv" delimiter="," firstobs=2;
input Deaths Total Center Treatment$;
RUN;

/*fit logistic regression*/
PROC GENMOD data= betablocker;
class Treatment(ref="Control");
model Deaths/Total= Treatment/dist= binomial link= logit;
RUN;

/*fit the Bayes regression model with 1000 burn-in*/
```

```
PROC GENMOD data= BetaBlocker;
class Treatment(ref="Control");
model Deaths/Total= Treatment/dist= binomial link= logit;
bayes nbi=1000 seed= 123 outpost= postbetablocker ;
RUN;

/*fit the Bayes regression model with multivariate normal
  prior*/
DATA prior;
input _type_ $ Intercept x;
datalines;
Var 1000 1000
Mean 0 0
;
RUN;

PROC GENMOD data= betablocker;
class Treatment(ref="Control");
model Deaths/Total= Treatment/dist= binomial link= logit;
bayes nbi=1000 seed= 123 outpost= postbetablocker
coeffprior=normal(input= prior);
RUN;

/****************************************************************
Section 9.4.3:Count Data - Bayesian Possion Regression
****************************************************************/
DATA Polyps;
infile "/home/ln23040/polyps.csv" delimiter="," firstobs=2;
input number treat$ age;
RUN;

/*fit Bayes poisson regression*/
PROC GENMOD data= Polyps;
class treat(ref= "placebo");
model number= treat age / dist= poisson;
bayes nbi=1000 seed= 123 outpost=postPolyps;
RUN;

/*print the quantiles*/
PROC UNIVARIATE data= postPolyps;
var Intercept Treatdrug Age;
output out= q  PCTLPRE=intercept treattdrug age
PCTLPTS= 2.5 25 50 75 97.5 PCTLPRE = q;
RUN;
```

Chapter 10

Bioequivalence Clinical Trials

In this chapter, we illustrate the use of R in the analysis of data collected in bioequivalence clinical trials. Similar to previous chapters, we describe two datasets from bioequivalence trials, the associated statistical analysis methods, and then step-by-step implementation of the methods in R .

10.1   Data from Bioequivalence Clinical Trials

10.1.1   Data from Chow and Liu (2009)

The first dataset is obtained from a bioequivalence clinical trial described in Chow and Liu (2009), Table 3.6.1, Page 71. Since Chow and Liu used SAS for statistical analyses, we use this dataset to illustrate the reproducibility of their results using the R system to analyze data from a bioequivalence clinical trial.

The trial utilized a standard two-sequence (i.e., RT and TR), two-period, two-formulation (T = Test; R = Reference) (i.e., $2 \times 2 \times 2$) crossover design to compare two oral formulations of a drug, and was conducted with 24 healthy volunteers (subjects). Volunteers were randomly assigned to either five 50 mg tablets (i.e., test formulation, T) or 5 mL of a suspension (i.e., 50 mg/mL, reference formulation, R) at the first period baseline, and then crossed over to the alternative formulation at the second period baseline. Blood samples were collected at 0 hour before dosing and at various times after dosing up through 32 hours post-dosing.

The trapezoid rule was applied to the drug concentrations in the samples to compute the bioavailability endpoint: area under the concentration-by-time curve (AUC) over the interval from 0 to 32 hours. The AUC data from Chow and Liu (2009) are reproduced here in Table 10.1 for easy reference.

10.1.2   Bioequivalence Trial on Cimetidine Tablets

The second dataset derives from a bioequivalence clinical trial described in Randolph et al. (1986). The trial utilized a standard $2 \times 2 \times 2$ crossover design to compare two oral formulations of Cimetidine, and was conducted

TABLE 10.1: AUC Data from Chow and Liu (2009)

Sequence	Period	Formulation	Subject	AUC
1	1	R	1	74.675
1	1	R	4	96.400
1	1	R	5	101.950
1	1	R	6	79.050
1	1	R	11	79.050
1	1	R	12	85.950
1	1	R	15	69.725
1	1	R	16	86.275
1	1	R	19	112.675
1	1	R	20	99.525
1	1	R	23	89.425
1	1	R	24	55.175
1	2	T	1	73.675
1	2	T	4	93.250
1	2	T	5	102.125
1	2	T	6	69.450
1	2	T	11	69.025
1	2	T	12	68.700
1	2	T	15	59.425
1	2	T	16	76.125
1	2	T	19	114.875
1	2	T	20	116.250
1	2	T	23	64.175
1	2	T	24	74.575
2	1	T	2	74.825
2	1	T	3	86.875
2	1	T	7	81.675
2	1	T	8	92.700
2	1	T	9	50.450
2	1	T	10	66.125
2	1	T	13	122.450
2	1	T	14	99.075
2	1	T	17	86.350
2	1	T	18	49.925
2	1	T	21	42.700
2	1	T	22	91.725
2	2	R	2	37.350
2	2	R	3	51.925
2	2	R	7	72.175
2	2	R	8	77.500
2	2	R	9	71.875
2	2	R	10	94.025
2	2	R	13	124.975
2	2	R	14	85.225
2	2	R	17	95.925
2	2	R	18	67.100
2	2	R	21	59.425
2	2	R	22	114.050

with 24 healthy volunteers (subjects). Volunteers were randomly assigned in balanced fashion to two sequences (TR or RT) of formulation administration, where the test formulation (T) is one 800 mg Cimetidine tablet and the reference formulation (R) is two 400 mg Cimetidine tablets. Blood samples were collected at 0 hour before dosing and at various times after dosing up through 24 hours post-dosing.

Bioavailability endpoints: Maximum Concentration (CMAX), Time-to-Maximum Concentration (TMAX) and area under the concentration-by-time curve (AUC) over the 0 to 24 hours interval, were computed from the drug concentration-by-time data. Bioavailability endpoints are summarized in Table 10.2.

The objective of this data analysis is to statistically assess whether the test formulation (one 800 mg tablet) and reference formulation (two 400 mg tablets) are bioequivalent in terms of the bioavailability endpoints using the R system.

10.2 Bioequivalence Clinical Trial Endpoints

In a bioequivalence trial comparing the bioavailability of oral formulations T (test) and R (reference) of a drug, blood samples are obtained at baseline (t_0) and at specified times $(t_1, t_2, \cdots, c_k)$ post-baseline (after ingesting each formulation). The blood (or plasma depending on assay) samples are then analyzed to determine the concentrations $(c_0, c_1, \cdots, c_k)$ of the drug in the samples. A concentration-by-time curve is a plot of the pairs $(t_0, c_0), (t_1, c_1), \cdots, (t_k, c_k)$.

The primary endpoints in the statistical assessment of bioequivalence are AUC, $CMAX$ and $TMAX$, and are directly calculated from the blood/plasma concentration-by-time curve. These endpoints are defined and calculated as follows:

1. AUC = the area under curve which is calculated by the trapezoid rule as:

$$AUC = \sum_{\tau=1}^{k} \frac{(c_\tau + c_{\tau-1}) \times (t_\tau - t_{\tau-1})}{2} \qquad (10.1)$$

This AUC is commonly denoted by AUC_{0-k}.

2. $CMAX$ = the maximum concentration from the curve defined as:

$$CMAX = max(c_0, c_1, \cdots, c_k) \qquad (10.2)$$

3. $TMAX$ = the time of sample collection at which maximum concentration is observed and is defined as:

$$Tmax = t_\tau \text{ at which } CMAX \text{ is observed} \qquad (10.3)$$

TABLE 10.2: AUC, CMAX, and TMAX Data from Cimetidine

Sequence	Period	Formulation	Subject	AUC	CMAX	TMAX
1	1	R	1	13.68	3.22	1.5
2	1	T	2	15.04	3.28	1.0
1	1	R	3	15.73	3.99	2.0
2	1	T	4	10.38	2.42	2.0
1	1	R	5	10.70	2.63	1.0
2	1	T	6	18.98	5.08	3.0
2	1	T	7	21.69	4.38	3.0
1	1	R	8	13.90	3.10	3.0
1	1	R	9	14.81	4.10	1.0
2	1	T	10	17.92	4.38	1.5
2	1	T	11	18.05	4.96	1.5
1	1	R	12	15.84	5.42	1.5
2	1	T	14	14.48	3.37	2.0
2	1	T	15	17.82	4.66	2.0
1	1	R	16	17.13	4.04	2.0
1	1	R	17	22.94	4.42	1.5
2	1	T	18	24.10	7.00	1.5
1	1	R	19	21.79	3.68	3.0
2	1	T	20	17.80	4.34	2.0
2	1	T	21	13.34	3.42	2.0
1	1	R	22	11.93	2.47	3.0
1	1	R	23	16.35	6.08	1.5
2	1	T	24	19.94	3.89	3.0
1	2	T	1	16.24	4.08	2.0
2	2	R	2	12.88	3.12	1.0
1	2	T	3	16.45	4.18	2.0
2	2	R	4	13.12	3.47	3.0
1	2	T	5	14.07	3.49	1.5
2	2	R	6	18.54	3.94	3.0
2	2	R	7	20.55	4.40	3.0
1	2	T	8	18.56	4.62	0.5
1	2	T	9	14.80	4.60	3.0
2	2	R	10	18.12	6.72	2.0
2	2	R	11	16.79	5.66	1.0
1	2	T	12	11.04	2.88	2.0
2	2	R	14	15.14	3.22	3.0
2	2	R	15	19.74	4.64	2.0
1	2	T	16	17.20	4.06	3.0
1	2	T	17	24.01	5.46	2.0
2	2	R	18	24.28	5.46	2.0
1	2	T	19	17.56	4.44	3.0
2	2	R	20	17.47	5.28	1.5
2	2	R	21	12.55	3.45	2.0
1	2	T	22	10.31	2.46	3.0
1	2	T	23	9.67	2.32	1.0
2	2	R	24	18.69	4.08	1.5

where t_τ is the τth time point of blood sample collection and c_τ is the τth blood or plasma concentrations and $\tau = 0, 1, 2, \cdots, k$ (the last sample collected). The time $t_0 = 0$ is the time at which the baseline sample is collected and $c_0 = 0$ is the concentration of the drug in the sample.

Note that the AUC computed from the observed concentration-by-time curve in Equation (10.1) is typically symbolized as AUC_{0-k} where k is the last time of sample collection.

Other bioavailability parameters of interest that can be estimated from the blood/plasma concentration-by-time curve are:

1. β_t = the terminal elimination rate. The terminal elimination rate β_t for each subject is estimated by the slope of a straight line fit to the log concentration-by-time data for the last "few" samples. Most calculations in the literature are performed to "eyeball" the curve and select the last few samples to fit a regression line which is highly variable and somewhat arbitrary.

   As discussed in Peace and Chen (2010), an approach to select the largest number of samples for which the fit of the straight line is best is obtained by using the measure of the coefficient of determination (R^2). Since a perfect fit is obtained from the last two samples, the last three samples are chosen initially and the value of R^2 (say R_3^2) noted. Then the last four samples are included and the value of R^2 noted (say R_4^2). If $R_4^2 \leq R_3^2$, then β_t is estimated from the last three samples. If $R_4^2 \geq R_3^2$, then the last five samples are included and the value of R^2 (say R_5^2) compared to R_4^2. If $R_5^2 \leq R_4^2$, then β_t is estimated from the last four samples, etc.

2. $t_{1/2}$ = the terminal half-life and is calculated as

$$t_{1/2} = -\frac{ln(2)}{\beta_t} \tag{10.4}$$

3. $AUC_{0-\infty}$ = the AUC extrapolated to infinity which is often called total exposure and is calculated as

$$AUC_{0-\infty} = AUC_{0-k} + \frac{c_k}{\beta_t} \tag{10.5}$$

10.3 Statistical Methods to Analyze Bioequivalence

In evaluating bioequivalence of two formulations, the commonly used statistical inference from usual hypothesis testing has long been criticized in pharmaceutical research to be inappropriate. It is now well known that confidence intervals (CI) provide a more appropriate inferential framework for assessing bioequivalence. We discuss the most commonly used CIs in assessing bioequivalence following the notations in Peace and Chen (2010). Readers are referred to Chow and Liu (2009) for more statistical methods.

10.3.1   Decision CIs for Bioequivalence

The Division of Biopharmaceutics at the FDA has specified a decision criterion for concluding bioequivalence of a test formulation (T) to a reference formulation (R): T is bioequivalent to R if the 90% confidence interval (CI) on the ratio of the mean of T to the mean of R is between 80% and 125% for bioequivalence endpoints $CMAX$, AUC_{0-t} and $AUC_{0-\infty}$.

The decision criterion for concluding bioequivalence is therefore:

$$90\%CI = (R_L, R_U) \in DecisionCI_{ratio} = (80\%; 125\%) \qquad (10.6)$$

where (R_L, R_U) is a 90% CI on the ratio $\frac{\mu_T}{\mu_R}$ of the mean (μ_T) of T to the mean of R (μ_R) for the evaluated endpoint (such as, $CMAX$, AUC_{0-t} and $AUC_{0-\infty}$). That is, the observed (used when referring to a quantity that is computed from the observed data) 90% CI of (R_L, R_U) for the ratio must be contained in the decision interval of $DecisionCI_{ratio} = (80\%; 125\%)$.

When evaluation is based on observed means and the mean difference, the above decision criterion based on ratio $\frac{\mu_T}{\mu_R}$ in interval $(80\%; 125\%)$ is converted to an interval on the mean difference of $\mu_T - \mu_R$. Then, the decision interval on the mean difference is

$$90\%CI = (M_L, M_U) \in DecisionCI_{mean} = (-0.2 \times \mu_R, 0.25 \times \mu_R) \quad (10.7)$$

where M_L and M_U denote the lower and upper CI limits for the mean difference.

There is a technical issue in this decision criterion since μ_R is the unknown population mean for the reference formulation. However, since the mean from reference of $\bar{Y}_R$ is a uniformly minimum variance unbiased (UMVU) estimator of μ_R, it may be used to replace the unknown μ_R. Therefore, an operational decision criterion for the mean difference can be obtained as:

$$
\begin{aligned}
90\%CI = (M_L, M_U) \in DecisionCI_{mean} &= (-0.2 \times \bar{Y}_R, 0.25 \times \bar{Y}_R) \\
&= (\theta_L, \theta_U) \qquad (10.8)
\end{aligned}
$$

Note for future reference that we introduced another notation (θ_L, θ_U) for this decision CI as $DecisionCI_{mean} = (\theta_L, \theta_U) = (-0.2 \times \bar{Y}_R, 0.25 \times \bar{Y}_R)$.

If the observed 90% CI (M_L, M_U) is completely contained in $DecisionCI_{mean}$ we conclude that the test formulation is bioequivalent to the reference formulation.

10.3.2   The Classical Asymmetric Confidence Interval

The classical (or shortest) asymmetric CI is based on the least squares means for the test and reference formulations using the t-statistic:

$$T = \frac{(\bar{Y}_T - \bar{Y}_R) - (\mu_T - \mu_R)}{\hat{\sigma}_d \sqrt{\frac{1}{n_1} + \frac{1}{n_2}}} \qquad (10.9)$$

which follows a t-distribution with $df = n_1 + n_2 - 2$ degrees of freedom where $\hat{\sigma}_d^2$ is the pooled (intrasubject) variance based upon within subject formulation differences from both sequences, and $\bar{Y}_T$ and $\bar{Y}_R$ are the means. Therefore, the classical $100(1 - 2\alpha)\%$ CI on the mean difference $\mu_T - \mu_R$ (hereafter referred to as CI_1) can be constructed as follows:

$$
\begin{aligned}
CI_1 &= (L_1, U_1) \\
&= \left((\bar{Y}_T - \bar{Y}_R) - t_{\alpha, df} \hat{\sigma}_d \sqrt{\frac{1}{n_1} + \frac{1}{n_2}}, (\bar{Y}_T - \bar{Y}_R) + t_{\alpha, df} \hat{\sigma}_d \sqrt{\frac{1}{n_1} + \frac{1}{n_2}} \right)
\end{aligned}
$$
$$(10.10)$$

where $t_{\alpha, df}$ is the α-percentile of t-distribution with degrees of freedom of df.

Since this CI is on the difference in means, bioequivalence of the test formulation to the reference formulation is concluded if the observed CI_1 is completely contained in $DecisionCI_{mean}$.

Alternatively, CI_1 on $\mu_T - \mu_R$ may be converted to an interval on the ratio of $\frac{\mu_T}{\mu_R}$ by adding the reference mean to both L_1 and U_1 and dividing the result by the reference mean $\bar{Y}_R$; i.e.,

$$CI_2 = \left(\frac{L_1}{\bar{Y}_R} + 1, \frac{U_1}{\bar{Y}_R} + 1 \right) \times 100\% \qquad (10.11)$$

If CI_2 is completely contained in the ratio decision interval $DecisionCI_{ratio}$, then formulation T is considered bioequivalent to the reference formulation R.

10.3.3   Westlake's Symmetric Confidence Interval

This classical CI_1 on $\mu_T - \mu_R$ is symmetric about $\bar{Y}_T - \bar{Y}_R$, but not 0, and its conversion to the interval CI_2 on the ratio $\frac{\mu_T}{\mu_R}$ is symmetric about $\frac{\bar{Y}_T}{\bar{Y}_R}$, but not about unity. Westlake (1976) suggested adjusting the CI_1 to be symmetric about 0 and the CI_2 to be symmetric about 1. This is accomplished by finding k_1 and k_2 such that

$$\int_{k_2}^{k_1} T \, dt = 1 - \alpha \text{ and } (k_1 + k_2) \times \sigma_d^2 \sqrt{\frac{1}{n_T} + \frac{1}{n_R}} = 2 \left(\bar{Y}_T - \bar{Y}_R \right) \qquad (10.12)$$

where $f(t)$ is the probability density function of T. A numerical algorithm is needed to solve these two equations for k_1 and k_2. The R system handles this type of calculation very well.

10.3.4   Two One-Sided Tests

Another method for assessing bioequivalence is the two one-sided test procedures originally proposed by Schuirmann (1987). The null (bioinequivalence) and alternative (bioequivalence) hypotheses are formulated against the $DecisionCI_{mean}$ in (10.8) as:

$$H_{01} : \mu_T - \mu_R \leq \theta_L \text{ v.s } H_{a1} : \mu_T - \mu_R > \theta_L$$

and

$$H_{02} : \mu_T - \mu_R \geq \theta_U \text{ v.s } H_{a2} : \mu_T - \mu_R \leq \theta_L$$

The method requires conducting two one-sided tests each at the pre-specified significance level $\alpha = 5\%$, and concluding bioequivalence of the test and reference formulations if and only if both null hypotheses H_{01} and H_{02} are rejected. Therefore, we reject the two null hypotheses and conclude bioequivalence of the test formulation T to reference formulation R if:

$$T_U = \frac{(\bar{Y}_T - \bar{Y}_R) - \theta_U}{\hat{\sigma}_d \sqrt{\frac{1}{n_1} + \frac{1}{n_2}}} > t(\alpha, n_T + n_R - 2)$$

$$T_L = \frac{(\bar{Y}_T - \bar{Y}_R) - \theta_L}{\hat{\sigma}_d \sqrt{\frac{1}{n_1} + \frac{1}{n_2}}} < -t(\alpha, n_1 + n_2 - 2) \qquad (10.13)$$

The decision regarding bioequivalence may also be based on the two one-sided P-values; i.e., reject H_{01} and H_{02} and conclude bioequivalence if $max(P_L, P_U) < 0.05$, where P_L and P_U are the one-sided P-values from testing H_{01} and H_{02}, respectively.

10.3.5   Bayesian Approaches

The above methods are so-called frequentist methods which fundamentally assume that the parameter of interest (such as the direct formulation effect) is unknown but fixed, and an inferential procedure (based on CI or two, one-sided tests) is derived based on the sampling distribution of the parameter estimate. Alternatively, a Bayesian inferential approach may be taken where the unknown direct formulation effect is a random variable with some distribution.

There are several Bayesian CI based methods for concluding bioequivalence. We illustrate the one proposed by Rodda and Davis (1980) for the bioequivalence trial datasets.

This method requires computing the probability that the difference of $\mu_T - \mu_R$ will be within the bioequivalence limits.

The fundamental conclusion is that the marginal posterior distribution of $\mu_T - \mu_R$ given the observed data is a non-central t-distribution with $df = n_1 + n_2 - 2$ degrees of freedom and non-centrality parameter $\bar{Y}_T - \bar{Y}_T$. Therefore, the posterior probability of $\mu_T - \mu_R$ being within the bioequivalence decision interval $DecisionCI_{mean}$ in (10.8) is computed as:

$$p_{RD} = P\left(\theta_L < \mu_T - \mu_R < \theta_U\right) = pt(t_U) - pt(t_L) \qquad (10.14)$$

where pt is the cumulative probability function for central t distribution with $df = n_1 + n_2 - 2$ degrees of freedom and

$$t_L = \frac{\theta_L - (\bar{Y}_T - \bar{Y}_R)}{\hat{\sigma}_d\sqrt{\frac{1}{n_1} + \frac{1}{n_2}}}$$

$$t_U = \frac{\theta_U - (\bar{Y}_T - \bar{Y}_R)}{\hat{\sigma}_d\sqrt{\frac{1}{n_1} + \frac{1}{n_2}}}$$

We then conclude that the test formulation T is bioequivalent to the reference formulation R if $p_{R.D.} = 90\%$. Essentially, this Bayesian method is equivalent to the classical CI_1 in Equation (10.9).

10.3.6 Individual-Based Bienayme-Tchebycheff (BT) Inequality CI

This is the method proposed by Peace (1986) to use within subject ratios rather than using within subject differences as the analysis unit in the assessment of bioequivalence. In addition to using the within subject ratios, he suggested constructing a two-sided 90% CI on the mean of the distribution of ratios using the Bienayme-Tchebycheff (BT) inequality as:

$$Pr\left(\bar{r} - K\sigma_{\bar{r}} \le \mu_r \le \bar{r} + K\sigma_{\bar{r}}\right) \ge 1 - \frac{1}{K^2} \qquad (10.15)$$

where r is the ratio of the endpoint of interest for the test formulation T to that of the reference formulation R for each subject. $\bar{r}$ and $\sigma_{\bar{r}}$ are the mean and standard deviation of sampling distribution of the ratios from $n = n_1 + n_2$ subjects. This inequality states that the probability that the mean of the sample ratios is within K standard error units of the true mean of the ratios is at least $1 - \frac{1}{K^2}$ regardless of the distribution of ratios. Setting the lower bound on the probability to be 90% yields $K = 3.1623$. Therefore, the 90% CI can be constructed as $(\bar{r} - K\sigma_{\bar{r}}, \bar{r} + K\sigma_{\bar{r}})$.

The advantage for this CI is that the BT based CI holds regardless of the true distribution of ratios. If the distribution of the ratios were known, K would be determined directly from that distribution to produce an interval that could be compared with the $DecisionCI_{ratio}$. It should be noted that the BT inequality brackets the true mean in a symmetric manner (-K to +K). The regulatory decision interval for concluding bioequivalence is asymmetric (80% to 125%), rather than symmetric (80% to 120%). The lower bound of the probability on the BT inequality, 1 - (1/K2), would actually be larger when accounting for the content of the sampling distribution of ratios between 120% and 125%.

Alternatively, resampling methods may be applied to the sample of ratios to determine a 90% confidence interval on the true mean of the ratios.

10.3.7   Individual-Based Bootstrap CIs

Following the discussion in Section 10.3.6, we propose a bootstrapping approach (hereafter referred to as $Bootstrap_1$) by resampling the n individual subject ratios r_i, $i = 1, 2, \cdots, n$ with replacement for a large number of times (say, N=1,000) to construct a resampling distribution for the mean of the individual ratios. The 90% CI based on the individual ratios is the interval ranging from the 5th to the 95th percentile of this resampling distribution, and may be compared to the $DecisionCI_{ratio}$ to conclude whether bioequivalence is achieved.

Extending this idea, we can alternatively perform bootstrapping by resampling the endpoint measures of interest (such as the AUC, CMAX) and determine the bootstrap resampling distribution (hereafter referred to as $Bootstrap_2$) of the ratio of means of $\frac{Y_T}{Y_R}$. Similarly the 90% CI based on the ratio of means of formulation T to formulation R is the interval ranging from the 5th to the 95th percentile of this resampling distribution, and may be compared to the $DecisionCI_{ratio}$ to conclude whether bioequivalence is achieved.

It should be noted that the $Bootstrap_2$ can act as a checkmark for those CI methods in previous sections to see whether the distribution assumption is reasonable.

10.4   Step-by-Step Implementation in R

10.4.1   Analyze the data from Chow and Liu (2009)

10.4.1.1   Load the data into R

The data can be loaded into the R system by `read.csv` as follows:

```
> dat = read.csv("ChowLiuTab361.csv", header=T)
```

Descriptive summary information for this data can be produced using the R command `aggregate` to check the sample size, the mean and variance table as:

```
> # use ``aggregate" to the sample size
> tab.n    = aggregate(dat$AUC,list(seq=dat$Sequence,
```

```
                             prd=dat$Period),length)
> n1         = tab.n[tab.n$seq==1 & tab.n$prd==1,]$x
> n2         = tab.n[tab.n$seq==2 & tab.n$prd==1,]$x
> n          = n1+n2
> # use ``aggregate" to get the mean
> tab.mean = aggregate(dat$AUC,list(seq=dat$Sequence,
                             prd=dat$Period),mean)
> # use ``aggregate" to get the variance
> tab.var  = aggregate(dat$AUC,list(seq=dat$Sequence,
                             prd=dat$Period),var)
> # make a dataframe for the summary data
> summaryTab = data.frame(Sequence=tab.mean$seq,
 Period=tab.mean$prd, numSample = tab.n$x,
 Mean = tab.mean$x, Var=tab.var$x)
> # print the summary table
> round(summaryTab,2)

  Sequence Period numSample Mean Var
1        1      1        12 85.8 246
2        2      1        12 78.7 539
3        1      2        12 81.8 389
4        2      2        12 79.3 635
```

In R, there is another set of functions called `apply` for making this type of calculation easy and efficient. To list a few, include:

- `tapply` = Apply a Function Over a "Ragged" Array

- `lapply` = Apply a Function over a List or Vector

- `sapply` = A user-friendly version of `lapply` by default returning a vector or matrix if appropriate

- `mapply` = Apply a function to multiple list or vector arguments and `mapply` is a multivariate version of `sapply`

- `rapply` = Recursively Apply a Function to a List and `rapply` is a recursive version of `lapply`.

For example, we can use `tapply` to produce the mean table using the following R code chunk:

```
> tapply(dat$AUC, dat[,c("Sequence","Period")], mean)

          Period
Sequence    1    2
       1 85.8 81.8
       2 78.7 79.3
```

From the summary table, we note that there are 12 subjects in each sequence. The sequence-by-period means and variances are reproduced exactly (see bottom of page 70 in Chow and Liu (2009)). The data derive from the two-sequence, two-period, two-formulation crossover design which is the most commonly used design in clinical trials designed to assess whether a new formulation (T) is bioequivalent to a reference formulation (R).

Before making an inference as to the bioequivalence of two formulations in terms of direct effect of the drug (in the formulations), there are other effects associated with this crossover design that may need to be tested; e.g., differential carryover and period effects. The most important of these is the differential carryover or residual drug effect. The presence of differential carryover effect may impact the inference as to bioequivalence and attendant statistical methods. We now illustrate the implementation in R for these tests.

10.4.1.2   Tests for Carryover Effect

We will illustrate the step-by-step implementation of the tests from Chapter 3 in Chow and Liu (2009) in the R system. Readers may refer to the referenced text for statistical details.

Following Section 3.2 of the referenced text, we first calculate the subject totals (addition across periods for each subject) for each sequence as

$$U_{ik} = Y_{i1k} + Y_{i2k} \qquad i = 1, 2, \cdots, n_k; \quad k = 1, 2 \qquad (10.16)$$

This can be done in R as:

```
> Uik             = aggregate(dat$AUC,
                   list(seq = dat$Sequence,sub=dat$Subject), sum)
> colnames(Uik) = c("seq", "sub","Uik")
```

In order to statistically test for differential carryover effect C, we first calculate the sample mean of the subject totals for each sequence as

$$\bar{U}_{.k} = \frac{1}{n_k} \sum_{i=1}^{n_k} U_{ik}, k = 1, 2 \qquad (10.17)$$

which is done in R as:

```
> mUk  = aggregate(Uik$Uik, list(seq=Uik$seq), mean)
> colnames(mUk) = c("seq", "mUk")
> print(mUk)

  seq mUk
1   1 168
2   2 158
```

Then the differential carryover effect C is estimated by the difference in sequence means as

$$\hat{C} = \bar{U}_{.2} - \bar{U}_{.1} \qquad (10.18)$$

which can be done in R code as:

```
> hatC = mUk[2,2]-mUk[1,2]
> hatC
```

`[1] -9.59`

Under the assumption of normality (the analyst should check this as functions of concentrations are often not normally distributed but their log transforms are) of the subject totals, $\hat{C}$ is normally distributed with mean C (see chapter 10, section 10.7.2.4.2.1, Tables 10.3 and 10.4 of Peace and Chen) and variance $Var(\hat{C})$ is estimated by

$$\widehat{Var}(\hat{C}) = \hat{\sigma}_u^2 \left(\frac{1}{n_1} + \frac{1}{n_2} \right) \tag{10.19}$$

where

$$\hat{\sigma}_u^2 = \frac{1}{n_1 + n_2 - 2} \sum_{k=1}^{2} \sum_{i=1}^{n_k} (U_{ik} - \bar{U}_{.k})^2 \tag{10.20}$$

which is implemented in R by merging the two dataframes Uik and mUk for calculation as follows:

```
> dU    = merge(Uik, mUk)
> sigu2 = sum((dU$Uik-dU$mUk)^2)/(n1+n2-2)
> sigu2
```

`[1] 1474`

Under the null hypothesis of no carryover effect, the statistical t-test statistic is:

$$T_C = \frac{\hat{C}}{\sqrt{\hat{\sigma}_u^2 \left(\frac{1}{n_1} + \frac{1}{n_2} \right)}} \tag{10.21}$$

which is calculated in R as:

```
> se.sigu = sqrt(sigu2*(1/n1+1/n2))
> TC      = hatC/se.sigu
> TC
```

`[1] -0.612`

Since $|T_C| = 0.612 < t(\alpha/2, n_1 + n2 - 2) = 2.074$, the null hypothesis of no differential carryover effect is not rejected.

The p-value associated with the test for no differential carryover effects is calculated by:

```
> pC = 2*(1-pt(abs(TC), n1+n2-2))
> pC
```

`[1] 0.547`

10.4.1.3   Test for Direct Formulation Effect

The calculation for testing the direct differential formulation effect begins by forming the difference in periods for each subject within each sequence as follows:

$$d_{ik} = \frac{1}{2}\left(Y_{i2k} - Y_{i1k}\right), i = 1, 2, \cdots, n_k;\ k = 1, 2 \qquad (10.22)$$

which is implemented in R as:

```
> dik           = aggregate(dat$AUC,
                  list(sub=dat$Subject,seq=dat$Sequence),diff)
> dik$x         = dik$x/2
> colnames(dik)= c("sub", "seq","dik")
> dik
```

	sub	seq	dik
1	1	1	-0.5000
2	4	1	-1.5750
3	5	1	0.0875
4	6	1	-4.8000
5	11	1	-5.0125
6	12	1	-8.6250
7	15	1	-5.1500
8	16	1	-5.0750
9	19	1	1.1000
10	20	1	8.3625
11	23	1	-12.6250
12	24	1	9.7000
13	2	2	-18.7375
14	3	2	-17.4750
15	7	2	-4.7500
16	8	2	-7.6000
17	9	2	10.7125
18	10	2	13.9500
19	13	2	1.2625
20	14	2	-6.9250
21	17	2	4.7875
22	18	2	8.5875
23	21	2	8.3625
24	22	2	11.1625

Then the direct differential formulation effect can be estimated as:

$$\hat{F} = \bar{d}_{.1} - \bar{d}_{.2} \qquad (10.23)$$

where $\bar{d}_{.k} = \frac{1}{n_k}\sum_{i=1}^{n_k} d_{ik}$ are the sample means for the period differences for each sequence. R can be implemented as follows:

```
> mdk            = aggregate(dik$dik, list(seq=dik$seq), mean)
> colnames(mdk)  = c("seq", "mdk")
> hatF           = mdk[1,2]-mdk[2,2]
> hatF
```

[1] -2.29

Under the assumption of no differential carryover effect, $\hat{F}$ is normally distributed with mean F and variance

$$Var(\hat{F}) = \sigma_d^2 \left(\frac{1}{n_1} + \frac{1}{n_2} \right) \tag{10.24}$$

which may be estimated by $\widehat{Var}(\hat{F}) = \hat{\sigma}_d^2 \left(\frac{1}{n_1} + \frac{1}{n_2} \right)$ and

$$\hat{\sigma}_d^2 = \frac{1}{n_1 + n_2 - 2} \sum_{k=1}^{2} \sum_{i=1}^{n_k} (d_{ik} - \bar{d}_{.k})^2 \tag{10.25}$$

which is implemented in R by merging the two dataframes `dik` and `mdk` for calculation as follows:

```
> dF     = merge(dik, mdk)
> sigd2  = sum((dF$dik-dF$mdk)^2)/(n1+n2-2)
> sigd2
```

[1] 83.6

Therefore, the t-statistic for testing no direct differential formulation effect can be constructed as:

$$T_F = \frac{\hat{F}}{\sqrt{\hat{\sigma}_d^2 \left(\frac{1}{n_1} + \frac{1}{n_2} \right)}} \tag{10.26}$$

which is calculated in R as:

```
> se.sigd = sqrt(sigd2*(1/n1+1/n2))
> TF      = hatF/se.sigd
> TF
```

[1] -0.613

Since $|T_F|=0.613 < t(\alpha/2, n_1 + n2 - 2) = 2.074$, we fail to reject the null hypothesis of no direct differential formulation effect suggesting that the two formulations are statistically bioequivalent. Similarly, we can make this conclusion using the observed p-value as calculated by:

```
> pF = 2*(1-pt(abs(TF), n1+n2-2))
> pF
```

`[1] 0.546`

We emphasize that the above test for equality of direct formulation effects is provided to show agreement between results of the test using R and those in Chow and Liu (2009). Usually, this test has little utility in the analysis of bioequivalence studies, rather bioequivalence is assessed using CIs or the two, one-sided tests procedure.

The test for equality of period effects can be implemented in exactly the same way and we leave the implementation on this test for the reader.

10.4.1.4   Analysis of Variance

The above t-tests also follow from an analysis of variance (ANOVA) of bioavailability endpoints. The principle underlying ANOVA is to analyze the variability of the observed endpoint by partitioning the total sum of squares (SS) into components reflecting fixed and random effects, followed by the statistical F-tests.

The detail mathematical derivations for ANOVA in bioequivalence appear in Chow and Liu (2009). We merely illustrate how easy it is to implement the ANOVA using the R system; i.e., with one line of R code as follows:

```
> # cat("We first re-format the data into R dataframe","\n")
> Data = data.frame(subj = as.factor(dat$Subject),
                    formu = as.factor(dat$Formulation),
                    seq  = as.factor(dat$Sequence),
                    prd  = as.factor(dat$Period),
                    AUC  = dat$AUC)
> # cat("Then call R function aov for ANOVA Table", "\n")
> summary(aov(AUC ~ seq*formu + Error(subj), data = Data))
```

```
Error: subj
           Df Sum Sq Mean Sq F value Pr(>F)
seq         1    276     276    0.37   0.55
Residuals 22  16211     737
```

```
Error: Within
           Df Sum Sq Mean Sq F value Pr(>F)
formu       1     63    62.8    0.38   0.55
seq:formu   1     36    36.0    0.22   0.65
Residuals 22   3679   167.2
```

It is observed that the p-values from the F-tests for differential carryover and direct formulation effects are identical to those from the t-tests in the previous sections.

In summary, we conclude that there are no statistically significant differential carryover, period, or direct formulation effects in this bioequivalence clinical trial.

We can now proceed to illustrate computation of the confidence interval methods discussed in Section 10.3.

10.4.1.5 Decision CIs

The 90% decision CI for the ratio of means is $DecisionCI_{ratio} = (80\%, 125\%)$ as indicated in Equation (10.6). The decision CI for the difference in means as defined in Equation (10.8) has to be calculated using the mean of the reference formulation. Since we will need the means for both formulations, we calculate both and denote them by $\bar{Y}_T$ and $\bar{Y}_R$. We denote the limits for this decision CI as θ_L and θ_U for future reference.

The implementation in the R system appears in the following R code chunk:

```
> # get the mean for AUC by Formulation
> mformu    = tapply(dat$AUC, list(formu=dat$Formulation), mean)
> # extract the means
> ybarT    = mformu["T"]
> ybarR    = mformu["R"]
> # make the decision CI
> dec2.low = theta.L = -0.2*ybarR
> dec2.up  = theta.U = 0.25*ybarR
> cat("DecisionCI.mean=(",dec2.low,",",dec2.up,")",sep="","\n")
```

```
DecisionCI.mean=(-16.5,20.6)
```

Therefore, the decision CI for mean difference is $DecisionCI_{mean} = (\theta_L, \theta_U) = (-16.512, 20.64)$.

It is noted that we are using the asymmetric interval of $(80\%, 125\%)$ in this book corresponding to Peace and Chen (2010) which is slightly different from Chow and Liu (2009), where they use the symmetric interval of $(80\%, 120\%)$. Parenthetically, the symmetric decision interval was originally proposed by FDA and later changed to the asymmetric one. This was due primarily to the fact that measures of bioavailability AUC and CMAX are most often lognormally distributed rather than normally distributed. It is noted that the log transform on the asymmetric interval is a symmetric interval $[\log(4/5); \log(5/4)]$. Therefore, calculations in this book associated with θ_U will differ from those in Chow and Liu (2009).

10.4.1.6 Classical Shortest 90% CI

The CI for the mean difference in Equation (10.10) is implemented using the following R code chunk:

```
> # the confidence coefficient: alpha
> alphaCI  = .1
> # the t-value
> qt.alpha = qt(1-alphaCI, n1+n2-2)
> qt.alpha
```

[1] 1.32

```
> # the lower and upper limits for CI1
> low1 = (ybarT-ybarR)-qt.alpha*sqrt(sigd2)*sqrt(1/n1+1/n2)
> up1  = (ybarT-ybarR)+qt.alpha*sqrt(sigd2)*sqrt(1/n1+1/n2)
> cat("The classical CI1=(", round(low1,3),",",
 round(up1,3),")", sep=" ","\n\n")
```

The classical CI1=(-7.22 , 2.64)

```
> # the lower and upper limits for CI2
> low2 = (low1/ybarR+1)*100
> up2  = (up1/ybarR+1)*100
> cat("The Ratio CI2=(", round(low2,3),",",
 round(up2,3),")", sep=" ","\n\n")
```

The Ratio CI2=(91.3 , 103)

Then, the CI for the difference in means $CI_1 = (-7.22, 2.645)$ and the CI for ratio of means $CI_2 = (91.255, 103.204)$. It is observed that they are identical to those in Chow and Liu (2009).

10.4.1.7   The Westlake CI

From the second part of Westlake Equation (10.12), we first calculate $k12 = k_1 + k_2$ as

```
> k12 = 2*(ybarR-ybarT)/sqrt( sigd2*(1/n1+1/n2))
```

We substitute $k_1 = k12 - k_2$ into the first part and numerically solve for k_2 using R command uniroot as follows:

```
> k2 = uniroot(function(k2) pt(k12-k2,n1+n2-2)- pt(k2,n1+n2-2)
 -(1-alphaCI),lower = -10, upper = 10, tol = 0.0001)$root
> k1 =k12-k2
> cat("The Westlake k1=",k1," and k2=",k2,sep=" ", "\n\n")
```

The Westlake k1= 2.6   and k2= -1.37

Then the lower and upper limits are calculated as:

```
> low.west = k2*sqrt(sigd2*(1/n1+1/n2))-(ybarR-ybarT)
> up.west  = k1*sqrt(sigd2*(1/n1+1/n2))-(ybarR-ybarT)
```

The Westlake CI for mu_T-mu_A is (-7.41 , 7.41)

Again, this reproduces the results in Chow and Liu (2009).

10.4.1.8   Two One-Sided Tests

The T_L and T_U in Equations (10.13) are implemented as:

```
> TL = (ybarT-ybarR-theta.L)/sqrt(sigd2*(1/n1+1/n2))
> TU = (ybarT-ybarR-theta.U)/sqrt(sigd2*(1/n1+1/n2))
```

Since $T_L = 3.81 > t(\alpha, n_1 + n_2 - 2) = 1.321$ and $T_U = -6.141 < -t(\alpha, n_1 + n_2 - 2) = -1.321$, we conclude bioequivalence.

Alternatively, the two, one-sided p-values are

```
> pL = 1-pt(abs(TL), n1+n2-2); pU = pt(TU,n1+n2-2)
> p1side = max(pL, pU)
```

The p-values are $p_L = 0.000479$ and $p_U = $ 2e-06. The maximum of these two, one-sided p-values is $max(p_L, p_U) = 0.00048$ which is less than 0.05. Again we conclude bioequivalence.

10.4.1.9   Bayesian Approach

Computation of the posterior probability in Equation (10.14) can be implemented in the R system as:

```
> tL  = (theta.L -(ybarT-ybarR))/sqrt(sigd2*(1/n1+1/n2))
> tU  = (theta.U -(ybarT-ybarR))/sqrt(sigd2*(1/n1+1/n2))
> pRD = pt(tU, n1+n2-2) - pt(tL, n1+n2-2);
> pRD

R
1
```

Since the posterior probability $p_{RD} = 0.9995 > 90\%$, we again conclude bioequivalence.

10.4.1.10   Individual-Based BT CI

The step-by-step implementation of the individual-based Bienayme-Tchebycheff Inequality CI in Section 10.3.6 is as follows:

1. Create the individual ratios:

```
> dR   = dat[dat$Formulation=="R",c("Subject","AUC")]
> dT   = dat[dat$Formulation=="T",c("Subject","AUC")]
> colnames(dR) = c("Subject","AUC4R")
> colnames(dT) = c("Subject","AUC4T")
> dRT  = merge(dR,dT)
> rT2R = dRT$AUC4T/dRT$AUC4R; rT2R

 [1]  0.987 2.003 1.673 0.967 1.002 0.879 1.132 1.196
 [9]  0.702 0.703 0.873 0.799 0.980 1.163 0.852 0.882
[17]  0.900 0.744 1.020 1.168 0.719 0.804 0.718 1.352
```

2. Get the mean and standard error:

```
> k       = 1/sqrt(1-.9);       rbar = mean(rT2R)
> sigrbar = sqrt(var(rT2R)/n); rbar

[1] 1.01

> sigrbar

[1] 0.0638
```

3. Calculate the lower and upper limits for BT CI:

```
> low.BT = rbar-k*sigrbar; up.BT  = rbar+k*sigrbar

The Tchebycheff CI for mu_T/mu_A is (0.807,1.21)
```

Then the CI from the individual-based Bienayme-Tchebycheff Inequality is (0.807, 1.211) which lies in the $DecisionCI_{ratio}$ =(80%, 125%). Again we conclude bioequivalence.

10.4.1.11 Bootstrap CIs

As outlined in Section 10.3.7, there are two bootstrap approaches. One is to bootstrap the individual ratios and calculate the mean. The other is to bootstrap the individual bioavailability endpoints and calculate the ratio of the means.

We create 2000 bootstrap samples, which is easily implemented using the R system as follows:

```
> # B=number of bootstrap
> B       = 2000
> # boota and bootb to keep track the bootstrap results
> boota = bootb = NULL
> for(b in 1:B){
 # Bootstrap the observed individual ratios
 boota[b] = mean(sample(rT2R, replace=T))
 # bootstrap the individuals and calculate the means
 tmp       = dRT[sample(1:n, replace=T),]
 bootb[b] = mean(tmp$AUC4T)/mean(tmp$AUC4R)
 }

> qxa = quantile(boota, c(0.05, 0.95)); qxa

   5%    95%
0.913 1.120

> qxb = quantile(bootb, c(0.05, 0.95)); qxb
```

```
  5%    95%
0.904  1.048
```

Again, we conclude bioequivalence from both approaches since both bootstrap 90% CIs are completely within the $DecisionCI_{ratio}$.

The bootstrap sampling distributions from the mean of the individual ratios and the ratio of the means can be generated using the following R code to produce Figures 10.1 and 10.2, respectively. In both figures, the two solid vertical segments indicate the limits for the 90% CI and the middle dashed vertical line indicates the means.

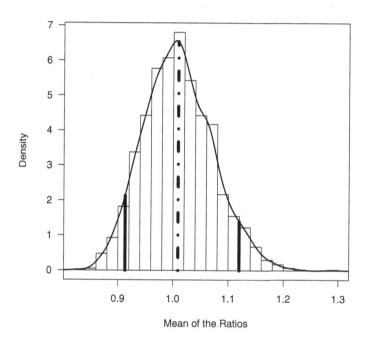

FIGURE 10.1: Bootstrap Distribution for the Mean of the Individual Ratios

```
> # R code for Figurwe 10.1
> hist(boota,nclass=30, freq=F,las=1,
 xlab="Mean of the Ratios", ylab="Density", main="")
> box()
> den = density(boota)
> lines(den, lwd=2)
> qya = approx(den$x, den$y, c(qxa,rbar))$y
> segments(qxa[1],0,qxa[1],qya[1], lwd=5)
```

```
> segments(qxa[2],0,qxa[2],qya[2], lwd=5)
> segments(rbar,0,rbar,qya[3],lty=4, lwd=5)

> # R code for Figure 10.2:
> hist(bootb,nclass=30, freq=F,las=1,
 xlab="Ratio of the Means", ylab="Density", main="")
> box()
> den = density(bootb)
> lines(den, lwd=2)
> rmean = mean(dRT$AUC4T)/mean(dRT$AUC4R)
> qyb = approx(den$x, den$y, c(qxb,rmean))$y
> segments(qxb[1],0,qxb[1],qyb[1], lwd=5)
> segments(qxb[2],0,qxb[2],qyb[2], lwd=5)
> segments(rmean,0,rmean,qyb[3],lty=4, lwd=5)
```

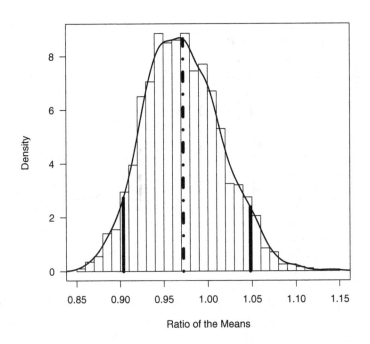

FIGURE 10.2: Bootstrap Distribution for the Ratio of the Means

We can use the bootstrap samples to test whether the distribution is normally distributed using the so-called *qqnorm* plot as seen in Figure 10.3. From this QQ-plot, we conclude that the distribution is heavy-tailed and we can test whether it is a normal distribution using the Shapiro test as

```
> shapiro.test(bootb)

        Shapiro-Wilk normality test

data:   bootb
W = 1, p-value = 4e-06
```

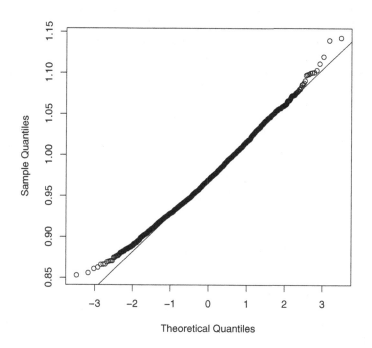

FIGURE 10.3: QQ-Plot for the Ratio of the Means

10.4.2 Analyze the data from Cimetidine Trial

10.4.2.1 Clinical Trial Endpoints Calculations

To illustrate the calculation of bioavailability endpoints, we take the concentration-by-time data from the first sequence and second period (i.e., formulation T = one 800 mg Cimetidine tablet).

The data is loaded into R using the following R code chunk as follows:

```
> datRaw0    = read.csv("CimetidineRaw.csv", header=T)
> print(datRaw0)
```

	Subject	HR0	HR05	HR10	HR15	HR20	HR30	HR40	HR60
1	1	0.00	2.81	2.39	2.96	4.08	2.72	1.88	0.94
2	3	0.00	0.25	2.25	2.64	4.18	3.97	2.25	0.94
3	5	0.00	1.80	3.16	3.49	2.85	2.71	1.52	0.75
4	8	0.10	4.62	4.06	3.31	3.88	3.19	1.73	0.94
5	9	0.11	1.72	1.67	2.45	2.63	4.60	2.00	0.69
6	12	0.00	1.48	1.82	1.84	2.88	2.12	1.22	0.58
7	16	0.00	1.02	1.68	2.95	3.30	4.06	2.17	1.11
8	17	0.00	2.48	4.02	3.98	5.46	4.80	3.20	1.39
9	19	0.00	1.12	1.65	1.57	1.71	4.44	3.06	1.33
10	22	0.00	0.21	1.91	1.11	1.64	2.46	1.55	0.75
11	23	0.00	0.81	2.32	2.19	2.16	1.24	0.94	0.51

	HR80	HR100	HR120	HR180	HR240
1	0.56	0.28	0.00	0	0
2	0.41	0.15	0.10	0	0
3	0.39	0.22	0.00	0	0
4	0.53	0.23	0.11	0	0
5	0.26	0.19	0.00	0	0
6	0.40	0.20	0.00	0	0
7	0.57	0.33	0.14	0	0
8	0.58	0.27	0.15	0	0
9	0.59	0.28	0.17	0	0
10	0.41	0.18	0.00	0	0
11	0.35	0.23	0.14	0	0

The original concentration-by-time data datRaw0 is in the "wide" format and we take advantage of R reshape to reshape this data into column format using the following R code chunk and we use head to show the first few observations:

```
> datRaw            = reshape(datRaw0, direction="long",
                        varying=-1,idvar = "Subject",sep="")
> datRaw$time       = datRaw$time/10
> colnames(datRaw)  = c("subj","time","conc")
> head(datRaw)
```

	subj	time	conc
1.0	1	0	0.00
3.0	3	0	0.00
5.0	5	0	0.00
8.0	8	0	0.10
9.0	9	0	0.11
12.0	12	0	0.00

Therefore, the subject-wise concentration-by-time curves can be graphically displayed in Figure 10.4 as follows:

```
> # load the library
> library(lattice)
> # call "xyplot"
> print(xyplot(conc~time,group=subj,datRaw,xlab="Time(HR)",
  xlim=c(0,13),auto.key = list(corner=c(1,1),lines = TRUE) ,
  ylab="Concentration(mCG/ML)",type=c("p","a")))
```

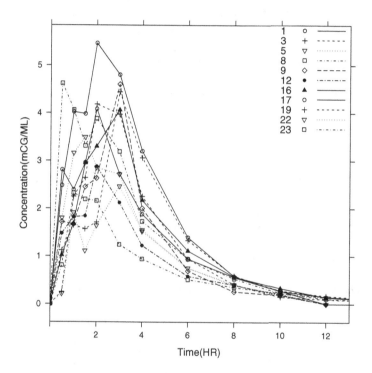

FIGURE 10.4: The Concentration-by-Time for First Sequence and Second Period.

As usual, the mean concentration-by-time curve can be obtained by calculating the mean concentration at each time of sample collection using **aggregate** and plot it in Figure 10.5 as follows:

```
> # make the mean concentration
> dat.mean= aggregate(datRaw$conc, list(time=datRaw$time), mean)
> # plot it with a line
> plot(conc~time,las=1,type="n",datRaw,xlab="Time",xlim=c(0,13),
```

```
  ylim=c(0, 4), ylab="Mean Concentration")
> lines(x~time,dat.mean, lty=1, lwd=3)
```

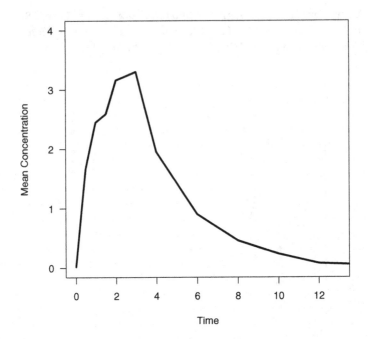

FIGURE 10.5: The Mean Concentration-by-Time for First Sequence and Second Period

From both Figures 10.4 and 10.5, we observe that the variability between or among subjects is large. We now calculate the endpoints.

As outlined in Section 10.2, we develop some functions to be called to calculate the endpoints for each subject. The first function call is to calculate the elimination rate β in Section 10.2 using the iterative approach:

```
> # function `make.beta' with argument `dt'
> make.beta = function(dt){
 # terminal elimination beta to find the slope for R2(k+1) <R2(k)
 n = length(dt$conc) # get the length of data

 # end the loop at tmax
 tmax = which.max(dt$conc)

 # loop over starting from the last time-conc point to tmax
```

```
for(k in n:tmax){
dt1 = dt[((k-2):n),] # start with last 3 pts and move on
dt2 = dt[((k-3):n),] # start with last 4 pts and move on
# some date have 0s at the end of t-c curve and make the lm crash
# so make this dataframe at least 3 data points
if( dim(dt1[dt1$conc>0,])[1]>= 3 ){
# fit log(conc) to time and track the r-square
m1     = lm(log(conc)~time, dt1[(dt1$conc>0),])
m2     = lm(log(conc)~time, dt2[(dt2$conc>0),])
betat = m1$coef[[2]]
#cat("Check=",summary(m1)$r.squared > summary(m2)$r.squared,"
#and Stopped at", k, "with beta=",betat,sep=" ","\n\n")
if(summary(m1)$r.squared > summary(m2)$r.squared) break
        } # end of if-loop
} # end of k-for-loop
#cat("final beta=",betat,"\n\n")
# return
betat
} # end of make-beta function
```

With this function, we can then develop a R function `make` to compute all the endpoints as defined in Section 10.2 as follows:

```
> make    = function(dt){
time    = dt$time; conc = dt$conc
#   calculate AUC
t.dif   = diff(time) # the t(i)-t(i-1)
c.mean = (conc[-1]+conc[-length(conc)])/2
auc     = sum(t.dif*c.mean)
# Cmax
cmax    = max(conc)
# tmax
tmax    = dt[which.max(dt$conc),]$time
# terminal elimination beta to find the slope for R2(k+1) <R2(k)
betat   = make.beta(dt)
# terminal halflife
t5      = round(-log(2)/betat*2.303,1)
# AUC infinite
aucinf = auc+ conc[length(conc)]/betat
# return the results.
c(auc,cmax,tmax, betat, t5, aucinf)
}
```

Then, we can call the `make`-function along with the concentration-by-time data to perform the calculations with output `endpts` as follows:

```
> name.subj    = sort(unique(datRaw$subj))
```

```
> num.subj    = length(name.subj)
> endpts      = matrix(0, nrow=num.subj, ncol=7)
> colnames(endpts) = c("subj","AUC","CMAX","TMAX",
          "betat","t5","AUCinf")
> for(id in 1:num.subj){
  tmp          = datRaw[(datRaw$subj == name.subj[id]),
                  c("time","conc")]
  endpts[id,] = c(name.subj[id],make(tmp))
  }
> endpts
```

```
       subj   AUC CMAX TMAX  betat   t5 AUCinf
 [1,]     1 16.24 4.08  2.0 -0.319  5.0  16.24
 [2,]     3 16.45 4.18  2.0 -0.419  3.8  16.45
 [3,]     5 14.07 3.49  1.5 -0.307  5.2  14.07
 [4,]     8 18.55 4.62  0.5 -0.393  4.1  18.55
 [5,]     9 14.80 4.60  3.0 -0.459  3.5  14.80
 [6,]    12 11.04 2.88  2.0 -0.290  5.5  11.04
 [7,]    16 17.20 4.06  3.0 -0.335  4.8  17.20
 [8,]    17 24.02 5.46  2.0 -0.338  4.7  24.02
 [9,]    19 17.56 4.44  3.0 -0.373  4.3  17.56
[10,]    22 10.31 2.46  3.0 -0.363  4.4  10.31
[11,]    23  9.67 2.32  1.0 -0.229  7.0   9.67
```

It is observed that this calculation re-produces the values in Table 10.2.

10.4.2.2   ANOVA: Tests for Carryover and Other Effects

For this data, we only illustrate the analysis of variance (ANOVA) approach with the F-test since it is equivalent to the t-test for two periods/formulations.

Again the clinical trial data is loaded into R system as follows:

```
> dat = read.csv("Cimetidine.csv",  header=T)
```

Then we re-format the data into a R dataframe and call the R functions lm and aov for a series of ANOVA as in the following R code chunk:

```
> Data = data.frame(subj  = as.factor(dat$Subject),
                    formu = as.factor(dat$Formulation),
                    seq   = as.factor(dat$Sequence),
                    prd   = as.factor(dat$Period),
                    AUC   = dat$AUC, lAUC= log(dat$AUC),
                          CMAX = dat$CMAX, lCMAX= log(dat$CMAX))
```

The number of subjects in the trial can be tracked as

```
> nsubj = tapply(dat$Subject, list(dat$Sequence), length)/2
> n1    = nsubj[1]
> n2    = nsubj[2]
> n     = n1+n2
```

We have total number of subjects in the trial as 23 with 11 in Sequence 1 and 12 in Sequence 2.

Specifically, we call `lm` for fixed effect ANOVA model to test "formulation" and "period" effects. However, this ANOVA model is not appropriate to test "carryover" effect as outlined in Section 3.5, Chow and Liu (2009) and Chapter 10 in Peace and Chen (2010). We need to call `aov` to test for "carryover" effect which is implemented as in the following R code chunk:

1. The ANOVAs for AUC:

```
> # the fixed model using lm for "formulation" and "period"
> mdAUC = lm(AUC ~ seq + subj:seq + prd + formu,data = Data)
> print(anova(mdAUC))

Analysis of Variance Table

Response: AUC
           Df Sum Sq Mean Sq F value  Pr(>F)
seq         1     34    34.1    9.62  0.0054 **
prd         1      1     0.9    0.26  0.6127
formu       1      0     0.3    0.08  0.7861
seq:subj   21    525    25.0    7.06 1.8e-05 ***
Residuals  21     74     3.5

> # the random effect model using aov for carryover
> # and other effects
> mdAUC.R = aov(AUC ~ prd * formu + Error(subj),
      data = Data)
> print(summary(mdAUC.R))

Error: subj
           Df Sum Sq Mean Sq F value Pr(>F)
prd:formu   1     34    34.1    1.36   0.26
Residuals  21    525    25.0

Error: Within
           Df Sum Sq Mean Sq F value Pr(>F)
prd         1    0.9    0.94    0.26   0.61
formu       1    0.3    0.27    0.08   0.79
Residuals  21   74.4    3.54
```

As seen from these ANOVA tables, the *p*-value for "carryover" effect is 0.256 indicating no statistically significantly "carryover" effect. In addition, the *p*-values for "period" and "formu (actually formulation)" are 0.786 and 0.613, respectively, from both the fixed linear model and random effect model.

The same analysis can be performed on log(AUC), CMAX and log(CMAX), etc. as follows:

2. The ANOVAs for log AUC:

```
> # the fixed effects model using lm for "formulation"
> # and "period"
> mdlAUC  = lm(lAUC ~ seq + subj:seq + prd + formu,data = Data)
> print(anova(mdlAUC))

Analysis of Variance Table

Response: lAUC
          Df Sum Sq Mean Sq F value  Pr(>F)
seq        1  0.145  0.1453    8.05 0.00987 **
prd        1  0.005  0.0048    0.27 0.61189
formu      1  0.003  0.0033    0.18 0.67236
seq:subj  21  1.924  0.0916    5.07 0.00023 ***
Residuals 21  0.379  0.0181

> # the random effect model using aov for carryover and
> # other effects
> mdlAUC.R = aov(lAUC~prd*formu+Error(subj),data=Data)
> print(summary(mdlAUC.R))
```

3. The ANOVAs for CMAX:

```
> # the fixed effects model using lm for "formulation"
> # and "period"
> mdCMAX = lm(CMAX ~ seq + subj:seq + prd + formu,data = Data)
> print(anova(mdCMAX))

Analysis of Variance Table

Response: CMAX
          Df Sum Sq Mean Sq F value Pr(>F)
seq        1    2.4   2.449    2.74   0.11
prd        1    0.1   0.063    0.07   0.79
formu      1    0.2   0.164    0.18   0.67
seq:subj  21   31.9   1.519    1.70   0.12
Residuals 21   18.8   0.895

> # the random effect model using aov for carryover
> # and other effects
> mdCMAX.R = aov(CMAX ~ prd * formu + Error(subj), data = Data)
> print(summary(mdCMAX.R))
```

```
Error: subj
           Df Sum Sq Mean Sq F value Pr(>F)
prd:formu  1    2.4    2.45    1.61   0.22
Residuals 21   31.9    1.52
```

```
Error: Within
           Df Sum Sq Mean Sq F value Pr(>F)
prd        1   0.06   0.063    0.07   0.79
formu      1   0.16   0.164    0.18   0.67
Residuals 21  18.79   0.895
```

4. The ANOVAs for log CMAX:

```
> # the fixed effects model using lm for "formulation"
> # and "period"
> mdlCMAX  = lm(lCMAX ~ seq + subj:seq + prd + formu,data = Data)
> print(anova(mdlCMAX))
```

```
Analysis of Variance Table
```

```
Response: lCMAX
           Df Sum Sq Mean Sq F value Pr(>F)
seq         1  0.152  0.1518    2.91   0.10
prd         1  0.005  0.0046    0.09   0.77
formu       1  0.010  0.0098    0.19   0.67
seq:subj   21  1.909  0.0909    1.74   0.11
Residuals  21  1.096  0.0522
```

```
> # the random effect model using aov for carryover
> # and other effects
> mdlCMAX.R = aov(lCMAX ~ prd * formu + Error(subj), data = Data)
> print(summary(mdlCMAX.R))
```

```
Error: subj
           Df Sum Sq Mean Sq F value Pr(>F)
prd:formu  1  0.152  0.1518    1.67   0.21
Residuals 21  1.909  0.0909
```

```
Error: Within
           Df Sum Sq Mean Sq F value Pr(>F)
prd        1  0.005  0.0046    0.09   0.77
formu      1  0.010  0.0098    0.19   0.67
Residuals 21  1.096  0.0522
```

From these ANOVAs, we can confidently conclude that there are no statistically significant carryover, period, or direct formulation effects in this bioequivalence clinical trial for Cimetidine.

We now proceed to the confidence interval methods in Section 10.3. Since we can just call the R code chunks in Section 10.4.1 exactly with minimal changes, we just illustrate the analysis for the Cimetidine data copying-and-pasting from Section 10.4.1. Readers can use the R code here in the same fashion for their own bioequivalence clinical trial data analysis.

10.4.2.3 Decision CIs

Similarly, the 90% decision CI for the ratio of the means is $DecisionCI_{ratio} = (80\%, 125\%)$ as indicated in Equation (10.6). The decision CI for the difference in means as defined in Equation (10.8) can be calculated using the mean of reference formulation. The implementation in the R system is in following R code chunk:

```
> mformu    = tapply(dat$AUC, list(formu=dat$Formulation), mean)
> ybarT   = mformu["T"]; ybarR = mformu["R"]
> dec2.low = theta.L = -0.2*ybarR
> dec2.up  = theta.U = 0.25*ybarR
> cat("DecisionCI.mean=(",dec2.low,",",dec2.up,")",sep="","\n")

DecisionCI.mean=(-3.33,4.16)
```

Therefore, the decision CI for the mean difference is $DecisionCI_{mean} = (\theta_L, \theta_U) = (-3.328, 4.159)$.

10.4.2.4 Classical Shortest 90% CI

The CI for the mean difference in Equation (10.10) can be implemented using the following R code chunk:

```
> # the confidence coefficient: alpha
> alphaCI  = .1
> # the t-value
> qt.alpha = qt(1-alphaCI, n1+n2-2); qt.alpha

[1] 1.32

> # the sigma using the ANOVA model instead
> sigd2 = anova(mdAUC)[5,3]/2
> # the lower and upper limits for CI1
> low1 = (ybarT-ybarR)-qt.alpha*sqrt(sigd2)*sqrt(1/n1+1/n2)
> up1  = (ybarT-ybarR)+qt.alpha*sqrt(sigd2)*sqrt(1/n1+1/n2)
> cat("The classical CI1=(", round(low1,3),",",
      round(up1,3),")", sep=" ","\n\n")
```

```
The classical CI1=( -0.875 , 0.595 )

> # the lower and upper limits for CI2
> low2=(low1/ybarR+1)*100; up2=(up1/ybarR+1)*100
> cat("The Ratio CI2=(", round(low2,3),",",
      round(up2,3),")", sep=" ","\n\n")

The Ratio CI2=( 94.7 , 104 )
```

Then, the CI for the difference in means $CI_1 = (-0.875, 0.595)$ and the CI for the ratio of means $CI_2 = (94.74, 103.577)$ concluding bioequivalence of the two Cimetidine formulations.

10.4.2.5 The Westlake CI

Again, we calculate $k12 = k_1 + k_2$ first as

```
> k12 = 2*(ybarR-ybarT)/sqrt( sigd2*(1/n1+1/n2))
```

We substitute $k_1 = k12 - k_2$ into the first part to numerically solve for k_2 using R command uniroot as follows:

```
> k2 = uniroot(function(k2) pt(k12-k2,n1+n2-2)- pt(k2,n1+n2-2)
 -(1-alphaCI),lower = -10, upper = 10, tol = 0.0001)$root
> k1 =k12-k2
> cat("The Westlake k1=",k1," and k2=",k2,sep=" ", "\n\n")

The Westlake k1= 2.02   and k2= -1.52
```

The lower and upper limits are calculated as:

```
> low.west = k2*sqrt(sigd2*(1/n1+1/n2))-(ybarR-ybarT)
> up.west  = k1*sqrt(sigd2*(1/n1+1/n2))-(ybarR-ybarT)

The Westlake CI for mu_T-mu_A is ( -0.983 , 0.983 )
```

Again, we conclude bioequivalence of the two Cimetidine formulations.

10.4.2.6 Two One-Sided CIs

Similary the T_L and T_U in Equations (10.13) can be implemented as:

```
> TL = (ybarT-ybarR-theta.L)/sqrt(sigd2*(1/n1+1/n2))
> TU = (ybarT-ybarR-theta.U)/sqrt(sigd2*(1/n1+1/n2))
```

Since $T_L = 5.737 > t(\alpha, n_1 + n_2 - 2) = 1.323$ and $T_U = -7.739 < -t(\alpha, n_1 + n_2 - 2) = -1.323$, we conclude bioequivalence.

We can look at this from the two, one-sided p-values as

```
> pL = 1-pt(abs(TL), n1+n2-2); pU = pt(TU,n1+n2-2)
> p1side = max(pL, pU)
```

The p-values are $p_L = $ 5e-06 and $p_U = 0$. The max of these two are $max(p_L, p_U) = $ 1e-05 which is less than 0.05. Again we conclude bioequivalence of the two Cimetidine formulations.

10.4.2.7   Bayesian Approach

The posterior probability in Equation (10.14) can be implemented in the R system as:

```
> tL  = (theta.L -(ybarT-ybarR))/sqrt(sigd2*(1/n1+1/n2))
> tU  = (theta.U -(ybarT-ybarR))/sqrt(sigd2*(1/n1+1/n2))
> pRD = pt(tU, n1+n2-2) - pt(tL, n1+n2-2); pRD
```

```
R
1
```

Since the posterior probability $p_{RD} = 1 > 90\%$, we again conclude bioequivalence of the two Cimetidine formulations.

10.4.2.8   Individual-Based BT CI

The step-by-step implementation of the individual-based Bienayme-Tchebycheff Inequality CI in Section 10.3.6 is as follows:

1. Create the individual ratios:

```
> dR   = dat[dat$Formulation=="R",c("Subject","AUC")]
> dT   = dat[dat$Formulation=="T",c("Subject","AUC")]
> colnames(dR) = c("Subject","AUC4R")
> colnames(dT) = c("Subject","AUC4T")
> dRT  = merge(dR,dT)
> rT2R = dRT$AUC4T/dRT$AUC4R; rT2R
```

```
 [1] 1.187 1.168 1.046 0.791 1.315 1.024 1.055 1.335
 [9] 0.999 0.989 1.075 0.697 0.956 0.903 1.004 1.047
[17] 0.993 0.806 1.019 1.063 0.864 0.591 1.067
```

2. Get the mean and standard error:

```
> k   = 1/sqrt(1-.9); rbar = mean(rT2R)
> sigrbar = sqrt(var(rT2R)/n); rbar
```

```
[1] 1
```

```
> sigrbar
```

```
     1
  0.0363
```

3. Calculate the lower and upper limits for BT CI:

```
> low.BT = rbar-k*sigrbar; up.BT = rbar+k*sigrbar
> cat("The Tchebycheff CI for mu_T/mu_A is
  (",low.BT,",",up.BT,")",sep="",  "\n\n")

The Tchebycheff CI for mu_T/mu_A is (0.885,1.11)
```

Then, the CI from the individual-based Bienayme-Tchebycheff Inequality is (0.885, 1.115) which lies in the $DecisionCI_{ratio}$ =(80%, 125%) and again we conclude bioequivalence, regardless of what the distribution of ratios is.

10.4.2.9   Bootstrap CIs

As outlined in Section 10.3.7, there are two bootstrap approaches. One is to bootstrap the individual ratios and calculate the mean, and another is to bootstrap the individual bioavailability endpoints and calculate the ratio of the means.

We create 2000 bootstrap samples using the R system as follows:

```
> # B=number of bootstrap
> B      = 2000
> # boota and bootb to keep track the bootstrap results
> boota = bootb = NULL
> for(b in 1:B){
 # Bootstrap the observed individual ratios
 boota[b] = mean(sample(rT2R, replace=T))
 # boottrap the individuals and calculate the means
 tmp = dRT[sample(1:n, replace=T),]
 bootb[b] = mean(tmp$AUC4T)/mean(tmp$AUC4R)
 }
```

The 90% bootstrap CIs for the mean ratios and the ratio of the means are:

```
> qxa = quantile(boota, c(0.05, 0.95)); qxa

   5%    95%
0.943 1.058

> qxb = quantile(bootb, c(0.05, 0.95)); qxb

   5%    95%
0.937 1.044
```

which again conclude bioequivalence from both approaches since both boot-strap 90% CIs are completely within the $DecisionCI_{ratio}$.

The bootstrap sampling distributions for the mean of the individual ratios and the ratio of the means are generated using the following R code to produce Figures 10.6 and 10.7, respectively. In both figures, the two solid vertical segments indicate the limits for the 90% CI and the middle dashed vertical line indicates the means.

```
> # For Figure 10.6
> hist(boota,nclass=30, freq=F,las=1,
 xlab="Mean of the Ratios", ylab="Density", main="")
> box()
> den = density(boota); lines(den, lwd=2)
> qya = approx(den$x, den$y, c(qxa,rbar))$y
> segments(qxa[1],0,qxa[1],qya[1], lwd=5)
> segments(qxa[2],0,qxa[2],qya[2], lwd=5)
> segments(rbar,0,rbar,qya[3],lty=4, lwd=5)
```

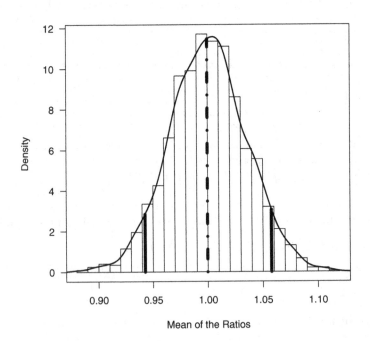

FIGURE 10.6: Bootstrap Distribution for the Mean of the Individual Ratios

```
> # For Figure 10.7
> hist(bootb,nclass=30, freq=F,las=1,
     xlab="Ratio of the Means", ylab="Density", main="")
> box()
> den = density(bootb)
> lines(den, lwd=2)
> rmean = mean(dRT$AUC4T)/mean(dRT$AUC4R)
> qyb = approx(den$x, den$y, c(qxb,rmean))$y
> segments(qxb[1],0,qxb[1],qyb[1], lwd=5)
> segments(qxb[2],0,qxb[2],qyb[2], lwd=5)
> segments(rmean,0,rmean,qyb[3],lty=4, lwd=5)
```

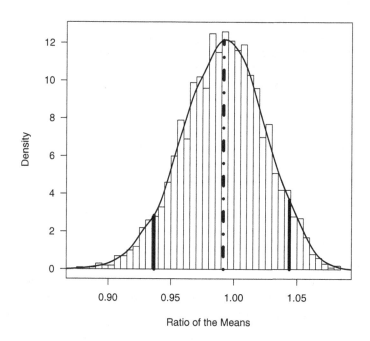

FIGURE 10.7: Bootstrap Distribution for the Ratio of the Means

10.5   Summary and Conclusions

We illustrated the analysis of bioequivalence clinical trials for the purpose of assessing bioequivalence using the R system applied to two datasets. For more methodological details, readers can refer to the seminal book by Chow and Liu (2009). The book by Peace and Chen (2010) describes the bioequivalence trials.

There is a R package *bear* made by Hsin-ya Lee and Yung-jin Lee which is available from

http://pkpd.kmu.edu.tw/bear

for average bioequivalence and bioavailability data analysis. This package includes sample size estimation, non-compartmental analysis (NCA), ANOVA (lm) for a standard RT/TR $2 \times 2 \times 2$ crossover design and linear mixed effect model (lme of nlme) for a two-treatment, two-sequence, with two periods or more (i.e., $2 \times 2 \times 3/2 \times 2 \times 4$) replicate design or a two-treatment, two-sequence, and one-period parallel ABE study ($2 \times 2 \times 1$). We encourage the readers to download this package for their bioequivalence clinical trial data analysis.

10.6   Appendix: SAS Program

Bioequivalence clinical trials have been commonly analyzed in SAS and there are many SAS programs online to be used. Therefore, we do not duplicate this effort in this chapter. Instead, we refer to following online link for the interested readers: http://onbiostatistics.blogspot.com/2012/04/cookbook-sas-codes-for-bioequivalence.html from Dr. Deng in his "Cookbook SAS Codes for Bioequivalence Test in $2 \times 2 \times 2$ Crossover Design", which is for the bioequivalence trials used in this chapter. In addition, there are extensive discussions on issues in biostatistics and clinical trials as seen in

http://onbiostatistics.blogspot.com/.

Chapter 11

Adverse Events in Clinical Trials

In this chapter, we illustrate the application of R to analyze adverse events (AEs) in clinical trials. Similarly to other chapters, we introduce clinical trial data in Section 11.1 and present the statistical models using confidence interval and significance level methods to analyze this type of data in Section 11.2. In Section 11.3, we show step-by-step implementation using R system to analyze AE data followed by a summary and discussion in Section 11.4. Much of the material in this chapter appears in Chapter 17 in our book Peace and Chen (2010). Readers may refer to that book for more detailed descriptions of the data and methods.

11.1 Adverse Event Data from a Clinical Trial

Data from a randomized, parallel, double blind clinical trial of two doses (D_1, D_2) of a new drug compared to a control (C) appear in Table 11.1.

TABLE 11.1: AE Data for Clinical Trial

	Stage	ND2	fD2	ND1	fD1	NC	fC
1	1	15	1	15	0	15	0
2	2	30	2	31	0	29	0
3	3	50	4	48	1	49	0
4	4	70	4	68	3	72	2
5	5	95	6	94	4	95	3
6	6	120	9	119	5	120	4
7	7	140	11	138	5	141	6
8	8	150	12	150	6	150	7

The trial was designed to detect a 20% difference in efficacy between a dose group $(n = 150)$ and the control with 95% power and a 5% Type-I error rate. Entry of patients into the clinical trial is staggered; i.e., occurs in stages (intervals of time). The data consist of the number of patients entered and

315

the number having a particular AE in each group totaled sequentially across stages. These data are used retrospectively to illustrate the methods in this chapter and how they may be used to monitor AEs in clinical trials.

The notations for columns are as follows:

- **Stage** is the stage in the clinical trial;

- **ND2** is the total number of patients in dose D_2;

- **fD2** is the total number of AEs in D_2;

- **ND1** is the total number of patients in D_1;

- **fD1** is the total number of AEs in D_1;

- **NC** is the total number of patients in the control group; and

- **fC** is the total number of AEs in the control group, respectively.

Since the exact time of AE occurrence is not available, the AE rate for each stage is the crude rate and is calculated as the ratio of the observed number of patients having the AE to the total number of patients [Table 11.1 for all ith $(i = 1, \cdots, 8)$]. Therefore, when these rates are plotted by treatment group and stage using the following R code chunk (which produces Figure 11.1), they may oscillate across stages.

```
> # plot the rate by stage
> plot(p2~Stage, type="n",dat,xlim=c(1,9),
     ylim=c(0,max(dat$p1, dat$p2, dat$pC)),
    xlab="Stage",las=1, ylab="AE Rate")
> # add lines for other rates
> lines(pC~Stage, dat,lwd=3, lty=8)
> lines(p1~Stage, dat,lwd=3, lty=4)
> lines(p2~Stage, dat,lwd=3, lty=1)
> # add legend
> legend("bottomright", legend = c("C","p1","p2"),
         lty = c(8,4,1),lwd=3,title = "Line Types")
```

The AE rates by accrual stage for the three treatment groups appear in Figure 11.1. It may be observed that the AE rates for dose group D_1 and the control group C are quite similar and lower than those of dose group D_2. However, the AE rates for D_2 are substantially higher than those in the control group. Therefore, analyses consistent with monitoring focus on comparing these two groups.

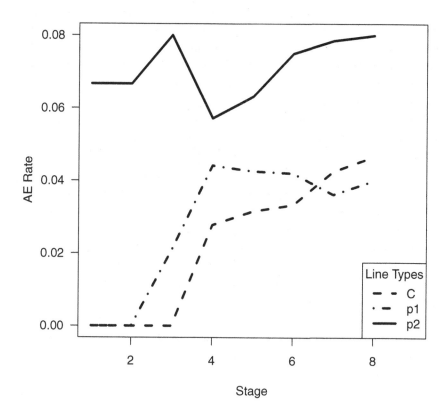

FIGURE 11.1: Plot of AE Rate for the Three Dose Treatments

11.2 Statistical Methods

In this section, we review the statistical methods in Chapter 17 of our book (Peace and Chen (2010)). Readers may refer to that book for greater methodological detail.

We describe two related confidence interval methods for comparing the observed AE rates for two groups where the confidence level (complement of the significance level) is determined so that the two groups are different at that level. A sampling-resampling approach is developed parallel to these two methods.

11.2.1   Confidence Interval (CI) Methods

One CI method is to use the usual, asymmetric CI on the difference in AE rates of two groups to *directly* compare the two groups. The other is an *indirect* comparison of the two groups, that is facilitated by comparing the lower confidence limit (LL) of the CI on the AE rate in one group to the upper confidence limit (UL) of the CI on the AE event rate in the other group.

11.2.1.1   Comparison Using Direct CI Method

Directly comparing two groups by using a CI on the difference in their AE rates is the more traditional approach in monitoring AEs in clinical trials. The direct, comparative CI on the difference is often based on the normal approximation to the binomial for AE events. This traditional confidence interval (CI) can be constructed as follows:

Let p_i and p_j be the true incidence rates of some AE in the populations to be treated with the ith and jth regimens, and let f_i, f_j, P_i and P_j denote the corresponding observed incidences and incidence rates among N_i and N_j treated patients, respectively. Then the observed difference, $\delta_{ij} = P_i - P_j$ is an unbiased estimate of the difference in true incidences where $P_i = \frac{f_i}{N_i}$ and $P_j = \frac{f_j}{N_j}$. The estimate of the variance of the observed difference is given by $V_i + V_j$ where V_i is the estimate of the variance of the observed incidence rates in the ith regimen given by $V_i = \frac{P_i(1-P_i)}{N_i}$ with similar definition for jth regimen.

Therefore, the traditional, direct, $100(1 - 2\alpha)\%$ can be represented as

$$L_{ij} \leq p_i - p_j \leq U_{ij}, \qquad (11.1)$$

where L_{ij} is the lower limit and U_{ij} is the upper limit and are given by:

$$
\begin{aligned}
L_{ij} &= P_i - P_j - Z_\alpha \sqrt{V_i + V_j} \\
U_{ij} &= P_i - P_j + Z_\alpha \sqrt{V_i + V_j}
\end{aligned}
$$

where Z_α is the upper percentile of the standardized distribution of $P_i - P_j$. The direct comparison of two regimens via $100(1 - 2\alpha)\%$ confidence intervals also permits concluding that two regimens are different.

The conclusion is based on the lower limit. If the lower limit L_{ij} is positive (presuming that the observed incidence rate in the ith regimen exceeded the observed incidence rate in the jth regimen), one may conclude that the two regimens are statistically different at the nominal significance level α.

11.2.1.2   Comparison Using Indirect CI Methods

We describe two indirect methods based upon per group CIs. One is based on the normal approximation to binomial distribution of AEs (hereafter referred as "IndirectCI1"), and the other is based on the exact binomial distribution from AEs (hereafter referred as "IndirectCI2").

Method "IndirectCI1" is a non-standard, indirect approach for comparing AE incidence rates from two regimens originally proposed by Peace (1987) as follows (using the same notation from Section 11.2.1.1).

A two-sided $100(1 - 2\alpha)\%$ CI on the true incidence p_i in the ith regimen is

$$L_i \leq p_i \leq U_i \tag{11.2}$$

where L_i and U_i are the lower and upper limits given by:

$$L_i = P_i - Z_\alpha \sqrt{V_i}$$
$$U_i = P_i + Z_\alpha \sqrt{V_i}$$

where Z_α is the $100(1 - \alpha)\%$ percentile of the distribution of P_i based on the normal approximation. In addition to such confidence intervals bracketing the true incidences in each regimen, they also permit two regimens to be indirectly compared. One could infer that regimens i and j are statistically different at the nominal significance level α if the lower limit of the $100(1 - 2\alpha)\%$ confidence interval on the true incidence of regimen i is greater than the upper limit of regimen j; that is, if $L_i > U_j$ where again the observed incidence in the ith regimen is greater than the observed incidence in the jth regimen.

Method "IndirectCI2" AEs follow a binomial distribution. We use the binomial distribution to construct the CI on the true AE rate. This binomial approach is based on the well-known fact that if f is binomially distributed with $binomial(N, p)$, then the exact $(1 - 2\alpha)\%$ confidence interval can be obtained by finding L and U such that $\sum_{k=0}^{L} Binom(k, N, p) \leq \alpha$ and $\sum_{k=U}^{N} Binom(k, N, p) \geq \alpha$. Therefore, the indirect CI2 comparison using the exact binomial distribution of AEs can be constructed to determine whether $L_i \geq U_j$ where L_i is determined from $\sum_{k=0}^{L_i} Binom(k, N_i, \hat{p}_i) \leq \alpha$ and U_j is determined from $\sum_{k=U_j}^{N} Binom(k, N_j, \hat{p}_j) \geq \alpha$. Note that $\hat{p}_i = \frac{f_i}{N_i}$ and $\hat{p}_j = \frac{f_j}{N_j}$.

11.2.2 Significance Level Methods (SLMs)

11.2.2.1 SLM using normal approximation

From method "IndirectCI1" in Section 11.2.1.2 based upon the normal approximation to the binomial, we conclude that $p_i \geq p_j$ if $L_i \geq U_j$ at the significance level α, where $P_i - z_\alpha \sqrt{V_i} \geq P_j + z_\alpha \sqrt{V_j}$. This is equivalent to

$$z_\alpha \leq \frac{P_i - P_j}{\sqrt{V_i} + \sqrt{V_j}} \tag{11.3}$$

at the significance level α. Consequently "IndirectCI1" gives rise to a decision rule based upon the significance level α. Consequently, the significance level method requires determining α from an appropriate distribution such that

$$CR_\alpha \leq \frac{P_i - P_j}{\sqrt{V_i} + \sqrt{V_j}} \tag{11.4}$$

where CR_α is the critical point such that there is α area in the tail of the distribution of P_i (or P_j) to the right of $\frac{P_i - P_j}{\sqrt{V_i} + \sqrt{V_j}}$. From the normal approximation to binomial distribution for AEs, Equation (11.4) is equivalent to Equation (11.3) and the significance level α is easily calculated by:

$$\alpha \geq pnorm\left(\frac{P_i - P_j}{\sqrt{V_i} + \sqrt{V_j}}\right) \tag{11.5}$$

where *pnorm* is the cumulative normal probability function.

11.2.2.2   SLM using exact binomial distribution

This method is also based on the fact that $p_i \geq p_j$ if $L_i \geq U_j$ at the significance level α, which can be determined as in Section 11.2.2.1. However, we use the exact binomial distribution of AEs to determine L_i and U_j where L_i is determined from $\sum_{k=0}^{L_i} Binom(k, N_i, \hat{p}_i) \leq \alpha$ and U_j is determined from $\sum_{k=U_j}^{N} Binom(k, N_j, p_j) \geq \alpha$. The equation $L_i = U_j$ is then solved numerically for the smallest α. This method involves extensive numerical analyses which are easily performed in R.

11.2.2.3   SLM using resampling from pooled samples

The methods considered thus far are geared toward comparing $p_i \geq p_j$ and making a statistical inference based the UL and LL of per groups CIs or to find the critical value CR_α for significance level α based on underlying distributions of the AEs.

Even though these methods are not constrained by $H_0 : p_i = p_j$, were we to test H_0 directly using significance testing and the randomization test, we would combine the data under H_0 with $(f_i + f_j)$ AEs in $(N_i + N_j)$ subjects. Therefore, a sampling-resampling approach can be developed as in following steps:

1. Draw a random sample of size N_i from the $(N_i + N_j)$ combined data and the rest would be N_j samples from the combined sample;

2. Compute a new set of incidence rates of P_i^{new} and P_j^{new}. If $P_i^{new} \leq P_j^{new}$, go back to Step 1, else compute a new critical value as

$$CR^{new} = \frac{P_i^{new} - P_j^{new}}{\sqrt{V_i^{new}} + \sqrt{V_j^{new}}}$$

3. Repeat Steps 1 and 2 for a significant number of times (say $N = 10000$) to construct a sampling-resampling distribution.

The significance level α would be the percentage of CR^{New} greater than the observed CR_α in (11.4) in these N samples.

11.2.2.4 SLM using resampling from pooled AE rates

Similar to the method in Section 11.2.2.3, a sampling-resampling approach can be proposed from the pooled incidence rates from the binomial AEs. Based on the null hypothesis that $H_0 : p_i = p_j = p$, we can then estimate the true p from the observed incidence rates of P_i and P_j as the pooled $\hat{p} = \frac{P_i + P_j}{2}$. The sampling-resampling approach can be implemented in the following steps:

1. Sample $f_i^s \sim Binom(N_i, \hat{p})$ and $f_j^s \sim Binom(N_j, \hat{p})$ and then calculate $P_i^s = \frac{f_i^s}{N_i}$ and $P_j^s = \frac{f_j^s}{N_j}$;

2. If $P_i^s \leq P_j^s$, then go back to Step 1; otherwise, calculate

$$CR^s = \frac{P_i^s - P_j^s}{\sqrt{V_i^s} + \sqrt{V_j^s}}$$

3. Repeat Steps 1 and 2 for a significant number of times (say $N = 10,000$) to construct a sampling-resampling distribution.

The significance level α would be the percentage of CRs greater than the observed CR in (11.4) in these N samples.

11.3 Step-by-Step Implementation in R

11.3.1 Clinical Trial Data Manipulation

Similarly to the previous chapters, we first read the data using R function `read.csv` as follows:

```
> dat = read.csv("datAE.csv", header=T)
```

This data is then shown as in Table 11.1. For further data manipulation, we calculate the AE rate as well as the associated variance as follows:

```
> # the AE rate
> dat$p2 = dat$fD2/dat$ND2
> dat$p1 = dat$fD1/dat$ND1
> dat$pC = dat$fC/dat$NC
```

```
> # The variance
> dat$V2 = dat$p2*(1-dat$p2)/dat$ND2
> dat$V1 = dat$p1*(1-dat$p1)/dat$ND1
> dat$VC = dat$pC*(1-dat$pC)/dat$NC
> len    = length(dat[,1])
```

where "len" is defined for the length of stages ("len"= 8) future use.

11.3.2   R Implementations for CI Methods

To implement the direct CI method in Section 11.2.1.1, we first make a R function (named as direct.CI) to be called to calculate the direct CI for any two regimens with input vector *(N1,f1,N2,f2,alpha)* where "alpha" is the desired significance level.

```
> # Function for direct comparison
> direct.CI = function(N1,f1,N2,f2,alpha){
        p1 = f1/N1; p2 = f2/N2
        v1 = p1*(1-p1)/N1;v2 = p2*(1-p2)/N2
        z.alpha = qnorm(1-alpha)
        low =(p1-p2)-z.alpha*sqrt(v1+v2)
        up  =(p1-p2)+z.alpha*sqrt(v1+v2)
        data.frame(testp=p1>p2,low=low,diff=p1-p2,
                    p1=p1,p2=p2,N1=N1,N2=N2)
}
```

The outputs for this function include:

1. testp to check whether the observed AE rate in regimen 1 is greater than that in regimen 2 as "TRUE" or "FALSE",

2. low to show the value of the lower limit to check whether L_{i2} is positive,

3. diff to show the difference of AE rate between regimens 1 to 2, and

4. p1,p2,N1,N2 are other relevant information for the regimens.

Using this function, we can calculate the direct CI by calling this function to compare dose 1 to control (named as **CI1toC**) and dose 2 to C (named as **CI2toC**) as follows:

```
> # call ``direct.CI" to compare dose 1 to control
> CI1toC = direct.CI(dat$ND1, dat$fD1, dat$NC, dat$fC, 0.025)
> # print the calculation
> CI1toC
```

```
    testp    low      diff    p1     p2    N1  N2
1 FALSE   0.0000  0.00000 0.0000 0.0000  15  15
```

```
2 FALSE  0.0000  0.00000 0.0000 0.0000  31  29
3  TRUE -0.0196  0.02083 0.0208 0.0000  48  49
4  TRUE -0.0455  0.01634 0.0441 0.0278  68  72
5  TRUE -0.0429  0.01097 0.0426 0.0316  94  95
6  TRUE -0.0396  0.00868 0.0420 0.0333 119 120
7 FALSE -0.0520 -0.00632 0.0362 0.0426 138 141
8 FALSE -0.0527 -0.00667 0.0400 0.0467 150 150
```

```
> # call ``direct.CI" to compare dose 2 to control
> CI2toC = direct.CI(dat$ND2, dat$fD2, dat$NC, dat$fC, 0.025)
> # print the calculation
> CI2toC
```

```
  testp    low   diff     p1     p2  N1  N2
1  TRUE -0.0596 0.0667 0.0667 0.0000  15  15
2  TRUE -0.0226 0.0667 0.0667 0.0000  30  29
3  TRUE  0.0048 0.0800 0.0800 0.0000  50  49
4  TRUE -0.0369 0.0294 0.0571 0.0278  70  72
5  TRUE -0.0287 0.0316 0.0632 0.0316  95  95
6  TRUE -0.0154 0.0417 0.0750 0.0333 120 120
7  TRUE -0.0196 0.0360 0.0786 0.0426 140 141
8  TRUE -0.0217 0.0333 0.0800 0.0467 150 150
```

It may be observed from these outputs that there is no positive lower limit for the comparison from D_1 to C indicating that D_1 and C are not statistically significantly different at any stage, whereas the positive lower limit (i.e., L_{3C} = 0.005) is achieved at stage 3 indicating D_2 and C are statistically different at this stage.

11.3.3   R Implementations for Indirect CI Methods

Similarly, we make an R function to facilitate this calculation. The "IndirectCI1" method using normal approximation to the binomial described in Section 11.2.1.2 can be programmed in R function `indirect.CI` to calculate the CI limit for each regimen as follows:

```
> # Function for indirect comparison: using normal approximation
> indirect.CI = function(N,f,alpha){
        p = f/N; v = p*(1-p)/N
        z.alpha = qnorm(1-alpha)
        low     = p-z.alpha*sqrt(v)
        up      = p+z.alpha*sqrt(v)
        data.frame(low=round(low,3),up=round(up,3),N=N,f=f,
            p=round(p,3))
}
```

Therefore, the associated lower and upper limits can be calculated and outputed as:

```
> CIC = indirect.CI(dat$NC, dat$fC, 0.025)
> CIC

     low    up    N f   p
1  0.000 0.000  15 0 0.000
2  0.000 0.000  29 0 0.000
3  0.000 0.000  49 0 0.000
4 -0.010 0.066  72 2 0.028
5 -0.004 0.067  95 3 0.032
6  0.001 0.065 120 4 0.033
7  0.009 0.076 141 6 0.043
8  0.013 0.080 150 7 0.047

> CI1 = indirect.CI(dat$ND1, dat$fD1, 0.025)
> CI1

     low    up    N f   p
1  0.000 0.000  15 0 0.000
2  0.000 0.000  31 0 0.000
3 -0.020 0.061  48 1 0.021
4 -0.005 0.093  68 3 0.044
5  0.002 0.083  94 4 0.043
6  0.006 0.078 119 5 0.042
7  0.005 0.067 138 5 0.036
8  0.009 0.071 150 6 0.040

> CI2 = indirect.CI(dat$ND2, dat$fD2, 0.025)
> CI2

     low    up    N f    p
1 -0.060 0.193  15  1 0.067
2 -0.023 0.156  30  2 0.067
3  0.005 0.155  50  4 0.080
4  0.003 0.112  70  4 0.057
5  0.014 0.112  95  6 0.063
6  0.028 0.122 120  9 0.075
7  0.034 0.123 140 11 0.079
8  0.037 0.123 150 12 0.080
```

We inspect these outputs to determine which stage $L_i \geq U_j$ is satisfied. The comparison for the doses D_1 and D_2 to Control can be printed as:

```
> # make a dataframe for dose 1 to control
> out1toC = data.frame(Stage= dat$Stage,
```

```
        indirect.test = CI1$low > CIC$up,
        low1=CI1$low, upC =CIC$up)
> # print it
> print(out1toC)
```

	Stage	indirect.test	low1	upC
1	1	FALSE	0.000	0.000
2	2	FALSE	0.000	0.000
3	3	FALSE	-0.020	0.000
4	4	FALSE	-0.005	0.066
5	5	FALSE	0.002	0.067
6	6	FALSE	0.006	0.065
7	7	FALSE	0.005	0.076
8	8	FALSE	0.009	0.080

```
> # make a dataframe for dose 2 to control
> out2toC = data.frame(Stage= dat$Stage,
        indirect.test = CI2$low > CIC$up,
        low2=CI2$low, upC =CIC$up)
> # print it
> print(out2toC)
```

	Stage	indirect.test	low2	upC
1	1	FALSE	-0.060	0.000
2	2	FALSE	-0.023	0.000
3	3	TRUE	0.005	0.000
4	4	FALSE	0.003	0.066
5	5	FALSE	0.014	0.067
6	6	FALSE	0.028	0.065
7	7	FALSE	0.034	0.076
8	8	FALSE	0.037	0.080

We identify stage 3 as the only stage for which the lower limit for D_2 (i.e., $L_{D_2} = 0.005$) is greater than the upper limit of control ($U_C = 0$). This confirms the conclusion from the direct comparison.

For the second indirect comparison (i.e., *IndirectCI2*) using exact binomial distribution described in Section 11.2.1.2 can be programmed in R function exact.CI to calculate the CI limit for each regimen as follows. This R function exact.CI will be used and called in later sections.

```
> # Function to calculate the CI for binomial
> exact.CI = function(N,f,alpha){
        p   = f/N
        low = qbinom(alpha, N, p)
        up  = qbinom(1-alpha,N,p)
 data.frame(N=N,p=p,f=f,low=low,up=up, plow =low/N, pup=up/N)
 }
```

Therefore, the associated lower and upper limits may be calculated and outputted as:

```
> # for control
> CIC = exact.CI(dat$NC, dat$fC, 0.025)
> CIC

    N       p f low up    plow    pup
1  15 0.0000 0   0  0 0.00000 0.0000
2  29 0.0000 0   0  0 0.00000 0.0000
3  49 0.0000 0   0  0 0.00000 0.0000
4  72 0.0278 2   0  5 0.00000 0.0694
5  95 0.0316 3   0  7 0.00000 0.0737
6 120 0.0333 4   1  8 0.00833 0.0667
7 141 0.0426 6   2 11 0.01418 0.0780
8 150 0.0467 7   2 12 0.01333 0.0800

> # for dose 1
> CI1 = exact.CI(dat$ND1, dat$fD1, 0.025)
> CI1

    N       p f low up    plow    pup
1  15 0.0000 0   0  0 0.00000 0.0000
2  31 0.0000 0   0  0 0.00000 0.0000
3  48 0.0208 1   0  3 0.00000 0.0625
4  68 0.0441 3   0  7 0.00000 0.1029
5  94 0.0426 4   1  8 0.01064 0.0851
6 119 0.0420 5   1 10 0.00840 0.0840
7 138 0.0362 5   1 10 0.00725 0.0725
8 150 0.0400 6   2 11 0.01333 0.0733

> # for dose 2
> CI2 = exact.CI(dat$ND2, dat$fD2, 0.025)
> CI2

    N      p  f low up   plow   pup
1  15 0.0667  1   0  3 0.0000 0.200
2  30 0.0667  2   0  5 0.0000 0.167
3  50 0.0800  4   1  8 0.0200 0.160
4  70 0.0571  4   1  8 0.0143 0.114
5  95 0.0632  6   2 11 0.0211 0.116
6 120 0.0750  9   4 15 0.0333 0.125
7 140 0.0786 11   5 18 0.0357 0.129
8 150 0.0800 12   6 19 0.0400 0.127
```

We inspect these outputs and determine the stages for which $L_i \geq U_j$ is satisfied. The comparison for the doses D_1 and D_2 to Control can be printed as:

```
> # dataframe for dose 1 to control
> out1toC = data.frame(Stage= dat$Stage,
          indirect.test = CI1$plow > CIC$pup,
          low1=CI1$plow, upC =CIC$pup)
> print(out1toC)
```

	Stage	indirect.test	low1	upC
1	1	FALSE	0.00000	0.0000
2	2	FALSE	0.00000	0.0000
3	3	FALSE	0.00000	0.0000
4	4	FALSE	0.00000	0.0694
5	5	FALSE	0.01064	0.0737
6	6	FALSE	0.00840	0.0667
7	7	FALSE	0.00725	0.0780
8	8	FALSE	0.01333	0.0800

```
> # dataframe for dose 2 to control
> out2toC = data.frame(Stage= dat$Stage,
          indirect.test = CI2$plow > CIC$pup,
          low2=CI2$plow, upC =CIC$pup)
> print(out2toC)
```

	Stage	indirect.test	low2	upC
1	1	FALSE	0.0000	0.0000
2	2	FALSE	0.0000	0.0000
3	3	TRUE	0.0200	0.0000
4	4	FALSE	0.0143	0.0694
5	5	FALSE	0.0211	0.0737
6	6	FALSE	0.0333	0.0667
7	7	FALSE	0.0357	0.0780
8	8	FALSE	0.0400	0.0800

We observe that stage 3 is the only stage for which the lower limit for D_2 (i.e., $L_{D_2} = 0.02$) is greater than the upper limit of control ($U_C = 0$). This again confirms the conclusion from the direct comparison.

11.3.4   R for Significant Level Methods

Since we have observed that D_1 is not statistically different from Control, We do not consider this dose regimen in the following analysis and focus on the comparison of D_2 to control.

11.3.4.1   R for SLM with normal approximation

The significance level method (SLM) using the normal approximation in Section 11.2.2.1 can be implemented in R to calculate the right bound in

Equation (11.4) and then use the cumulative normal probability function to calculate the significant level α.

We make an R function `bound.CI` first since this function will be called for other methods as follows:

```
> # Function to calculate bounds
> bound.CI = function(N1,f1,N2,f2){
        p1 = f1/N1
        p2 = f2/N2
        v1 = p1*(1-p1)/N1
        v2 = p2*(1-p2)/N2
 data.frame(bound= (p2-p1)/(sqrt(v1)+sqrt(v2)),
        N1=N1,f1=f1,p1=p1,N2=N2,f2=f2,p2=p2)
 }
```

We can then use the function to calculate the bound and compute the significance level as:

```
> # call function ``bound.CI" and make the calculation
> d0               = bound.CI(dat$NC,dat$fC,dat$ND2,dat$fD2)
> # calculate the alpha from normal approximation
> d0$alpha.normal = 1-pnorm(d0$bound)
> # print it
> round(d0,4)
```

	bound	N1	f1	p1	N2	f2	p2	alpha.normal
1	1.035	15	0	0.0000	15	1	0.0667	0.1503
2	1.464	29	0	0.0000	30	2	0.0667	0.0716
3	2.085	49	0	0.0000	50	4	0.0800	0.0185
4	0.623	72	2	0.0278	70	4	0.0571	0.2665
5	0.736	95	3	0.0316	95	6	0.0632	0.2308
6	1.031	120	4	0.0333	120	9	0.0750	0.1514
7	0.906	141	6	0.0426	140	11	0.0786	0.1824
8	0.847	150	7	0.0467	150	12	0.0800	0.1986

It can be seen that only at stage 3, is the significance level $\alpha = 0.019$ less than 0.05. We can plot the αs using following R code to produce Figure 11.2.

```
> plot(dat$Stage, d0$alpha.normal,type="o", xlab="Stage",
  ylab=expression(alpha), las=1, main="")
> text(dat$Stage, d0$alpha.normal,round(d0$alpha.normal,3))
```

11.3.4.2   R for SLM with exact binomial

The principle for this method in Section 11.2.2.2 is to search for a smallest α so that $L_{D_2} - U_C = 0$ (i.e., $L_{D_2} = U_C$). We will re-use the R function `exact.CI` we created before and call R built-in function `uniroot` to find the one-dimensional root for each stage using a R for-loop structure.

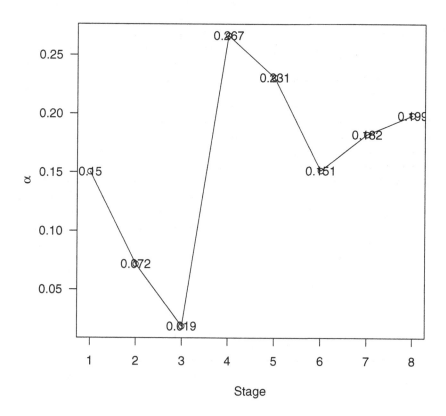

FIGURE 11.2: The Estimated Significance Level α for Each Stage

```
> # make a funtion for L_D2-UC
> fn = function(alpha, stage){
 LD2 = exact.CI(dat$ND2,dat$fD2,alpha)$plow[stage]
 UC  = exact.CI(dat$NC,dat$fC,alpha)$pup[stage]
 LD2-UC
 }
> # call R function ``uniroot" to solve equation
> est.alpha = NULL
> for(s in 1:len)
 est.alpha[s]=uniroot(fn, c(0,0.8), stage=s)$root
> est.alpha
```

```
[1] 0.3529 0.0986 0.0112 0.2296 0.1988 0.1860 0.1483
[8] 0.1977
```

It can be seen that only at stage 3, is the significance level $\alpha=0.011$ less than 0.05. The reader may wish to generate a plot similar to that in 11.2 for this method, by following the code in Section 11.3.4.1.

11.3.4.3 R for SLM using Sampling-Resampling

The significance level method using the sampling-resampling approach from pooled samples in Section 11.2.2.3 is implemented with a for-loop for each stage under the null hypothesis of $H_0 : p_C = p_{D_2}$ as in the following R code chunk with further explanations.

At each stage, we create two vectors, named as *x1* and *x2*, for control and D_2 to mimic the observed AEs from "fC" and "fD2" from Table 11.1. Under the H_0, we combine "fC+fD2" AEs from "NC+ND2" subjects which is the data-frame x in the R code.

Now as in Step 1, we draw a random sample of size N_C from the $(N_C+N_{D_2})$ using the R function `sample` applied to the frequencies for control and D_2, named as "'f1" and "f2" in the chunk.

In Step 2, we calculate the new AE rates P_C^{new} and $P_{D_2}^{new}$ (denoted as "p1" and "p2" in the chunk). If $P_{D_2}^{new} \leq P_C^{new}$, we compute the new critical value as

$$CR^{new} = \frac{P_C^{new} - P_{D_2}^{new}}{\sqrt{V_C^{new}} + \sqrt{V_{D_2}^{new}}} \tag{11.6}$$

by calling the R function `bound.CI` to calculate the new bound.

```
> # set.seed to fix the seed for random number generation
> set.seed(123)
> # number of simulation
> num.sim = 1000
> # matrix to hold the output "bound"
> bound3 = matrix(0, ncol=len, nrow=num.sim)
> for(stage in 1:len){
        ds = d0[stage,]
      # make the 0 and 1's from the data from control
        x1 = c( rep(1, ds$f1), rep(0, ds$N1-ds$f1))
      # from D2
        x2 = c( rep(1, ds$f2), rep(0, ds$N2-ds$f2))
      # combine them
    x   = data.frame(id = 1:(ds$N1+ds$N2),c(x1,x2))

  tsim=0
  repeat{
          # sample it and sum the freq
          f = sample(x$id, ds$N1)
          f1 = sum(x[f,2])
```

```
        f2 = sum(x[-f,2])
        p1 = f1/ds$N1
        p2 = f2/ds$N2
if(p2 > p1){
   tsim=tsim+1
   bound3[tsim,stage] = bound.CI(ds$N1,f1,ds$N2,f2)$bound
                } # end of if
if(tsim ==num.sim) break
            } # end of repeat
} # end of stage
```

Repeat Steps 1 and 2 for *num.sim* = 1000 times to create a sampling-resampling distribution denoted by *bounds3* which has 8 (number of stages) columns and 1000 rows (number of sampling-resampling). We can check it by R command dim:

```
> dim(bound3)
```

[1] 1000   8

The implementation to the sampling-resampling from pooled AE rates in Section 11.2.2.4 is similar to the method in Section 11.2.2.3 and is briefly explained as follows. The only difference is that the pooled AE rate is calculated as $\hat{p} = \frac{P_i + P_j}{2}$ and draws binomial samples with this pooled AE rate.

```
> bound4 = matrix(0, ncol=len, nrow=num.sim)
> for(stage in 1:len){
        ds = d0[stage,]
 tsim=0
 repeat{
        f1 = rbinom(1, ds$N1, (ds$p1+ds$p2)/2)
        f2 = rbinom(1, ds$N2, (ds$p1+ds$p2)/2)
        p1 = f1/ds$N1
        p2 = f2/ds$N2
if(p2 > p1){
   tsim=tsim+1
   bound4[tsim,stage] = bound.CI(ds$N1,f1,ds$N2,f2)$bound
                } # end of if
if(tsim ==num.sim) break
        } # end of repeat
} # end of stage
> dim(bound4)
```

[1] 1000   8

The significance level α is then calculated by tracking the percentage of these simulated 1000 samples CR^{new} in *bound3* or *bound4* which are greater than the observed CR_α, using Equation (11.4) the following R code:

```
> est.alpha3 = NULL
> est.alpha4 = NULL
> for(i in 1:len){
        regimen3 = bound3[,i]
        regimen4 = bound4[,i]
#calculate how many simulations > the obs bound in d0$bound
        est.alpha3[i] = sum(regimen3 > d0$bound[i])/num.sim
        est.alpha4[i] = sum(regimen4 > d0$bound[i])/num.sim
 }
> est.alpha3

[1] 0.000 0.000 0.000 0.160 0.164 0.078 0.119 0.151

> est.alpha4

[1] 0.204 0.081 0.010 0.312 0.337 0.171 0.186 0.235
```

As a final summary for the significance level method (SLM), we put all the αs together and make a unified plot to display them using following R code chunk:

```
> # make the alpha plot
> d0$alpha.binom = est.alpha
> d0$alpha.samp1 = est.alpha3
> d0$alpha.samp2 = est.alpha4
> # keep track of the max values for alpha for y-axis limit
> max.alpha = max(d0$alpha.normal, d0$alpha.binom,
                  d0$alpha.samp1, d0$alpha.samp2)
> # plot the alpha
> plot(dat$Stage, d0$alpha.normal,type="n", ylim=c(0,max.alpha),
    xlab="Stage", ylab=expression(alpha), las=1, main="")
> # add lines to the plots
> lines(dat$Stage, d0$alpha.normal,lwd=3,lty=1)
> lines(dat$Stage, d0$alpha.binom,lwd=3,lty=3)
> lines(dat$Stage, d0$alpha.samp1,lwd=3,lty=4)
> lines(dat$Stage, d0$alpha.samp2,lwd=3,lty=8)
> # add the reference line
> abline(h=0.025, lwd=4, lty=1)
> # add legend
> temp <- legend("topright", legend = c(" ", " "," "," "),
                text.width = strwidth("Normal Approx"),
                lty = c(1,3,4,8),lwd=3,xjust = 1, yjust = 1,
                title = "Line Types")
> text(temp$rect$left + temp$rect$w, temp$text$y,
    c("Normal Approx", "Exact Binomial","Resampling 1",
    "Resampling 2"), pos=2)
```

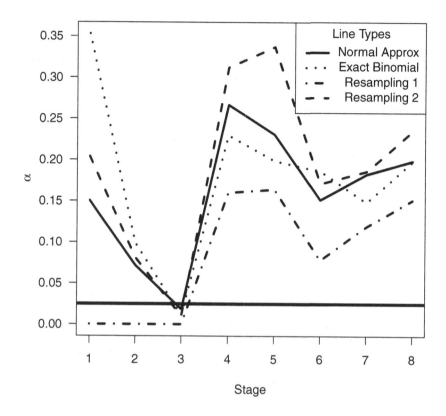

FIGURE 11.3: The Estimated αs for Each Stage Under All Four Methods

It can be observed from Figure 11.3 that all four methods identify stage 3 as the only stage at which there is a significant difference between the high dose group and control.

11.4 Summary and Discussions

In this chapter, we presented an array of statistical methods to monitor AEs in clinical trials. These methods are intended to serve as an alerting mechanism in the usual monitoring of adverse events in clinical trials. Their attractiveness is their simplicity and the fact that they represent little effort beyond what is usually done in monitoring AEs as they accumulate. The methods were applied to AE data from a completed clinical trial. Therefore, they were applied to the crude rate AE data across all stages of entry for illustration. Had they been applied prospectively as the trial was ongoing and the AE was serious, the significant excess of the AE in the highest dose group as compared to control (if placebo) at stage 3 would have led to serious discussions about possibly stopping the trial or at least dropping the high dose group from further enrollment.

Statistical procedures involving confidence intervals were suggested for monitoring AEs in clinical trials. Further per group confidence intervals on the true AE rates are recommended as they permit easier comparative interpretation, particularly in trials with a large number of treatment groups. The significance level based methods presented in this chapter would be in addition to these methods.

Readers should review Chapter 17 of our "Clinical Trial Methodology" book (Peace and Chen (2010)) for more in depth presentation and discussion of the methods and issues.

11.5   Appendix: SAS Programs

There is no SAS procedure specifically designed for this calculation. We then programmed the calculations in this chapter using SAS `proc iml` and `proc model` for illustration purposes.

```
/***************************************************
Section 11.3.1. Data manipulation
***************************************************/
Data datAE;
infile "Your file path/datAE.csv" delimiter="," firstobs=2;
input Stage ND2 fD2 ND1 fD1 NC fC;;
proc print; RUN;
proc iml;
* Read data into IML ;
  use datAE;
  read all ;

/* the AE rate*/
p2 = fD2/Nd2; p1 = fD1/ND1; pC=fC/NC;
/* the variance*/
V2 = p2#(1-p2)#(1/ND2);
V1 = p1#(1-p1)#(1/ND1);
```

```
VC = pC#(1-pC)#(1/NC);
len=8;

/**********************************************************
Section 11.3.2. CI method
**********************************************************/
/* just for D1 to Control, same for D2 to Control*/
alpha      = 0.025;
zalpha     = quantile('NORMAL',1-alpha);
lowCI      = (p1-pC)-zalpha*sqrt(v1+vC);
upCI       = (p1-pC)+zalpha*sqrt(v1+vC);
testp      = p1>pC;
diffD1toC = p1-pC;
All        = testp||round(lowCI,0.001)||round(upCI,0.001)
||round(diffD1toC,0.001)||round(p1,0.001)
||round(pC,0.001)||ND1||NC;
print "Direct Comparison for D1 to Control";
print All;


/**********************************************************
Section 11.3.3. Indirect CI
**********************************************************/
/* 1. Using normal Approximation */
/*  Calculate CI for Control*/
ClowCI    = pC-zalpha*sqrt(vC);
CupCI     = pC+zalpha*sqrt(vC);
/* CI for Dose 1 */
d1lowCI   = p1-zalpha*sqrt(v1);
d1upCI    = p1+zalpha*sqrt(v1);
/* CI for Dose 2 */
d2lowCI   = p2-zalpha*sqrt(v2);
d2upCI    = p2+zalpha*sqrt(v2);
/* Indirect test for d1/d2 to Control*/
Indirecttest_d1toC = d1lowCI - CupCI;
Indirecttest_d2toC = d2lowCI - CupCI;
print Indirecttest_d1toC;
print Indirecttest_d2toC;

/* 2. Using Exact binomial */
/*  Calculate CI for Control*/
ClowCI    = quantile('BINOM',alpha,pC,nC);
CupCI     = quantile('BINOM',1-alpha,pC,nC);
/* CI for Dose 1 */
d1lowCI   = quantile('BINOM',alpha,p1,nD1);
```

```
d1upCI     = quantile('BINOM',1-alpha,p1,nD1);
/* CI for Dose 2 */
d2lowCI    = quantile('BINOM',alpha,p2,nD2);
d2upCI     = quantile('BINOM',1-alpha,p2,nD2);
/* Indirect test for d1/d2 to Control*/
Exact_d1toC = d1lowCI - CupCI>0;
Exact_d2toC = d2lowCI - CupCI>0;
print Exact_d1toC;
print Exact_d2toC;


/* Conclusion for both method: Stage 3*/


/*****************************************************
Section 11.3.4
Only for "SLM with Normal Approximation"
*****************************************************/
proc model data=datAE;
/* the AE rate*/
p2 = fD2/Nd2; pC=fC/NC;
/* the variance*/
V2 = p2*(1-p2)/ND2;
VC = pC*(1-pC)/NC;
/* the z-values */
zalpha = quantile('NORMAL',alpha);
/* low CI for control */
ClowCI = (pC-zalpha*sqrt(vC));
/* upper CI for dose 2 */
d2upCI = (p2+zalpha*sqrt(v2));
/* solve the diff =0*/
eq.diff    = ClowCI-d2upCI;
solve alpha/ out=sol4Norm solveprint;
id fc nc fd2 nd2;
run;

proc print data=sol4Norm; run;
```

Chapter 12

Analysis of DNA Microarrays in Clinical Trials

In this chapter, we discuss the analysis of microarray data derived from samples collected in clinical trials. In recent years, microarray technologies have been used extensively to study molecular differences among different types of cancer and these have played a fundamental role in identifying new drug leads for further development by the biotech industry. Along with the development of microarray technology, many new statistical methods and models have been developed in parallel and incorporated in software to analyze high-throughput data.

Although there are many software packages for analysis of microarray data we introduce `bioconductor` in this chapter – which is widely used and publicly available from `http://www.bioconductor.org`. In Section 12.1, we briefly introduce some basic concepts in bioinformatics specifically for gene, gene expression, and microarray. We use data derived from breast cancer patients in Section 12.2 to illustrate the application of `bioconductor` with a step-by-step approach. Concluding remarks appear in Section 12.3.

12.1 DNA Microarray

12.1.1 Introduction

DNA Microarray experiments are conducted in many areas of biomedical, biological, and biopharmaceutical research and development. Microarray techniques are applied to problems arising in gene discovery, diagnosis of disease, pharmacogenomics, and toxicogenomics among others. Gene discovery is the process of finding genes that are differentially expressed between patients with different diseases. When given reference gene expression profiles from diseased tissue and non-diseased tissue, diagnosis of an unknown tissue sample can be made by measuring its expression profile and comparing it with reference profiles.

Microarrays are designed to simultaneously measure expression levels of thousands of genes in a particular tissue or disease cell type. There are several different microarray technologies, including the cDNA arrays developed at Stanford and the high density oligonucleotide arrays produced by Affymetrix.

The Affymetrix GeneChip system is a commercial high-density oligonucleotide microarray platform which measures gene expression using hundreds of thousands of 25-mer oligonucleotide probes. This chapter serves as an introduction for microarray data analysis using `bioconductor` and we focus on data from the Affymetrix technology. Other microarray platforms can also be analyzed using `bioconductor`.

12.1.2   DNA, RNA, and Genes

We begin with some basic concepts in molecular biology such as DNA, RNA, and gene. The basic genetic material is known as *deoxyribonucleic acid* (DNA) which consists of nucleotides. Each nucleotide has three components: a base, a sugar, and a phosphate that are joined together to form long chains. The fundamental structure of these chains is formed by the sugar and phosphates with individual bases tied to each sugar. There are four different bases known as *adenine, cytosine, guanine*, and *thymine*. These are commonly denoted by the letters A, C, G, and T in molecular biology where the bases A and T bind together as do C and G. DNA strands have a typical length of millions of nucleotides. Each strand has polarities with the 5'-hydroxyl group at the beginning and 3'-hydroxyl group at the end of the nucleotide in the strand. A strand of DNA encloses many different genes with each gene containing a sequence of DNA to code a *protein*. The protein in turn controls a trait of the biological cell such as eye or hair color in humans.

Different from DNA, the *ribonucleic acid* (RNA) molecules are single-stranded with a length of only 75-5000 nucleotides. In addition, the base thymine (T) in DNA is replaced by *uracil* (U) in RNA and the sugar in RNA is ribose, rather than deoxyribose in DNA. There are several types of RNA in cells, such as messenger RNA (mRNA), transfer RNA (tRNA), and ribosomal RNA (rRNA).

12.1.3   Central Dogma of Molecular Biology

According to the central dogma in molecular biology, proteins are synthesized from DNA in two stages: transcription and translation. In the first stage, **transcription** transfers information from the double-stranded DNA molecule to the single-stranded RNA. The RNA polymerase moves from the 5' to the 3' direction along with the DNA strand to encode the complementary sequence as an RNA strand. This encoded DNA strand is called the "antisense" strand and the other is called the "sense" strand where the mRNA is complementary to the "antisense" strand and the base T is changed to U. Transcription begins at regions of the sequence known as "promoter sites" and ends at regions known as "terminator sites". Transcribed RNA molecules are edited and modified to produce messenger RNAs (mRNA).

In the second stage, **translation** mRNA is translated into a protein in the ribosome with the help of tRNA and rRNA. The tRNA molecules attach amino acids to the chain as a rRNA molecule moves along the mRNA. The process continues until one of the stop codons is reached. At this point, the protein is complete and can serve its purpose in the cell.

Gene expression in microarrays is then the process of converting a DNA sequence to a protein. For a particular organism, such as the human, the DNA content of cells is the same. However, the amount of mRNA and mRNA translated into proteins might differ among different types of cells or human cells under different disease conditions.

For example, consider two disease types A and B. If genes 1 and 2 in disease A are transcribed into mRNA and then translated into proteins, but only gene 2 in disease B is transcribed into mRNA and translated into protein and at a slower rate than in disease A, then we could conclude that gene 1 is expressed in disease A, but not in disease B, and that gene 2 is expressed at a slower rate in disease B than in disease A.

Microarray technology was developed to study different levels of gene expression under different diseases to learn the function of human cells that result in diseases. However, different from traditional technologies (such as RT-PCR and Northern blots) that study one gene at a time, microarray technology permits thousands of genes to be studied simultaneously. This leads to a new era in gene discovery, disease diagnosis, pharmacogenomics, and toxicogenomics, among others.

12.1.4 Probes, Probesets, Mismatch, and Perfectmatch

In the development of gene technology, many organisms have now been completely sequenced and others are currently being sequenced. Without the information of the whole genome, DNA microarrays can be designed based on expressed sequences. For each known sequence, a specific number of 25-mer sequences denoted by **probes** are chosen to complement the sequence for target genes. Typically 11 to 20 probes interrogate a given gene. This group of probes is usually called a **probeset** and there are between 12,000 to 22,000 probesets on one microarray. Usually, there are two types of probes: perfect match (PM) and mismatch (MM), where a PM probe complements exactly the sequence of interest and a MM probe complements the sequence of interest except at the central base. In theory, MM probes are used to quantify and remove non-specific hybridization. A PM probe and its corresponding MM probe are referred to as a probepair. PM and MM probe intensities for each probeset are combined to produce a summary value to be used for microarray statistical analysis.

12.1.5   Microarray and Statistical Analysis

The primary function of microarrays is to measure the amount of mRNA in thousands or more probes simultaneously to see which genes are being expressed in disease cell types. The primary measurements are the array intensities to be statistically analyzed to detect differences in gene expression for different disease types.

The associated statistical questions are focused on image analysis (for quality control), background noise correction, normalization among arrays, and detection of significantly expressed genes. Additional statistical questions arise in the design and planning of microarray experiments such as sample size, classification of microarray samples and genes, as well many others.

12.1.6   Software: R/Bioconductor

There are many software packages to analyze microarray data from Affymetrix. An early version of this package is called the "Affymetrix GeneChip Operating Software (GCOS)" which has been more or less updated and replaced by a newer software called Affymetrix GeneChip Command Console Software (AGCC) (http://www.affymetrix.com/). The most commonly used package associated with R is the bioconductor – considered as a gold standard in microarray data analysis. Since bioconductor is a package in the R system, it is therefore free. We illustrate the application of R/Bioconductor in this chapter.

The easiest way to download and install bioconductor from R is by typing:

```
> source("http://bioconductor.org/biocLite.R")
> biocLite()
```

The web browser will then link to the bioconductor homepage to download all necessary software.

12.2   Breast Cancer Data

Breast cancer (BRCA) is one of the most common cancers affecting women. The American Cancer Society estimates that there were 192,370 new cases of invasive breast cancer and 40,170 deaths from breast cancer in the United States in 2009 (http://www.cancer.org/).

BRCA can be both genetically and histopathologically heterogeneous with unknown underlying mechanisms. With the limitations of traditional treatments, recently developed microarray gene expression technology offers unprecedented opportunities to obtain molecular signatures from diseased cells and patients. In recent years, microarray technology has been utilized extensively to study molecular differences among different types of breast cancer and these differences have been successfully shown to relate to clinical features as commented in Chang et al. (2005) and Gruvberger-Saal et al. (2006).

A case in point is HER2-positive BRCA which is characterized by aggressive tumor growth. It is caused by the over-expression of the HER2/neu gene in tumor cells. Herceptin, a monoclonal antibody, manufactured by Genentech received FDA approval in late 2006 (`http://www.cancer.gov/cancertopics/druginfo/fda-trastuzumab`). It is administered to breast cancer patients whose cancer cells carry extra copies of the HER2/neu gene. Herceptin has been shown to dramatically slow the aggressive growth of HER2-positive BRCA and help women live longer (`http://www.cancer.org/`). Not only were microarray techniques used in the research and clinical development of Herceptin, they are used in determining which women diagnosed with BRCA are candidates for treatment with Herceptin.

Microarray technology allows for the simultaneous analysis of many thousands of individual genes from patient samples and makes it possible to study the complex biology of breast cancer in a more comprehensive manner. This has revolutionized basic biological sciences and hence biomedical and biopharmaceutical sciences.

12.2.1 Data Source

There are many publicly available datasets deposited in the National Center for Biotechnology Information (NCBI). Microarray gene expression data reside in the functional genomics data repository, called Gene Expression Omnibus (GEO), and is accessible via

$$\text{http://www.ncbi.nlm.nih.gov/geo/}$$

The GEO supports MIAME (Minimum Information About a Microarray Experiment)-compliant data submissions. The MIAME guidelines outline the minimum information that should be included when describing a microarray experiment. Many journals and funding agencies require microarray data to comply with MIAME. GEO deposited procedures enable and encourage submitters to supply MIAME compliant data. Further in GEO, tools are provided to help users query and download experiments and curated gene expression profiles. Additional information about the features and functionalities of GEO may be found by accessing the link:

$$\text{http://www.ncbi.nlm.nih.gov/geo/}$$

From the "GEO navigation" interface, we can use "Query" to search any dataset by key words, and "Browse" may be used to browse the entire GEO database. We searched for clinical trials of breast cancer by typing "breast cancer" and "clinical trial" and found eight accessions. The microarray sample names and their associated tumor types are seen from Table 12.1.

TABLE 12.1: Experimental Design and Data

Samples	Tumor Type	Samples	Tumor Type
GSM26878	apocrine	GSM26804	luminal
GSM26883	apocrine	GSM26867	luminal
GSM26886	apocrine	GSM26868	luminal
GSM26887	apocrine	GSM26869	luminal
GSM26903	apocrine	GSM26870	luminal
GSM26910	apocrine	GSM26872	luminal
GSM26871	basal	GSM26873	luminal
GSM26880	basal	GSM26874	luminal
GSM26882	basal	GSM26875	luminal
GSM26884	basal	GSM26876	luminal
GSM26888	basal	GSM26877	luminal
GSM26889	basal	GSM26879	luminal
GSM26892	basal	GSM26881	luminal
GSM26893	basal	GSM26885	luminal
GSM26895	basal	GSM26890	luminal
GSM26898	basal	GSM26891	luminal
GSM26900	basal	GSM26894	luminal
GSM26902	basal	GSM26896	luminal
GSM26905	basal	GSM26897	luminal
GSM26906	basal	GSM26899	luminal
GSM26908	basal	GSM26901	luminal
GSM26912	basal	GSM26904	luminal
		GSM26907	luminal
		GSM26909	luminal
		GSM26911	luminal
		GSM26913	luminal
		GSM26914	luminal

From this table, we note that there are 6 patients with apocrine, 16 patients with basal, and 27 patients with luminal tumor types.

For illustration, we use the first dataset available in the list, which has accession number GDS1329. These data derive from testing tumor samples obtained from 49 patients with large operable or locally advanced breast cancers using Affymetrix U133A gene expression microarrays [contributed by Farmer et al. (2005)]. Tumors were classified into luminal and basal classes, and a novel molecular apocrine class. Apocrine tumors are estrogen receptor negative (ER-) and androgen receptor positive (AR+), while luminal tumors are ER+ and AR+, and basal tumors are ER- and AR-. The 49 cel (i.e., file for measured intensities and locations for an array that has been hybridized) files may be downloaded from ftp://ftp.ncbi.nih.gov/pub/geo/

DATA/supplementary/series/GSE1561/, which is over 181 MB of data after zipping!

These zipped raw chip image files have to be unzipped; the unzipped files account for 573 MB of disk space. The data in these `cel` files represent the cell intensities to be used for microarray data analysis. This table can be loaded into R for future reference as follows:

```
> # Read the data into R
> dat = read.csv("BreastMicroarray.csv", header=T)
> # print it
> dat
```

```
   Samples    Tumor
1  GSM26878 apocrine
2  GSM26883 apocrine
3  GSM26886 apocrine
4  GSM26887 apocrine
5  GSM26903 apocrine
6  GSM26910 apocrine
7  GSM26871    basal
8  GSM26880    basal
9  GSM26882    basal
. . .
20 GSM26906    basal
21 GSM26908    basal
22 GSM26912    basal
23 GSM26804  luminal
24 GSM26867  luminal
25 GSM26868  luminal
. . . .
47 GSM26911  luminal
48 GSM26913  luminal
49 GSM26914  luminal
```

We note from the R output that there are 49 samples representing 49 patients with the corresponding tumor types.

There are usually two levels: low- and high-level of microarray data analysis. Their characterizations and distinctions are explained in the following subsections: Low-Level Data Analysis and High-Level Data Analysis.

12.2.2   Low-Level Data Analysis

12.2.2.1   Introduction

The low-level analysis of Affymetrix arrays involves the manipulation and modeling of probe intensity data. The goal of this analysis is to produce more biologically meaningful expression values. A motivation for low-level analysis is that information may be lost when moving from probe-level data to expression measures. Ideally, expression values should be both precise (low variance) and accurate (low bias). Obviously, these are desirable characteristics to permit determination of which genes are differentially expressed between treatment conditions – a primary goal of high-level analysis.

Other topics in low-level analysis include determining whether a gene is being expressed in a given tissue (presence/absence), as well as microarray quality assessment diagnostics.

A low-level analysis does not typically attempt to directly answer a question of biological interest; e.g., determining gene function; nor does it include more complex methods inherent in cell cycle studies and pathway analysis. Instead these are usually addressed by high-level analysis. As noted previously, a low-level analysis of the data should provide better expression measures to be used in higher-level analyses.

At the low-level, the most common operation is to convert probe level data to expression values. Typically, this is achieved through the following sequence:

- Reading in probe level data.

- Background correction.

- Normalization.

- Summarizing the probeset values into one expression measure and, in some cases, a standard error for this summary.

12.2.2.2   Library `affy`

In `bioconductor`, the low-level analysis is facilitated by the `affy` library. First, load the library into the R system:

```
> library(affy)
```

With the `affy` library, we read the breast cancer microarray data into R using function `ReadAffy`. This function is quite flexible and allows the user to specify the filenames, phenotype, and MIAME information. We make use of the data structure in Table 12.1 with `ReadAffy` to read the 573 MB *cel* intensity files from the 49 breast cancer patients as follows:

```
> # read the microarray cel files
> Dat = ReadAffy(filenames=paste(dat$Samples,".cel",sep=""))
```

To view the relevant information about these *cel* intensity files, we use `print` to print the `AffyBatch` object as:

```
> Dat
```

```
AffyBatch object
size of arrays=712x712 features (18 kb)
cdf=HG-U133A (22283 affyids)
number of samples=49
number of genes=22283
annotation=hgu133a
```

We note that the data object `Dat` consists of 49 samples (i.e., 49 patients) with microarray size 712×712 and with 22,283 genes in each sample. With this `Dat` object, we may observe further characteristics, such as the annotation:

```
> annotation(Dat)
```

```
[1] "hgu133a"
```

and description of the target samples hybridized to the arrays:

```
> phenoData(Dat)
```

```
An object of class "AnnotatedDataFrame"
  sampleNames: GSM26878.cel, GSM26883.cel, ..., GSM26
  914.cel  (49 total)
  varLabels and varMetadata description:
    sample: arbitrary numbering
```

Since the sample names are long, we change them into the tumor type for future analysis:

```
> # the original sample name
> sampleNames(Dat)
```

```
 [1] "GSM26878.cel" "GSM26883.cel" "GSM26886.cel"
 [4] "GSM26887.cel" "GSM26903.cel" "GSM26910.cel"
 [7] "GSM26871.cel" "GSM26880.cel" "GSM26882.cel"
[10] "GSM26884.cel" "GSM26888.cel" "GSM26889.cel"
[13] "GSM26892.cel" "GSM26893.cel" "GSM26895.cel"
[16] "GSM26898.cel" "GSM26900.cel" "GSM26902.cel"
[19] "GSM26905.cel" "GSM26906.cel" "GSM26908.cel"
[22] "GSM26912.cel" "GSM26804.cel" "GSM26867.cel"
[25] "GSM26868.cel" "GSM26869.cel" "GSM26870.cel"
[28] "GSM26872.cel" "GSM26873.cel" "GSM26874.cel"
[31] "GSM26875.cel" "GSM26876.cel" "GSM26877.cel"
[34] "GSM26879.cel" "GSM26881.cel" "GSM26885.cel"
[37] "GSM26890.cel" "GSM26891.cel" "GSM26894.cel"
[40] "GSM26896.cel" "GSM26897.cel" "GSM26899.cel"
[43] "GSM26901.cel" "GSM26904.cel" "GSM26907.cel"
```

```
[46] "GSM26909.cel" "GSM26911.cel" "GSM26913.cel"
[49] "GSM26914.cel"
```

```
> # change it to tumor type
> sample.names = dat$Tumor
> colnames(exprs(Dat)) = sample.names
```

The expression matrix should have columns corresponding to the numbers of arrays (49 in this example) and rows corresponding to the number of individual probes (which is $712 \times 712 = 506,944$ probes) on the array.

```
> e = exprs(Dat)
> dim(e)
```

```
[1] 506944    49
```

```
> nrow(Dat)*ncol(Dat)
```

```
[1] 506944
```

Note that the values in the array are the raw values for the probe expression in the *cel* files. We can also identify the gene names using the R function *geneNames()*. We only print the first 20 of the 22,283 genes for illustration purposes:

```
> # gene numbers
> gnames = geneNames(Dat)
> # the total number of genes
> length(gnames)
```

```
[1] 22283
```

```
> # print the first 20 genes
> gnames[1:20]
```

```
 [1] "1007_s_at" "1053_at"   "117_at"    "121_at"
 [5] "1255_g_at" "1294_at"   "1316_at"   "1320_at"
 [9] "1405_i_at" "1431_at"   "1438_at"   "1487_at"
[13] "1494_f_at" "1598_g_at" "160020_at" "1729_at"
[17] "177_at"    "1773_at"   "179_at"    "1861_at"
```

The length of *gnames* is 22,283 indicating that there are that many probesets on the chip.

12.2.2.3 Quality Control

After reading the data into R, quality control checks of the data should be conducted. First create an image plot:

1. **Image plot**, Image plot looks at the chips' image using `image(Dat)` to detect spatial artifacts. This can be done using the function `image` from the `affy` library. We do not show the output here because of its exceedingly large file size.

2. **Distribution plots for intensities**.

   Now several plots can be generated to provide information about the intensity distribution, such as histograms or boxplots. We show the boxplots for the 49 patients in Figure 12.1 using following R code chunk:

```
> # call "boxplot" to plot the data
> boxplot(Dat,col=c(rep("Green",6),rep("Blue",16),
                     rep("red",27)))
```

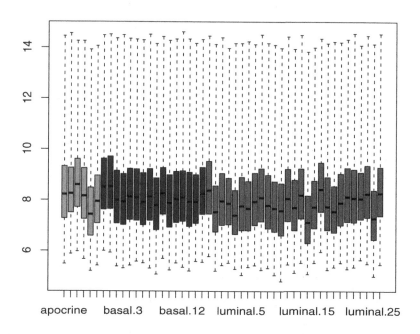

FIGURE 12.1: Boxplot for Original Expression Data

In Figure 12.1 generated with `boxplot`, the boxplot for each patient appears vertically. We note that the first 6 are for the patients with apocrine tumor, the middle 16 are for patients with basal tumor, and the last 27 are for patients with luminal tumor. In this figure, the line in the center of each patient's boxplot represents the median, and the boxes show the range of the middle 50% of the expression data. The additional lines reflect the overall range of the data, and the extreme values are depicted as individual lines or dots at the end of each boxplot. We note from the boxplots in Figure 12.1 that the gene expression intensity data are not normalized.

3. **MA-plot**. Another plot that has become widely used in microarray analysis is the MA-plot. It has been applied routinely as a part of a number of normalization procedures. MA-plots are typically used to compare two arrays or two groups of arrays. In a MA-plot, the vertical axis is the difference between the logarithms of the signals (i.e., the log ratio) and the horizontal axis is the average of the logarithms of the signals; "M" denotes minus and "A" denotes average.

In constructing a MA-plot, let X_{ij} be the intensity of gene g on array i. To compare two arrays i and j, the M and A values are computed by:

$$
\begin{aligned}
M_g &= log2(X_{gi}) - log2(X_{gj}) \\
A_g &= \frac{log2(X_{gi}) + log2(X_{gj})}{2}
\end{aligned}
$$

Parenthetically, the base 2 logarithm is used for convenience in microarray analysis so that a unit change in M represents 2 fold-change in expression, and a unit change in A represents a doubling of brightness. Because the probe-intensities are measured using a 16 bit image, the maximum possible value of A is 16.

For illustration, we compare an array from the first patient with apocrine tumor type with an array from the first patient with basal tumor type. This would be a huge file if we plotted all array pairs. We plot the two arrays using a MA-plot which gives Figure 12.2.

```
> # call "MAplot" to make the plot
> MAplot(Dat[,c(1,8)], pair=T)
```

While there is a visible difference between the two arrays of the two patients, a trend is not apparent. Since there are more probes with low intensities than probes with high intensities, the log transformation allows us to more easily assess the behavior across all intensities.

The MA-plot makes the relationship between the arrays much easier to visually assess.

We use MA-plots to compare the performance of various methods of

MVA plot

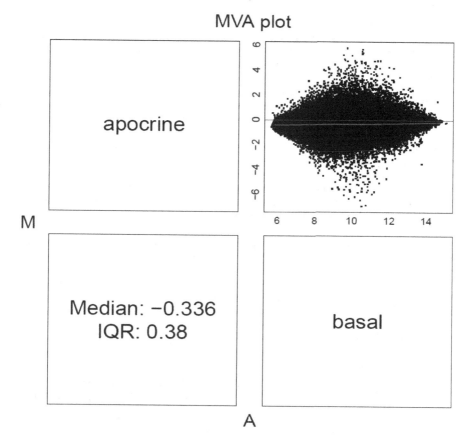

FIGURE 12.2: MA Plot for Two Arrays

computing expression measures. For non-differentially expressed probe-sets, ideally the MA-plot will be tight around $M = 0$ across all intensities. A lowess curve fitted to an MA-plot shows whether the M values are centered around 0 at each intensity value. The spread of the point cloud around the lowess curve allows us to measure the variability.

4. **Conclusion.** The boxplot and the MA-plot show that the object `Dat` needs normalization. Arrays that should be the same are different. Arrays that should be different are similar.

12.2.2.4 Background, Normalization, and Summarization

Following the low-level explorations in the previous section, the next step is to correct background noise, normalize, and summarize the probes' intensity data into gene expression values. There are several methods. The first one is *MAS5* which was developed by Affymetrix. The most commonly used, more robust and efficient method, is the "Robust Multi-array Average" (RMA) developed by Irizarry et al. (2003) where the expression measure can be computed as:

```
> # call RMA function
> eset = rma(Dat)

Background correcting
Normalizing
Calculating Expression
```

The rma is a code in C language which made the process extremely efficient and fast. As pointed in the manual, the rma function will process the expression data in the following fashion:

1. Probe specific correction of the PM probes using a model based on observed intensity being the sum of signal and noise.

2. Normalization of corrected PM probes using quantile normalization developed by Bolstad et al. (2003).

3. Calculation of expression measure using median polish.

Specifically, as in the affy manual, rma is implemented as:

1. **Background adjustment** to adjust raw PM probe intensities using a model based on observed intensity being the sum of signal and noise. The term "background correction", also referred to as "signal adjustment", describes a wide variety of methods. In addition, a background correction method performs some or all of the following:

   - Corrects for background noise and processing effects.

   - Adjusts for cross-hybridization which is the binding of non-specific DNA (i.e., non-complementary binding) to the array.

   - Adjusts expression estimates so that they fall on the proper scale, or are linearly related to concentration.

   The rma background correction is motivated by looking at the distribution of probe intensities. The observed intensity is modeled as the sum of a signal and a background component as $S = X + Y$, where X is signal and Y is background. Assume that X is distributed $exp(\alpha)$ and that Y is distributed $N(\mu, \sigma^2)$, with X and Y independent. Under this model, the background corrected intensities are $E(X|S = s)$.

2. **Quantile Normalization**. Normalization is the process of removing unwanted non-biological variation that might exist between chips in a microarray experiment. It has long been recognized that variability can exist between arrays, some of which are of biological interest and the

other of non-biological interest. These two types of variation are classified as either interesting or obscuring. The aim in normalizing arrays is to remove the obscuring variation. Sources of obscuring variation can include scanner setting differences, the quantities of mRNA hybridized, as well as many other factors.

The goal of quantile normalization is to give the same empirical distribution of intensities to each array. If two data vectors have the same distribution, a quantile-quantile plot will have a straight diagonal line with slope 1 and intercept 0. Thus, if the quantiles of two data vectors are plotted against each other and each of these points is then projected onto the 45-degree diagonal line, we have a transformation that gives the same distribution to both data vectors.

In summary, the aim of quantile normalization (Bolstad et al., 2003) of corrected PM probes is

- to make distribution of probe intensities the same for every chip, and

- to average each quantile across chips.

3. **Summarization.** This is the final step in the production of summary gene expression measures from probe intensities using median polish; i.e., use the multi-chip linear model:

$$y_{ij}^g = log_2\left(PM_{ij}^g\right) = \alpha_i^g + \beta_j^g + \epsilon_{ij}^g \tag{12.1}$$

where g denotes the probeset (or gene), and α_i^g is the probe effect and β_j^g is the log2 expression value. The median polish uses an algorithm from Tukey (1977) to fit the model robustly. Note that expression values from this method will be in the log2 scale.

After the `rma`, we can check the dimension of the expression sets (eset) and some of the gene expression values using the following R code chunk:

```
> # dimension
> dim(exprs(eset))

[1] 22283    49

> # print the first 20 genes for three patients
> exprs(eset)[1:20,1:3]
```

	GSM26878.cel	GSM26883.cel	GSM26886.cel
1007_s_at	11.29	11.04	11.02
1053_at	7.79	8.01	7.87
117_at	7.49	7.53	7.44

121_at	9.59	9.52	9.61
1255_g_at	5.00	5.13	4.95
1294_at	8.36	8.40	8.26
1316_at	7.19	6.65	6.45
1320_at	5.65	5.77	5.77
1405_i_at	7.14	7.49	7.38
1431_at	4.70	4.72	4.80
1438_at	7.43	8.11	7.58
1487_at	8.65	8.54	8.75
1494_f_at	7.50	7.68	7.66
1598_g_at	10.32	10.93	10.50
160020_at	8.53	8.74	8.62
1729_at	9.11	8.77	8.73
177_at	6.54	6.45	6.52
1773_at	6.22	6.44	6.17
179_at	9.91	9.88	9.76
1861_at	6.59	7.03	6.37

We see that the dimension of this object is 22,283 by 49, which means that there are 22283 genes from 49 patients. For brevity, we print only the first 20 genes from the first three patients in the above R code.

Following the *rma* procedure, diagnostic plots, such as the **image** plot, **hist** for histograms and **boxplot** for boxplots may be produced to permit a visual assessment of the normalized and background corrected summary gene expression data. For brevity, we only illustrate use of the boxplot with the following code chunk:

```
> # boxplot after RMA
> boxplot(data.frame(exprs(eset)),
    col=c(rep("Green",6),rep("Blue",16), rep("red",27)))
```

Figure 12.3 contains the boxplots for the 49 patients, and shows that all distributions are normalized after background correction.

12.2.3   High-Level Analysis

The primary aim of high-level microarray analysis is to find genes that are differentially expressed. Discovering genes that are differentially expressed between two groups (tumor, tissue, or disease types) may be the most common motivation for microarray experiments. We begin to describe the attendant statistical methods.

The typical naive microarray analysis is a simple fold-change to

1. calculate the average expression for each population and take the difference; i.e., in microarray terms, the fold-change;

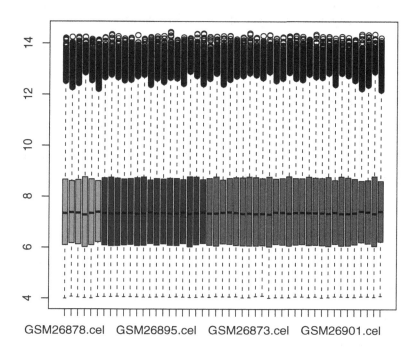

GSM26878.cel GSM26895.cel GSM26873.cel GSM26901.cel

FIGURE 12.3: Boxplot after RMA

2. rank the genes based on the fold-change;

3. select a cut-off point which is entirely up to the researcher, but typically chosen to pick up changes that are at least 2-fold; and

4. output those genes with fold-changes larger than the cut-off point.

Problems with this approach are

1. the simple differences in average log expressions do not include any information about variation;

2. one does not know whether the observed differences are small or large unless they are compared to other factors; and

3. the fold-change approach does not enable one to determine whether genes have different variances.

These problems may lead to erroneous conclusions regarding which genes are differentially expressed.

Therefore, additional and more appropriate statistical methods are needed to perform high-level analyses of microarray data. The limma package in bioconductor was developed for this purpose by Smyth (2004). We briefly describe this approach for a two-group (tumor, tissue, or disease type) comparison. Details may be found in referenced Smyth's paper.

12.2.3.1   Statistical t-test

First, we review some relevant statistical terms for comparisons in a two-group microarray experiment.

For each gene with samples $X_1, \cdots, X_m$ from one group, such as control, and $Y_1, \cdots, Y_n$ from another group, such as treated, we have

- Averages: $\bar{X} = \frac{\sum_{i=1}^{m} X_i}{m}$ and $\bar{Y} = \frac{\sum_{i=1}^{n} Y_i}{n}$

- Sample variance: $s_X^2 = \frac{\sum_{i=1}^{m}(X_i - \bar{X})^2}{m-1}$ and $s_Y^2 = \frac{\sum_{i=1}^{n}(Y_i - \bar{Y})^2}{n-1}$

- t-test statistic: $t = \frac{\bar{Y} - \bar{X}}{s_{\bar{Y} - \bar{X}}} = \frac{\bar{Y} - \bar{X}}{\sqrt{\frac{s_Y^2}{n} + \frac{s_X^2}{m}}}$ where s is the pooled sample

  standard error.

Then

1. Usual t-test with false discovery rate.

   Now rank the genes based on the values t of the t-test statistic or based on the corresponding p-values (which are most often used). Recall that a p-value, also called the *observed significance level*, is defined as the probability of realizing the value of the t-test statistic or one more extreme under the null hypothesis H_0 of no differential expression. One may also think of a p-value as a measure of the strength of evidence against the null hypotheses. The smaller the p-value, the more evidence we have against H_0 and the greater the departure.

   The p-value is associated with the Type-I error (i.e., the significance level α) in testing some null hypothesis. A Type-I decision error occurs if the null hypothesis is rejected when it is actually true. The Type-I error is also called a false-positive error and its magnitude is usually denoted by α (which is sometimes referred to as a rate). It is desirable that α is chosen to be small. If $\alpha = 0.05$ and if $p \leq \alpha$, we reject the H_0 of no differential expression. This means that we have a 5% probability of concluding that genes are significantly differentially expressed even when they are not. This level of control of the false positive rate is fine when conducting a test of a single null hypothesis for a single comparison.

   However, if one applies this type of testing to microarray analyses where thousands or even tens of thousands of genes are being compared, a

5% false positive rate could translate to hundreds or thousands of false-positive differentially expressed genes and lead to reporting hundreds or thousands of falsely discovered genes.

So we need statistical methods for controlling false discovery rates; e.g., as in Benjamini and Hochberg (1995).

2. Moderated t-test.

   In a typical microarray experiment, the sample sizes m and n are small. Thus the standard error in t-statistical $t = \frac{\bar{Y} - \bar{X}}{s}$ is very unstable leading to an unstable statistical t-test.

   Many methods have been developed that borrow strength across genes to increase the stability of variance estimates; e.g., the *moderated t-test* which is defined as:

$$t_g = \frac{\bar{Y}_g - \bar{X}_g}{\tilde{s}_g} \qquad (12.2)$$

   for each gene g where $\bar{Y}_g$ = mean of the group 1 samples, $\bar{X}_g$ = mean of the group 2 samples and $\tilde{s}_g$ = posterior standard deviation for gene g from the empirical Bayesian approach defined in Smyth (2004) as $\tilde{s}_g = \frac{d_0 s_0^2 + d_g S_g^2}{d_0 + d_g}$ where d_g and s_g^2 are from each gene g, but d_0 and s_0^2 are from the prior distribution estimated by the empirical Bayes approach. This approach is implemented in `limma` as function `ebayes`.

3. Linear Models for Microarray Analysis (LIMMA).

   The moderate t-test with Empirical Bayes approach for several experimental designs are now in LIMMA. We load `limma` into R as follows:

   ```
   > library(limma)
   ```

12.2.3.2 Model Fitting

We now consider investigating differential expression among the three tumor types: apocrine, basal, and luminal from the GEO dataset `GDS1329` found in Table 12.1. First, we specify the design matrix using the following R code chunk:

```
> # make the design matrix
> design <- model.matrix(~ 0+factor(c(rep("apocrine",6),
       rep("basal",16), rep("luminal",27))))
> # label the design
> colnames(design) <- c("apocrine", "basal", "luminal")
> # print the design
> design
```

	apocrine	basal	luminal
1	1	0	0
2	1	0	0
3	1	0	0
4	1	0	0
5	1	0	0
6	1	0	0
7	0	1	0
8	0	1	0
9	0	1	0
10	0	1	0
11	0	1	0
12	0	1	0
13	0	1	0
14	0	1	0
15	0	1	0
16	0	1	0
17	0	1	0
18	0	1	0
19	0	1	0
20	0	1	0
21	0	1	0
22	0	1	0
23	0	0	1
24	0	0	1
25	0	0	1
26	0	0	1
27	0	0	1
28	0	0	1
29	0	0	1
30	0	0	1
31	0	0	1
32	0	0	1
33	0	0	1
34	0	0	1
35	0	0	1
36	0	0	1
37	0	0	1
38	0	0	1
39	0	0	1
40	0	0	1
41	0	0	1
42	0	0	1
43	0	0	1
44	0	0	1

```
45         0     0      1
46         0     0      1
47         0     0      1
48         0     0      1
49         0     0      1
attr(,"assign")
[1] 1 1 1
attr(,"contrasts")
attr(,"contrasts")$`factor(c(rep("apocrine", 6),
      rep("basal", 16), rep("luminal", 27)))`
[1] "contr.treatment"
```

The design matrix is 49 by 3 where "1" corresponds to the available tumor samples. With this design matrix, we fit a linear model. Based on the model fit, we construct a contrast for pair-wise comparisons of different gene expressions by calling ebayes to borrow information from all genes using the empirical Bayesian model as follows:

```
> # fit the linear model for all genes
> fit = lmFit(eset, design)
> # make a contrast for pair-wise comparisons
> cont.matrix = makeContrasts(Comp2to1=basal-apocrine,
  Comp3to1=luminal-apocrine,Comp3to2=luminal-basal,levels=design)
> # then contrast fit
> fit2 = contrasts.fit(fit, cont.matrix)
> # then call ebayes
> fit2 = eBayes(fit2)
```

After fitting the model, we may observe the ranking of the genes with the function of topTable as follows:

```
> options(digits=3)
> topTable(fit2, coef=1, adjust="BH")
```

	ID logFC	AveExpr	t	P.Value	dj.P.Val	B
214243_s_at	-5.33	8.02	-11.33	3.68e-15	8.19e-11	23.9
204667_at	-2.56	8.71	-10.97	1.14e-14	8.90e-11	22.9
217284_x_at	-4.41	8.17	-10.95	1.20e-14	8.90e-11	22.8
217276_x_at	-4.28	8.16	-10.74	2.39e-14	1.33e-10	22.2
209787_s_at	1.86	10.04	10.17	1.48e-13	6.59e-10	20.5
202579_x_at	1.18	10.29	9.80	4.96e-13	1.65e-09	19.3
214404_x_at	-1.56	9.26	-9.79	5.17e-13	1.65e-09	19.3
206155_at	-1.11	6.16	-9.59	1.00e-12	2.79e-09	18.7
209616_s_at	-1.88	7.65	-9.47	1.48e-12	3.67e-09	18.3
209786_at	1.98	10.07	9.43	1.68e-12	3.74e-09	18.2

The default for `topTable` prints the first 10 genes and the input `coef=1` specifies the first contrast for comparing the "basal" and "apocrine" tumor types. The same can be done for the other two comparisons using `coef=2` and 3. The `adjust="BH"` provides adjustment for multiple comparisons as explained below.

Some explanations for the output from fitting the model are

1. **ID** is the gene IDs.

2. **logFC** is the log2 fold-change, i.e., the M-value. Positive M-values mean that the gene is up-regulated and negative values mean that it is down-regulated.

3. **AveExpr** is the average log2-intensity value for the probeset; i.e., the A value.

4. **t** is the value for the moderated *t*-statistic.

5. **P.Value** is the associated *p*-value from the moderate t-statistic.

6. **adj.P.Val** is the adjusted *p*-value (adjusted for multiple testing).

   The most popular adjustment is the "BH" by Benjamini and Hochberg (1995) to control the false discovery rate. This adjusted *p*-value is called "*q*-value" in microarray analysis if the intention is to control or estimate the false discovery rate.

   The meaning of "BH" *q*-values is as follows. If all genes with *q*-value below a threshold, say 0.05, are selected as differentially expressed, then the expected proportion of false discoveries in the selected group is controlled to be less than the threshold value, in this case 5%. This procedure is equivalent to the procedure of Benjamini and Hochberg, although the original paper did not formulate the method in terms of adjusted *p*-values.

7. **B** is the *B*-statistic which is the log-odds that the gene is differentially expressed.

   Suppose, for example, that $B = 1.5$. The odds of differential expression is $\exp(1.5) = 4.48$; i.e., about four and a half to one. The probability that the gene is differentially expressed is $4.48/(1+4.48)=0.82$; i.e., the probability is about 82% that this gene is differentially expressed. A *B*-statistic of zero corresponds to a 50-50 chance that the gene is differentially expressed. The *p*-values and *B*-statistics will normally rank genes in the same order. In fact, if the data contains no missing values or quality weights, the order will be exactly the same.

The *p* or *B*-values can reveal statistical significance, but say nothing about the size of an effect. The commonly used fold-change reveals the magnitude of the differential expression but not significance. A combined illustration to put both together is called a "volcano plot" `Volcano Plots`, as shown in Figure 12.4.

```
> # Call the "volcanoplot"
> volcanoplot(fit2,coef=2, highlight=10)
> # Add the vertical reference lines
> abline(v=c(-1,1),col="red")
> # add the horizontal reference line
> ilogit = function(p) exp(p)/(1+exp(p))
> abline(h=ilogit(0.05), col="blue")
```

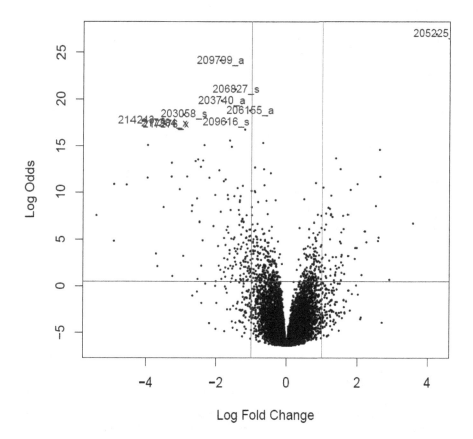

FIGURE 12.4: Volcano Plot for Gene Expression Data

In this figure, the two vertical lines denote the two-fold (on log 2 scale) changes with points outside the two vertical lines representing those genes that have more than two-fold changes in gene expressions. More specifically, the points above the right vertical line reflect those genes with positive two-fold changes and the points below the left vertical line represent negative two-fold changes. The horizontal line represents 5% q-values in log odds scale which means that those points above this line reflect genes that are statistically significantly expressed. The intersection of the q-value and two-fold change represents those genes of interest and can be pinpointed to export for further bioinformatics analysis.

12.2.3.3 Number of Significantly Expressed Genes

The output from `topTable` can show the significantly expressed genes from each comparison. This list can be quite long. Another way to display all three contrasts is to use a Venn diagram to show the number of genes in different categories.

To do so, we first call the `decisionTests` which is a function used for multiple testing across genes and contrasts in order to classify a series of related t-statistics as up, down, or not significant while adjusting for multiple testing. The following code chunk illustrates how this is done:

```
> # call decideTests function
> results = decideTests(fit2)
> # classification counts in a Venn diagram
> venn     = vennCounts(results)
> # print the venn table
> print(venn)
```

	Comp2to1	Comp3to1	Comp3to2	Counts
[1,]	0	0	0	15970
[2,]	0	0	1	2894
[3,]	0	1	0	298
[4,]	0	1	1	427
[5,]	1	0	0	596
[6,]	1	0	1	1334
[7,]	1	1	0	612
[8,]	1	1	1	152

```
attr(,"class")
[1] "VennCounts"
```

The Venn counts may be graphically displayed using `vennDiagram` as follows to produce Figure 12.5. Those genes of interest may be saved or outputted for further bioinformatics analysis, such as gene function analysis.

```
> # call "vennDiagram" to plot the Venn-Diagram
> vennDiagram(results,include=c("up","down"),
                counts.col=c("red","green"))
```

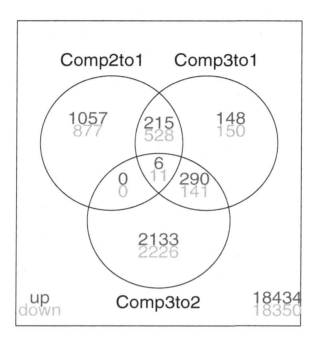

FIGURE 12.5: Venn Diagram

12.2.4 Functional Analysis of Gene Lists

When genes are identified, the next step is to analyze them for their functions. Readers are referred to

http://david.abcc.ncifcrf.gov/

which provides bioinformatics resources and tools for functional annotation and classification, etc.

12.3 Concluding Remarks

In this chapter, we briefly presented analysis of microarray data using bioconductor. In summary, for any microarray data analysis, the first step is to load the trial data into `bioconductor` and make preliminary pre-processing using low-level analysis methods to correct background noise and to normalize the array distributions using `rma`. We can then proceed with high-level analyses to identify significantly expressed gene lists for further bioinformatics analysis.

Other analyses not presented in this chapter include hierarchical cluster analysis and heatmap displays. We refer readers to the 2010 special issue of the *Journal of Biopharmaceutical Statistics*, Volume 20, Number 2, where extensive discussions on new methodologies appear for gene expression analysis, pharmacogenetics, systems biology, and predictive models, as well as linkage disequilibrium analysis and QTL mapping.

Further references may be found in the collection of papers on gene expression data analyses in the book by Parmigiani et al. (2003). The book by Gentleman et al. (2005) compiles an extensive list of papers in using R and `bioconductor` for bioinformatics and computational biology. The books by Hahne et al. (2008) and Gentleman (2008) use R and `bioconductor` for bioinformatics and include case studies for easy applications of newly developed methods. Other references and online documents can be found from the homepage of the `bioconductor` project at `http://www.bioconductor.org` which provides open source software for bioinformatics. For microarray design and sample size, readers are referred to Chapter 12 in Chow et al. (2008).

12.4   Appendix: SAS Programs

There is some SAS development for microarray gene expression data analysis. An SAS experimental procedure `proc HPMIXED` can be used to analyze microarray expression data to specify a linear mixed model with variance component structure. Then, this SAS procedure can estimate the covariance parameters by restricted maximum likelihood, and perform confirmatory inference. The details for this SAS procedure can be found at `https://support.sas.com/documentation/cdl/en/statug/63033/HTML/default/viewer.htm#hpmixed_toc.htm`. Example SAS programs can be found from `https://support.sas.com/documentation/cdl/en/statug/63033/HTML/default/viewer.htm#statug_hpmixed_sect035.htm`.

To analyze microarray gene expression data to identify significantly differentiated genes, the data should be first pre-processed. Drs. Don Li and Lei Qin from Queen's University summarized the data pre-processing using SAS macros in an online document from `http://www.lexjansen.com/pharmasug/2005/posters/po34.pdf`.

Based on our experience, we highly recommend using R Bioconductor from `http://www.bioconductor.org` described in this chapter for microarray data analysis.

Bibliography

Agresti, A. (2002). *Categorical Data Analysis, 2nd Edition*. Hoboken, NJ, USA: John Wiley & Sons Inc.

Albert, J. (2007). *Bayesian Computation with R*. New York, USA: Springer.

Alosh, M. and M. F. Huque (2009). A flexible strategy for testing subgroups and overall population. *Statistics in Medicine 28(1)*, 3–23.

Anderson, T. W. (1994). *An Introduction to Multivariate Statistical Analysis*. Wiley.

Begg, C. B. and M. Mazumdar (1994). Operating characteristics of a rank correlation test for publication bias. *Biometrics 50*, 1088–1101.

Benjamini, Y. and Y. Hochberg (1995). Controlling the false discovery rate: a practical and powerful approach to multiple testing. *Journal of the Royal Statistical Society. Series B 57*, 289–300.

Berry, S. M., B. P. Carlin, J. J. Lee, and P. Muller (2010). *Bayesian Adaptive Methods for Clinical Trials*. Chapman & Hall/CRC Biostatistics Series.

Besag, J. and P. D. Clifford (1991). Sequential monte carlo p-values. *Biometrika 78*, 301–304.

Bock, J. (1998). Bestimmung des stichprobenumfangs fuer biologische experimente und kontrollierte klinische studien. *Wien: Oldenbourg*.

Bolstad, B. M., R. A. Irizarry, M. Astrand, and T. P. Speed (2003). A comparison of normalization methods for high density oligonucleotide array data based on variance and bias. *Bioinformatics 19(2)*, 185–193.

Chalmers, T. C. (1987). Meta-analysis in clinical medicine. *Transactions of the American Clinical and Climatological Association. 99*, 144–150.

Chalmers, T. C., J. Berrier, H. S. Sacks, H. Levin, D. E. Reitman, and R. Nagalingam (1987a). Meta-Analysis of Clinical Trials as a scientific discipline: I. Control of bias and comparison with large cooperative trials. *Statistics in Medicine. 6(3)*, 315–328.

Chalmers, T. C., J. Berrier, H. S. Sacks, H. Levin, D. E. Reitman, and R. Nagalingam (1987b). Meta-Analysis of Clinical Trials as a scientific discipline: I. Replicate variability and comparison of studies that agree and disagree. *Statistics in Medicine. 6(3)*, 733–744.

Chalmers, T. C., H. Smith, B. Blackburn, B. Silverman, B. Schroeder, D. Reitman, and A. Ambroz (1981). A method for assessing the quality of a randomized control trial. *Controlled Clinical Trials 2*, 31–49.

Chambers, J. M. (1998). *Programming with Data*. New York, USA: Springer.

Chambers, J. M. (2008). *Software for Data Analysis: Programming with R*. New York, USA: Springer.

Chang, J. C., S. G. Hilsenbeck, and S. A. Fuqua (2005). The promise of microarrays in the management and treatment of breast cancer. *Breast Cancer Research. 7(3)*, 100–104.

Chen, D. G. and Y. Lio (2010). Parameter estimations for generalized exponential distribution under progressive type-i interval censoring. *Computation Statistics and Data Analysis. 54(6)*, 1581–1591.

Chen, D. G. and K. E. Peace (2013). *Applied Meta-analysis with R*. Chapman & Hall/CRC: Biostatistics Series. Boca Raton, FL.

Chen, D. G., J. Sun, and K. E. Peace (2012). *Interval-censored Time-to-Event Data: Methods and Applications*. Chapman & Hall/CRC: Biostatistics Series. Boca Raton, FL.

Chen, M.-H. and S. Kim (2009). Cure Rate Models with Application to Melanoma and Prostate Cancer Data. In *Design and Analysis of Clinical Trials with Time-to-Event Endpoints (Peace, KE Editor)*, pp. 349–370. Chapman & Hall/ Biostatistics Series/ Taylor & Francis, Boca Raton.

Chow, S. C. and J. P. Liu (2009). *Design and Analysis of Bioavailability and Bioequivalence Studies*. Chapman & Hall/CRC. Third Edition.

Chow, S. C., J. Shao, and H. S. Wanf (2008). *Sample Size Calculations in Clinical Research*. Chapman & Hall/CRC. Second Edition.

Cochran, W. G. (1937). Problems arising in the analysis of a series of similar experiments. *Journal of the Royal Statistical Society 4*, 102–119.

Cochran, W. G. (1943). The comparison of different scales of measurement for experimental results. *Annals of Mathematical Statistics 14*, 205–216.

Cochran, W. G. (1954). The combination of estimates from different experiments. *Biometrics*, 101–129.

Cohen, J. (1988). *Statistical power analysis for the behavioral sciences (2nd ed.)*. Hillsdale, NJ: Lawrence Erlbaum.

Collett, D. (2003). *Modeling Survival data in Medical Research, Second Edition.* Chapman & Hall/ CRC.

Connor, J. T. and S. M. Berry (2005). Bayesian analysis for medical device trials. *The American Journal of Gastroenterology 100*, 1732–1735.

Cook, J. D. (2005). Exact calculation of beta inequalities. *Technical Report UTMDABTR-005-05.*

Cox, D. R. (1972). Regression models and life-tables. *Journal of Royal Statistical Society, Series B 34*, 187–202, with discussion.

Cox, D. R. (1975). Partial likelihood. *Biometrika 62(2)*, 269–276.

DerSimonian, R. and N. Laird (1986). Meta-analysis in clinical trials. *Controlled Clinical Trials 7*, 177–188.

Draper, N. R. and H. Smith (1998). *Applied Regression Analysis, Third Edition.* John Wiley & Sons Inc.

Duncan, D. B. (1957). Multiple range tests for correlated and heteroscedastic means. *Biometrics 13(2)*, 164–176.

Everitt, B. and T. Hothorn (2006). *A Handbook of Statistical Analyses Using R.* Boca Raton, FL: Chapman & Hall/CRC.

Faraway, J. J. (2004). *Linear Models with R.* Boca Raton, FL: Chapman & Hall/CRC.

Faraway, J. J. (2006). *Extending Linear Models with R: Generalized Linear, Mixed Effects and Nonparametric Regression Models.* Boca Raton, FL: Chapman & Hall/CRC.

Farmer, P., H. Bonnefoi, V. Becette, M. Tubiana-Hulin, P. Fumoleau, D. Larsimont, G. Macgrogan, J. Bergh, D. Cameron, D. Goldstein, S. Duss, A. Nicoulaz, C. Brisken, M. Fiche, M. Delorenzi, and R. Iggo (2005). Identification of molecular apocrine breast tumours by microarray analysis. *Oncogene 24(29)*, 4660–4671.

Farrington, C. and G. Manning (1990). Test statistics and sample size formulae for comparative binomial trials with null hypothesis of non-zero risk difference or non-unity relative risk. *Statistics in Medicine 9*, 1447–1454.

Fay, M. P. and P. A. Shaw (2010). Exact and asymptotic weighted logrank tests for interval censored data: The interval R package. *Journal of Statistical Software 36(2)*, 1–34.

Finkelstein, D. M. (1986). A proportional hazard model for interval-censored failure time data. *Biometrics 42*, 845–854.

Fitzmaurice, G. M., N. M. Laird, and J. H. Ware (2004). *Applied Longitudinal Analysis*. John Wiley & Sons, Inc.

Gelfand, A. E. and A. F. M. Smith (1990). Sampling based approaches to calculating marginal densities. *Journal of the American Statistical Association*. *85*, 398–409.

Gelman, A., J. B. Carlin, H. S. Stern, and D. B. Rubin (2009). *Bayesian Data Analysis, Second Edition*. Chapman & Hall/CRC.

Geman, S. and D. Geman (1984). Stochastic relaxation, gibbs distribution and the bayesian restoration of images. *IEEE Transactions on Pattern Analysis and Machine Intelligence 6*, 721–741.

Gentleman, R. (2008). *R Programming for Bioinformatics*. Chapman & Hall/CRC Press.

Gentleman, R., V. J. Carey, W. Huber, R. A. Irizarry, and S. Dudoit (2005). *Bioinformatics and Computational Biology Solutions Using R and Bioconduction*. Springer.

Giardiello, F. M., S. R. Hamilton, A. J. Krush, S. Piantadosi, L. M. Hylind, P. Celano, S. V. Booker, C. R. Robinson, and G. J. A. Offerhaus (1993). Treatment of colonic and rectal adenomas with sulindac in familial adenomatous polyposis. *New England Journal of Medicine 328*, 1313–1316.

Giles, F. J., H. M. Kantarjian, J. E. Cortes, G. Garcia-Manero, S. Verstovsek, S. Faderl, D. A. Thomas, A. Ferrajoli, S. O'Brien, J. K. Wathen, L.-C. Xiao, D. A. Berry, and E. H. Estey (2003). Adaptive randomized study of idarubicin and cytarabine versus rroxacitabine and cytarabine versus troxacitabine and idarubicin in untreated patients 50 years or older with adverse karyotype acute myeloid leukemia. *Journal of Clinical Oncology*. *21*, 1722–1727.

Gruvberger-Saal, S. K., H. E. Cunliffe, K. M. Carr, and I. A. Hedenfalk (2006). Microarrays in breast cancer research and clinical practice-the future lies ahead. *Endocrine-Related Cancer*. *13*, 1017–1031.

Hahne, F., R. Huber, W. Gentleman, and S. Falcon (2008). *Bioconductor Case Studies*. Springer.

Hand, D. J. and C. C. Taylor (1987). *Multivariate Analysis of Variance and Repeated Measures*. Chapman & Hall.

Hardin, J. and J. Hilbe (2003). *Generalized Estimating Equation*. Boca Raton, FL: Chapman & Hall/CRC Press.

Hartung, J., G. Knapp, and B. K. Sinha (2008). *Statistical Meta-Analysis with Applications*. John Wiley & Sons, Inc.: Hoboken, New Jersey.

Hastings, W. K. (1970). Monte carlo sampling methods using markov chains and their applications. *Biometrika 57*, 977–1109.

Hedges, L. V. and I. Olkin (1985). *Statistical Methods for Meta-Analysis*. Academic Press, Inc.

Herson, J. (2009). *Data and Safety Monitoring Committees in Clinical Trials*. Chapman & Hall/CRC, VA.

Irizarry, R., B. Hobbs, F. Collin, Y. D. Beazer-Barclay, K. J. Antonellis, U. Scherf, and T. P. Speed (2003). Exploration, normalization, and summaries of high density oligonucleotide array probe level data. *Biostatistics 4*, 249–264.

Jennison, C. and B. W. Turnbull (1984). Repeated confidence intervals for group sequential clinical trials. *Controlled Clinical Trials 5*, 33–45.

Jennison, C. and B. W. Turnbull (2000). *Group Sequential Methods with Applications to Clinical Trials*. Chapman & Hall/CRC, Boca Raton, FL.

Kalbfleisch, J. D. and R. L. Prentice (2002). *The Statistical Analysis of Failure Time Data*. New York: John Wiley.

Kaplan, E. L. and P. Meier (1958). Nonparametric estimation from incomplete observations. *Journal of the American Statistical Association 53*, 457–481.

Krzanowski, W. J. (1998). *Principles of Multivariate Analysis. A User's Perspective*. Oxford.

Kutner, M. H., C. J. Nachtsheim, and J. Neter (2004). *Applied Linear Regression Models, Fourth Edition*. McGraw-Hill/Irwin.

Lachin, J. M. and M. A. Foulkes (1986). Evaluation of sample size and power for analyses of survival with allowance for nonuniform patient entry, losses to follow-up, noncompliance, and stratification. *Biometrics 42*, 507–519.

Lan, K. K. G. and D. L. DeMets (1983). Discrete sequential boundaries for clinical trials. *Biometrika 70*, 659–670.

Lawless, J. (1982). *Statistical Models and Methods for Lifetime Data*. New York: John Wiley & Sons.

Li, Y., L. Shi, and H. D. Roth (1994). The bias of the commonly-used estimate of variance in meta-analysis. *Communications in Statistics-Theory and Methods 23*, 1063–1085.

Liang, K. and S. L. Zeger (1986). Longitudinal data analysis using generalized linear models. *Biometrika 73*, 13–22.

Lindsey, J. C. and L. M. Ryan (1998). Tutorial in biostatistics: methods for interval-censored data. *Statistics in Medicine 17*, 219–238.

Mann, H. B. and D. R. Whitney (1947). On a test of whether one of two random variables is stochastically larger than the other. *Annals of Mathematical Statistics 18*, 50–60.

Mantel, N. and W. Haenszel (1959). Statistical aspects of the analysis of data from retrospective studies of disease. *Journal of the National Cancer Institute 22(4)*, 719–748.

McCullagh, P. and J. A. Nelder (1995). *Generalized Linear Models, 2nd Edition*. Chapman & Hall.

McLachlan, G. and D. Peel (2000). *Finite Mixture Models*. John Wiley & Sons Inc.

Metropolis, N., A. W. Rosenbluth, M. N. Rosenbluth, A. H. Teller, and E. Teller (1953). Equations of state calculations by fast computing machines. *Journal of Chemical Physics 21*, 1087–1091.

Miettinin, O. and M. Nurminen (1980). Comparative analysis of two rates. *Statistics in Medicine 4*, 213–226.

Murrell, P. (2005). *R Graphics*. Boca Raton, Florida, USA: Chapman & Hall/CRC.

Muss, H. B., D. A. Berry, C. T. Cirrincione, M. Theodoulou, A. M. Mauer, A. B. Kornblith, A. H. Partridge, L. G. Dressler, H. J. Cohen, H. P. Becker, P. A. Kartcheske, J. D. Wheeler, E. A. Perez, A. C. Wolff, J. R. Gralow, H. J. Burstein, A. A. Mahmood, G. Magrinat, B. A. Parker, R. D. Hart, D. Grenier, L. Norton, C. A. Hudis, and E. P. Winer (2009). Adjuvant chemotherapy in older women with early-stage breast cancer. *NEJM 30(20)*, 2055–2065.

Ntzoufras, I. (2009). *Bayesian Modelling Using WinBUGS*. Wiley.

O'Brien, P. and T. Fleming (1979). A multiple testing procedure for clinical trials. *Biometrics 35*, 549–556.

Pan, W. (1999). Extending the iterative convex minorant algorithm to the cox model for interval-censored data. *Journal of Computational and Graphical Statistics 78*, 109–120.

Parmigiani, G., E. S. Garrett, R. A. Irizarry, and S. L. Zeger (2003). *The Analysis of Gene Expression Data: Methods and Software*. Springer.

Peace, K. E. (1986). Estimating the degree of equivalence and non-equivalence: An alternative to bioequivalence testing. *In: Proceedings of Biopharmaceutical Section of the American Statistical Association*, 63–69.

Peace, K. E. (1987). Design, monitoring, and analysis issues relative to adverse events. *Drug Information Journal 21*, 21–28.

Peace, K. E. (1991a). Meta-analysis in ulcer disease. In *Ulcer Disease: Investigation and basis for Therapy. Swabb and Szabo (Ed.)*, pp. 407–430. Marcel Dekker, Inc.

Peace, K. E. (1991b). One-sided or two-sided p-values: Which most appropriately address the question of drug efficacy? *Journal of Biopharmaceutical Statistics. 1(1)*, 133–138.

Peace, K. E. (1992). The impact of investigator hetereogeneity in clinical trials on detecting treatment differences. *Drug Information Journal 26*, 463–469.

Peace, K. E. (1995). Considerations concerning subpopulations in the clinical development of new drugs. *Annual DIA Meeting on Statistical Issues in Clinical Development, Hilton Head, S.C.*.

Peace, K. E. (2009). *Design and Analysis of Clinical Trials with Time-to-Event Endpoints*. Chapman & Hall/CRC.

Peace, K. E. and D. G. Chen (2010). *Clinical Trial Methodology*. Chapman & Hall/CRC.

Peace, K. E. and R. E. Flora (1978). Size and power assessment of tests of hypotheses on survival parameters. *Journal of the American Statistical Association 73*, 129–132.

Piantadosi, S. (1997). *Clinical Trials: A Methodologic Perspective*. New York, USA: John Wiley & Sons.

Piantadosi, S. (2005). *Clinical Trials: A Methodologic Perspective*. New York, USA: John Wiley & Sons.

Pinheiro, J. C. and D. M. Bates (2000). *Mixed-Effect Models in S and SPLUS*. New York: Springer.

PMA (1993). PMA Biostatistics and Medical Ad Hoc Committee on Interim Analysis: Interim analysis in the pharmaceutical industry. *Controlled Clinical Trials 14*, 160–173.

Pocock, S. (1977). Group sequential methods in the design and analysis of clinical trials. *Biometrika 64*, 191–199.

Proschan, M., K. K. G. Lan, and J. T. Wittes (2006). *Statistical Monitoring of Clinical Trials: A Unified Approach*. Springer, NY.

R Development Core Team (2005). *R: A Language and Environment for Statistical Computing*. Vienna, Austria: R Foundation for Statistical Computing.

Randolph, W. C., K. E. Peace, J. J. Seaman, B. Dickson, and K. Putterman (1986). Bioequivalence of a new 800 mg cimetidine tablet with commercially available 400 mg tablets. *Current Therapeutic Research 39(5)*, 767–772.

Rizzo, M. L. (2008). *Statistical Computing with R*. Boca Raton, FL: Chapman & Hall/CRC.

Robert, C. and G. Casella (2009). *Introducing Monte Carlo Methods with R*. Springer.

Rodda, B. E. and R. L. Davis (1980). Determining the probability of an important difference in bioavailability. *Clinical Pharmacology and Therapeutics 28*, 247–252.

Sarkar, D. (2008). *Lattice: Multivariate Data Visualization with R*. New York: Springer.

Schoenfeld, D. A. (2001). A simple algorithm for designing group sequential clinical trials. *Biometrics 57*, 972–974.

Schuirmann, D. J. (1987). A comparison of the two one-sided tests procedure and the power approach for assessing the equivalence of average bioavailability. *Journal of Pharmacokinetics and Biopharmaceutics 15(6)*, 657–680.

Simon, R. (1989). Optimal two-stage designs for phase ii clinical trials. *Control Clin Trials 10(1)*, 1–10.

Smyth, G. K. (2004). Linear models and empirical bayes methods for assessing differential expression in microarray experiments. *Statistical Applications in Genetics and Molecular Biology 3(1) Article 3*.

Spiegelhalter, D. J., A. Thomas, and N. G. Best (2003). *WinBUGS Version 1.4 Users Manual*. Cambridge.

Spiegelhalter, D. J., A. Thomas, N. G. Best, and D. Lunn (2004). *WinBUGS Version 2.0 Users Manual*. Cambridge.

Sturtz, S., U. Ligges, and A. Gelman (2005). R2WinBUGS: A Package for Running WinBUGS from R. *Journal of Statistical Software 12(3)*, 1–16.

Sun, J. (2006). *The Statistical Analysis of Interval-Censored Failure Time Data*. Springer, London.

Tan, S.-B., D. Machin, B.-C. Tai, K.-F. Foo, and E.-H. Tan (2002). A Bayesian re-assessment of two Phase II Trials of Gemcitabine in Metastatic Nasopharyngeal cancer. *British Journal of Cancer 86*, 843–850.

Thall, P. F. and J. K. Wathen (2007). Practical bayesian adaptive randomization in clinical trials. *European Journal of Cancer. 43(5)*, 859–866.

Tukey, J. W. (1977). *Exploratory Data Analysis*. Addison-Wesley.

Turnbull, B. W. (1976). The empirical distribution function with arbitrarily grouped, censored and truncated data. *Journal of the Royal Statistical Society, Series B. 38*, 290–295.

VA Study Group (1967). Veterans administration cooperative study group on antihypertensive agents: Effects of treatment on morbidity in hypertension: Results in patients with diastolic blood pressures averaging 115 through 129 mm hg. *Journal of the American Medical Association 202(11)*, 1028–1034.

Venables, W. N. and B. D. Ripley (2002). *Modern Applied Statistics with S-PLUS. 4th Edition.* Springer-Verlag.

Welch, B. L. (1947). The generalization of "student's" problem when several different population variances are involved. *Biometrika 34*, 28–35.

Westlake, W. J. (1976). Symmetric confidence intervals for bioequivalence trials. *Biometrics 32*, 741–744.

Whitehead, A. (2003). *Meta-Analysis of Controlled Clinical Trials.* John Wiley & Sons, Inc.: New York, NY, USA.

Wilcoxon, F. (1945). Individual comparisons by ranking methods. *Biometrics Bulletin 1*, 80–83.

Yates, F. and W. G. Cochran (1938). The analysis of groups of experiments. *J of Agricultural Science. 28*, 556–590.

Yusuf, S., R. Peto, J. Lewis, R. Collins, and P. Sleight (1985). Beta blockade during and after myocardial infarction: an overview of the randomized trials. *Progress in Cardiovascular Diseases. 27*, 335–371.

Zhao, Y., D. Rahardja, and Y. Qu (2008). Sample size calculation for the Wilcoxon-Mann-Whitney test adjsuting for ties. *Statistics in Medicine. 27*, 462–468.

Index